Ethical Issues in Biomedical Publication

Ethical Issues in Biomedical Publication

Edited by

Anne Hudson Jones

and

Faith McLellan

The Johns Hopkins

University Press

Baltimore & London

The Johns Hopkins University Press
2715 North Charles Street
Baltimore, Maryland 21218-4363
www.press.jhu.edu

Library of Congress Cataloging-in-Publication Data will be found
at the end of this book.
A catalog record for this book is available from the British Library.

ISBN 0-8018-6314-7
ISBN 0-8018-6315-5 (pbk.)

Contents

Foreword

I approach the subject of this book wearing a number of hats. In my professional lifetime, I have been a clinical investigator, an academic physician, a subspecialty division director, a department head, and a medical school dean. At present, I have the privilege of leading a national organization that represents the field to which I have dedicated my professional life, academic medicine. So I've had the opportunity to consider the many facets of research ethics from different perspectives, and I welcomed the invitation from the editors of this important new collection to write the foreword.

My research mentor at Tufts-New England Medical Center, William B. Schwartz, was a fabulous role model. No one I've ever known adhered to higher ethical standards in doing research and publishing scientific papers. Laboratory data were scrupulously recorded. Every single number—and there were literally thousands per study—was checked by someone uninvolved in the particular experiment. Manuscripts were drafted and redrafted countless times to ensure accuracy and to avoid drawing conclusions beyond what the data permitted. Credit was always given to previous work in the field, and the sequence of authorship in multiauthored studies was openly discussed and fairly determined.

Bill Schwartz brooked no cutting of ethical corners. But I don't think his commitment was particularly unusual for his time. Indeed, my distinct impression is that virtually all of his peers in the 1950s, 1960s, and 1970s shared a common view of their ethical responsibilities. They saw themselves as members of a virtual priesthood, sworn to uphold scientific integrity at all costs. They were certainly no less ambitious or competitive than today's scientists are, but opportunities for personal advancement, as far as I could tell, rarely if ever superseded adherence to the shared code of conduct that grounded their professional behavior.

One of the things I learned from Bill Schwartz is that research does not stop when you run the last assay or write the last case note, nor do our ethical imperatives in the conduct of research end when a study is concluded. The tapestry of ethical issues related to any given research study extends through publication and continues for as long as the work remains cited in the literature. When you add something to the scientific literature, you create a legacy; the responsibility for the integrity of that research is timeless because others will be building upon the foundation of your work. As Frank Davidoff points out in his excellent chapter on the relationship between research and publishing, "Science does not exist until it is published."

But the public conversation on the ethics of clinical research tends to focus on one part of the process—the actual conduct of a study, most particularly the ethical questions involved when human subjects participate in clinical research. Less attention has been given to the ethical conundrums—and there are many—that surround the publication stage of the scientific process.

Many of the ethical problems involved in publishing biomedical research stem from intense pressure to publish in order to achieve professional advancement and reward. Sadly, we must admit that the sheer quantity of a scientist's publications is often valued more than are the quality and importance of the work. Resulting shortcuts, lapses, and outright violations of ethical responsibilities are, unfortunately, common enough that they have spawned their own vocabulary: "salami science" is the slicing of one large research project into its "LPUs" (least publishable units), the better to pad one's list of publications. Other problems include outright plagiarism (the direct theft of text) and more subtle "intellectual plagiarism" (the theft of ideas), inappropriate or "gift" authorship, failure to declare conflicts of interest, and "vanity" publication (i.e., publication without adequate peer review). The latter is becoming ever more of a concern with the growth of electronic publication, but it has always been with us.

The "publish or perish" environment is not unique to biomedical research, of course; it can be found in academic fields from English literature to Hegelian philosophy. But ethical breaches in medical research, I would argue, carry far more serious consequences than similar violations in, say, the study of applied sociolinguistics. If, for example, the results of a large multisite study are written up twice, using slightly different angles, in order to yield two publication credits rather than one, meta-analyses may miss the duplication—and one study may be given double the weight. In determining whether or not a new drug is safe and effective, it's easy to see the potential harm. But until we succeed in revising our institutional systems of professional recognition and reward to focus on quality rather than quantity, we cannot expect much change in this situation.

Given the current state of affairs, what is the responsibility of the editor of a medical journal? Many journal editors lament that their responsibility for maintaining ethical standards in publishing has never been made clear. In 1997, the editors of several leading British medical journals formed the Committee on Publication Ethics (COPE) in hopes of addressing their growing concerns over the lack of clear guidelines as to how editors should deal with ethical breaches that come to their attention during the publication process. Editors in the United States confront many of the same dilemmas. Does the journal editor play the role of gatekeeper or cop? How should an editor respond when plagiarism is brought to his or her attention? What about falsified data? How far are editors obligated to go in order to ferret out misconduct, and what must they do when misconduct is detected? What is the editor's responsibility upon discovering that a study published in his or her journal involved a breach of research ethics? What sanctions can an editor legitimately impose?

Researchers and editors alike are badly in need of some guidance—and the leaders of academic and scientific institutions must be willing to tackle the tough issues raised by breaches of publication ethics. As the editors of this book point out in their preface, while other aspects of laboratory work—including ethics in the conduct of research—are taught as part of a scientist's education, publication ethics is frequently assumed to be absorbed by osmosis. Not true. An understanding of the ethics involved in publication of one's research is an essential element of professional training and professionalism in science, and it must be inculcated in scientists early on, not left as something they will "pick up along the way."

Hence, educators, administrators, scientists, editors, and students should all welcome this comprehensive new book. Anne Hudson Jones and Faith McLellan have gathered a veritable who's who in the field of publication ethics for biomedical research. All those with a stake in biomedical research will surely want this volume on their bookshelf.

Jordan J. Cohen, M.D.
President
Association of American Medical Colleges

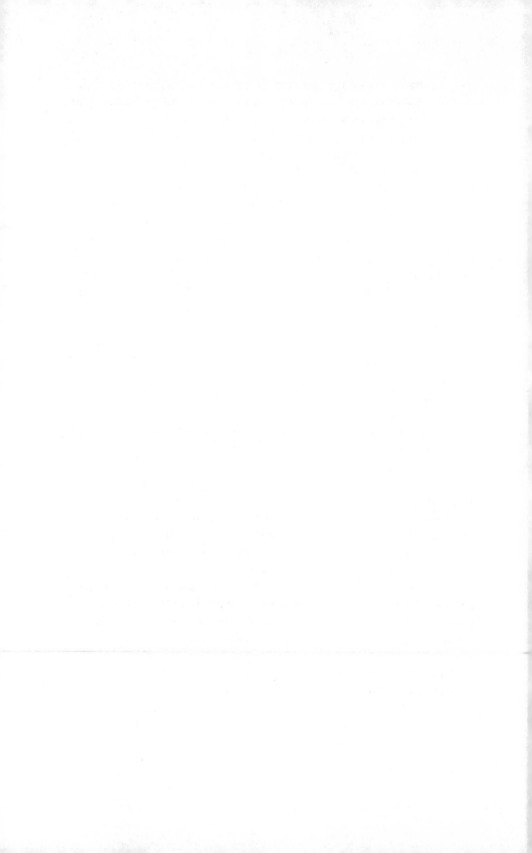

Preface

The idea for this book emerged from our involvement in issues of publication ethics in our roles as editors and teachers of research ethics and scientific writing. As editors, we have been active in professional organizations such as the American Medical Writers Association, the Council of Biology Editors, the European Association of Science Editors, and the European Medical Writers Association, at whose meetings we have listened to presentations, participated in debates, and led workshops about such issues as authorship, peer review, repetitive publication, conflict of interest, and the challenges of electronic publication. As teachers of junior researchers, we have led discussions of these issues in several venues, including the research ethics course at the University of Texas Medical Branch at Galveston (UTMB), which was established to fulfill the National Institutes of Health mandate of ethics education for all students funded by training grants. At UTMB, as at many other universities, this requirement has been extended to include *all* graduate students.

From our conversations with members of both the editing and the research communities, we have become increasingly concerned over the years that the standards of the editorial community are not well known among researchers. Scientists' understanding of issues in publication ethics varies widely, often across disciplines, occasionally (but not always predictably) by experience and seniority, and frequently even within a single department, division, clinic, or laboratory. Junior researchers, graduate students, and residents are often confused about the "rules" and standards in regard to publication. Their confusion is exacerbated by the prevalent notion that, although trainees obviously must be taught laboratory techniques and statistical methods, they should simply absorb the conventions of ethical publication practices through their work with mentors and other senior researchers. Given the wide range of understanding of the issues among more experienced researchers, however, simply following the example set by one's teachers and colleagues may not be enough. Nor may one short session of a research ethics course suffice.

The purpose of this volume, then, is to identify the important ethical matters that arise in biomedical publication, to trace something of their history and development, to set them in the larger context of the ethical conduct of research, to explain the evolution of current standards, and to outline the current debates about these issues. The articulating and communicating of these standards has in the past fallen largely to the editorial community; thus, many of our contributors are editors of major biomedical journals. We hope this book will encourage more members of the research community to become knowledgeable about current standards and to participate in debates about changing them. To be effective, standards for ethical publication must be consonant with the values of good science as understood and practiced by researchers. Inevitably, institutions—medical schools, research universities, and governmental agencies—will become involved with these issues, as they fulfill their obligation to investigate breaches of ethical standards. This book recommends that leaders of such institutions take an active role in supporting education that can help prevent disputes about authorship, for example, or incidents of scientific misconduct.

Our focus in this book is biomedical. Many forces in medicine have brought these issues to the forefront, especially the increasing emphasis on large, multicenter, multinational clinical trials and an awareness that public health and patients' lives may be directly affected by what is published in the biomedical literature. Whatever their genesis, however, the issues discussed here clearly cross disciplinary lines: physicists, for example, are more than passingly familiar with issues of multiple authorship, and basic scientists of all types, as industry and academia increasingly overlap, confront questions about conflict of interest and competing commitments.

The book also has an Anglo-American focus, simply because of the background and experience of the writers. We have made a serious effort, however, to identify international developments affecting the issues, in recognition of the global nature of the underlying concerns. While the United States may have the longest experience in organized responses to many problems of research and publication ethics, other countries are developing ways to address these problems. Where we are aware of these efforts, we have included them. Our hope is that the information we provide here will lead to further international discussions and creative solutions to these cross-disciplinary, transnational problems.

Our focus is also on the peer-reviewed journal article, rather than books or book chapters or grant applications, because it is the customary means of publishing scientific research, as well as the usual measure of academic scientists' achievements when they are reviewed for rewards such as tenure and promotion. The process of writing a journal article and then having it peer reviewed and published is central to scientific work and progress. So much so, in fact, that the process of creating a book may be unfamiliar even to many who are experts in biomedical publishing.

Thus, we think the process of making this book may be of some interest to our readers, as it has been to our contributors. To bring our idea to fruition, we followed a model that has been practiced with considerable success at the Institute for the Medical Humanities since 1983. First we identified the issues that we thought would be important to include, and then we set out to identify the persons we thought were best suited by previous work and interest to address each of those topics. Those who accepted our invitation were asked to prepare a draft of their chapters to be circulated to the other contributors before the group convened for a meeting in Galveston. At the meeting, each chapter received careful critique. The interchanges at that meeting helped direct the revision of chapters and shape the initial book manuscript. In its final form, the book is largely as we had originally conceived it, but it has been enriched and improved by the comments and suggestions of many reviewers.

Part 1 presents the major ethical issues of biomedical publication. Chapters 1 and 2 deal with authorship, arguably the most contentious and controversial problem in scientific publishing for both researchers and editors. Anne Hudson Jones examines traditions of authorship and gives historical background that explains the evolution of the most important current criteria for authorship; then, in the next chapter, Richard Horton dissects the problems of the current criteria and explains why the *Lancet* has abandoned authorship for a new model of contributors. Chapters 3 and 4 deal with the ethical practice of peer review: Fiona Godlee discusses the evolution of ethical standards for peer review as it is practiced now; Craig Bingham suggests how the practice of peer review is changing as a result of electronic publication. In chapter 5, Edward J. Huth examines the problems of repetitive and divided publication. Annette Flanagin takes up in chapter 6 the increasingly thorny question of conflict of interest—what it is and how researchers and editors ought to deal with it. And in chapter 7, Faith McLellan explores the many ethical challenges electronic publication poses for the scientific community.

Part 2 is both a cautionary and a hopeful tale. Debra M. Parrish and C. K. Gunsalus tell the interrelated stories of what happens, in the legal system (chap. 8) and on an institutional level (chap. 9), when ethical practice falters. Susan Eastwood and Addeane S. Caelleigh suggest ways to prevent those problems by educating junior researcher-authors (chap. 10) and academic leaders, who may wear many hats in the research community—as teachers, mentors, senior investigators, deans or other academic officials, leaders of professional societies, and editors of journals (chap. 11).

Part 3 offers two commentaries and an epilogue from the overlapping perspectives of three people who have been involved in all aspects of research and publication. In chapter 12, Paul J. Friedman reminds us of the larger context of ethical publication and of the continuum of practices that may lead to serious scientific misconduct and violations of ethical standards of publication. In chapter 13, Douglas S. DeWitt provides a reality check from the perspective of a researcher on the issues set forth and discussed in previous chapters. And in his epilogue (chap. 14), Frank Davidoff not only responds to previous chapters but also lays out a future path that may resolve tensions between the two cultures of research and publication.

Finally, we offer a list of selected key resources that will provide more information on specific topics and issues for researchers and teachers.

The goals of a book like this one are to educate and inform, to suggest where changes are needed, and to demonstrate ways of bringing about those changes. More discussion is clearly needed to resolve disagreements between those who are doing science and those who are publishing it. The end result of this critical, ongoing conversation, in which innovative solutions are created through the informed dialogue of diverse communities, will be a scientific literature of unparalleled integrity and quality, one that professionals and the public alike can trust.

Editors' note: Scientific research and publication are dynamic and evolving practices. For example, while this book was in press, the U.S. government was considering a proposal from the Office of Science and Technology Policy to modify the federal definition of research misconduct. If the proposal is accepted, all federal agencies will be expected to implement this new policy, thus establishing a uniform definition of research misconduct, as well as uniform guidelines for handling allegations of research misconduct. Two other developments need special mention: The proposed E-biomed is now called PubMed Central, and on January 1, 2000, the Council of Biology Editors became the Council of Science Editors.

Acknowledgments

Just as the process of research and publication involves a host of people, some with less visible but crucial responsibilities, so has the preparation of this book involved the generous contributions of many colleagues. Foremost among them is Ronald A. Carson, Harris L. Kempner Professor in Humanities in Medicine and Director of the Institute for the Medical Humanities, the University of Texas Medical Branch at Galveston, who provided, from the Jesse H. Jones Endowment in the Medical Humanities, financial support for the collaborative research seminar that made this book possible. We are also grateful to Dr. Donald S. Prough, Professor and Rebecca Terry White Distinguished Chair of Anesthesiology, for his support of Faith McLellan's work on this project. Institute staff members Sharon Goodwin and Beverly Claussen assisted ably in the preparations for the seminar meeting in Galveston. We are grateful to Professors Ellen Singer More and Douglas S. DeWitt, who served as respondents to the papers presented at the seminar. Dr. Larry Jenkins and Dana Fox Jenkins generously hosted a dinner for the seminar participants, and we thank them for their hospitality. We also thank Joal Hill, Faith Lagay, Thu Tram T. Nguyen, and Kayhan Parsi for their assistance with both the organizational details and the substantive issues of the seminar. Finally, there are two people whose work and enthusiasm for this project have been indispensable: We thank C. Jordan Kicklighter for his excellent research and editorial assistance and Donna A. Vickers for her superb preparation of the final manuscript.

Contributors

Craig Bingham, B.A., Dip.Ed., is communications development manager of the *Medical Journal of Australia* and coordinator of the *eMJA* Internet Peer Review Trial. The *eMJA*'s first trial was a joint project with the University of Sydney Library, partly funded by the Australian University Vice-Chancellors' Committee as one of several national projects in developing new models of electronic scholarly publication. The *Medical Journal of Australia* is now engaged in a second trial, in which the review process is conducted over the Internet as an open exchange between the journal editors, reviewers, authors, and a small panel of consultants.

Addeane S. Caelleigh, M.A., is the editor of *Academic Medicine,* published by the Association of American Medical Colleges (AAMC), in Washington, D.C. With a background in the social sciences, she has special interests in policy issues and medical education research involving academic medicine from the perspectives of science and the history and sociology of medicine. Before moving to positions in biomedical publication with academic societies, she did research, writing, and editing at the Center for Strategic and International Studies (Washington, D.C.) and at the University of Sydney (Australia).

Frank Davidoff, M.D., is the editor of *Annals of Internal Medicine.* His training is in internal medicine, and he has done research and teaching in the areas of diabetes and general internal medicine. He has held medical school faculty appointments at Harvard, the University of Connecticut, and the University of Pennsylvania. Before becoming editor of *Annals,* he was the director of education programs at the American College of Physicians.

Douglas S. DeWitt, Ph.D., is an associate professor of anesthesiology and the director of the Charles R. Allen Research Laboratories of the University of Texas Medical Branch at Galveston. He is secretary-treasurer of the National Neurotrauma Society, serves on the Department of Veterans Affairs National Merit Review Subcommittee for Neurobiology, and has served on site visit teams for the National Institutes of Health. He also is a regular reviewer for the *Journal of Neurotrauma,* the *American Journal of Physiology, Stroke,* and several other scientific publications in his field. He has received research support from the National Institutes of Health, the American Heart Association, and the Department of Defense.

Susan Eastwood, E.L.S.(D.), is the director of Publications and Grants Writing and an associate of the Brain Tumor Research Center in the Department of Neurological Surgery, University of California, San Francisco, where she also serves ex officio on the Dean's Committee on Ethical Conduct in Research. She is a recent president of the Council of Biology Editors (CBE), an international educational organization in which she has developed many programs, including CBE Retreats on critical issues affecting biological and biomedical publishing. She is also a diplomate of the Board of Editors in the Life Sciences and a fellow of the American Medical Writers Association.

Annette Flanagin, R.N., M.A., is managing senior editor, *JAMA* (the *Journal of the American Medical Association*), and the director of *JAMA* Programs and International Activities. Previously the editor of the *Journal of Obstetric, Gynecologic, and Neonatal Nursing,* she has written and spoken about many issues in biomedical publication. She serves as Congress Coordinator for the international congresses on biomedical peer review and is an active member of the Council of Biology Editors. She is also a co-author of the ninth edition of the *AMA Manual of Style: A Guide for Authors and Editors.*

Paul J. Friedman, M.D., is a professor, Department of Radiology, and former dean for academic affairs, University of California, San Diego. Previously on the Executive Council of the Association of American Medical Colleges, he chaired the Committee on Research Integrity. He was a member of the Institute of Medicine's (National Academy of Sciences)

Committee on the Responsible Conduct of Research and of the Advisory Committee on Research Integrity of the Department of Health and Human Services.

Fiona Godlee, M.B., M.R.C.P., is an assistant editor of the *BMJ* (*British Medical Journal*), the executive editor of *Clinical Evidence,* and the president of the World Association of Medical Editors. A general physician, she also has a degree in the history of medicine. She has written about the role of the World Health Organization and about the dissemination of evidence in clinical practice. She is actively involved in research into peer review and is the coordinator of the international network for research into peer review and dissemination of information in health sciences, Locknet.

C. K. Gunsalus, J.D., is an associate provost, University of Illinois at Urbana-Champaign, where she was formerly Associate Vice-Chancellor for Research. She served on the Association of American Medical College's Committee on Research Integrity, and she chaired the Committee on Scientific Freedom and Responsiblity of the American Association for the Advancement of Science. She was a member of the U.S. Commission on Research Integrity.

Richard Horton, M.B., F.R.C.P., is the editor of the *Lancet.* His background is in general medicine. His research interests include the study of communication in science, especially the influence of literary critical theory, the investigation of rhetorical devices in the scientific literature, and interpretive processes in epidemiological research. He is past president of the World Association of Medical Editors, a member of the International Committee of Medical Journal Editors, and a frequent contributor to literary and review journals.

Edward J. Huth, M.D., M.A.C.P., F.R.C.P., the editor of *Annals of Internal Medicine* for nineteen years, is now editor emeritus of that journal. An internist, he was a founding member of the International Committee of Medical Journal Editors and the founding editor of the *Online Journal of Current Clinical Trials.* He is the author of *Medical Style and Format: An International Manual for Authors, Editors, and Publishers* and of *Writing and Publishing in Medicine,* now in its third edition. He served as chair of the Council of Biology Editors committee that produced the sixth edition of the CBE style manual, *Scientific Style and Format.*

Anne Hudson Jones, Ph.D., is a professor at the Institute for the Medical Humanities of the University of Texas Medical Branch at Galveston, where she has taught courses in medical and scientific writing, medical ethics, and literature and medicine. She was a founding editor of the journal *Literature and Medicine,* which she served as editor-in-chief for more than a decade. Her current interests lie in the areas of authorship, author-editor relations, the theory and practice of literature and medicine, and narrative ethics. In 1999, she received the McGovern Award for Excellence in Medical Communication from the Southwest Chapter of the American Medical Writers Association.

Faith McLellan, Ph.D., is the managing editor of the Physicians Information and Education Resource (PIER) project of the American College of Physicians–American Society of Internal Medicine. For seven years she was Faculty Associate and Director, Manuscript and Grant Preparation Service, Department of Anesthesiology, the University of Texas Medical Branch at Galveston (UTMB). She received the Ph.D. degree from UTMB's Institute for the Medical Humanities, where her dissertation was on electronic narratives of illness. She has done research on authorship practices and awareness of issues in publication ethics. She is an active member of the Council of Biology Editors, for which she has developed educational programs in many areas of scientific publication.

Debra M. Parrish, J.D., is a partner in the Pittsburgh law firm of Titus & McConomy. She was formerly employed by the Office of the General Counsel, Department of Health and Human Services, Office of Research Integrity, where she worked closely with congressional staff, the Office of the Inspector General, and the Department of Justice on matters involving scientific misconduct. Her practice is concentrated in the areas of health law and intellectual property law, with a particular emphasis on science law.

Ethical Issues in Biomedical Publication

I

The Major Ethical Issues

Anne Hudson Jones

The concept of authorship once seemed clear: an author was a person who wrote something (DeBakey and DeBakey 1975). The written work could be a letter, a report, an essay, a poem, a novel, a judicial opinion, or a scientific paper. Neither the subject matter nor the genre determined authorship; the activity of writing did. Even now, if you ask someone on the street, What is an author?, you will almost certainly be told, A writer. Although that answer has been called simplistic (Huth 1990a), it is an answer that would be given not only by members of the general public but also by members of many, if not most, academic disciplines (Stumpf 1993; Lundberg 1998). In contemporary science, however, the concept of authorship has become separable from the act of writing (Conrad 1990; McLellan 1995). This separation is the source of much confusion and ethical difficulty.

An important basis for justifying contemporary claims to scientific authorship as residing in something other than the act of writing is the historical concept of creation or invention as an older definition of authorship (*Oxford English Dictionary* 1971), as exemplified in such expressions as "the Creator authored the universe" or "the father authored the child." Adopting this definition makes intellectual creativity or originality the primary basis for scientific authorship. The acceptance of originality as a necessary component of scientific authorship underlies several ethical claims about scientific publication. Authors are expected to make a new and significant contribution to knowledge in each research publication (DeBakey and De-Bakey 1975). By extension, therefore, both plagiarism and unacknowledged repetitive publication, sometimes called *self-plagiarism,* may be considered unethical practices (de Solla Price 1964; Commission on Research Integrity 1995; see chap. 5), as may reporting "salami science" in fragmented publications referred to as *least publishable units* (LPUs) (Broad 1981; Huth 1986c).

As long as the creator or originator of an idea or a research design or study participates in the writing of a publication about it, there is no conflict between the concept of author-as-creator and that of author-as-writer. Even when creators do not participate in the writing, the concept of author-as-creator in science presumably entitles them to authorship if others develop and write about their ideas. If this practice were the only kind of separation between the act of writing and claims to authorship of scientific publications, it might well be defended as an example of praiseworthy intellectual acknowledgment and generosity. Originators of ideas in other disciplines rarely get more than an acknowledgment, if that, from those who take up their ideas and write about them. Anecdotal examples of people writing up and publishing someone else's ideas as presented in classes, workshops, and professional meetings are not uncommon. Indeed, an argument could be made that other academic disciplines might well emulate the scientific norm of respecting the originality of others' ideas.

Unfortunately, the situation is often not so simple and straightforward as this line of reasoning assumes. The question, Whose idea is it, anyway? may not have an easy answer. Ideas are sometimes said to be "in the air" (Kennedy 1985, 3), and there have been many examples in the history of science of researchers coming up with the same ideas and same discoveries almost simultaneously, although they might have been working on different continents and have had no communication with each other. A more troubling situation occurs when a group of people who work closely together begins to brainstorm and comes up with important new ideas about how to proceed with a research project; assigning credit for the resulting ideas to a single designated creator may be difficult, if not unjust. For reasons perhaps reflected in these examples, the legal protection of copyright extends only to ideas that have been given "fixed expression" (see chap. 8). This stipulation of the law privileges the concept of author-as-writer over that of author-as-creator.

Although scientists must obey the law or face the legal consequences of breaking it, the concept of scientific authorship need not reduce itself to copyright law. The enduring importance of the concept of author-as-creator as a component of scientific authorship lies in its emphasis on intellectual rather than technical contributions (Alexander 1953). It is the quality of mind that has traditionally distinguished scientists from technicians. Developing this scientific quality of mind and thought is at the heart of graduate education in the sciences. Nonetheless, the separation between the act of writing and claims for scientific authorship has become much more complex and troubling than this concept of author-as-creator can justify. Understanding the more troubling aspects of the breach requires a brief historical look at how the act of writing became separable from the concept of authorship in science.

Historical Overview

The Emergence of Big Science and Multiple Authorship

The emergence after World War II of federally funded grants for research in the United States, especially in biomedical sciences, helped usher in an era of Big Science, which many believe led, both directly and indirectly, to the proliferation of multiple authors on scientific papers (de Solla Price 1963). This proliferation is dramatically more apparent in some disciplines than in others. At one extreme of the continuum is high-energy physics, in which papers with hundreds of authors have become routine, culminating (perhaps) in the spring of 1995, with publication in *Physical Review Letters* of two articles about the discovery of the "top quark"; between them, the two papers had a total of 831 authors (Schwitters 1996). Physicists defend this extreme example of multiple authorship because their research has become so complex that large teams of researchers at universities around the globe are necessary to carry it out. The proliferation of multiple authorship in the discipline, they claim, is a direct result of bigger and more expensive research equipment, techniques, and experiments. Yet it seems implausible that 831 people could all have participated in the writing of two papers.

Such long lists of authors defeat the expressed goal of giving credit to everyone who participated in a project by fragmenting credit so extensively that no one, especially not junior researchers, gets enough credit to make much difference in advancing an academic career. Using Derek J. de Solla Price's suggestion that credit for a publication be divided according to the number of co-authors, for example, would produce infinitesimal credit for each author of the top quark papers (de Solla Price 1981). Later modification of de Solla Price's scheme that would weight credit more heavily according to position in the order of authorship could not justly be applied in these cases because the ordering of authors is alphabetical (Hodge and Greenberg 1981). Although the practice of massive multiple authorship reflects the reality of Big Science in physics, the result may be self-defeating at the level of the individual researcher. Meanwhile, at the other end of the continuum, even in some scientific disciplines (such as mathematics), the norms of authorship have not changed much, and single authorship of papers is still routine (Huth 1990b).

The situation in the biomedical sciences falls between the extremes of high-energy physics and mathematics and has been the topic of several studies (de Solla Price 1963; Strub and Black 1976; Broad 1982; Burman 1982; Zook 1987; Huth 1990b; Epstein 1993; Onwude, Staines, and Lilford 1993). For example, Kenneth D. Burman (1982) contrasted averages of 1.3 authors on original articles published in *Annals of Internal Medicine* and 1.2 authors on such articles published in the *New England Journal of Medicine* during the 1930s with averages of 4.7 and 5.2 authors, respectively, on articles published by these same journals in 1979. Edward J. Huth (1990b, 176) ascertained the average number of authors for papers published in the *New England Journal of Medicine* and *Annals of Internal Medicine* between 1915 and 1985 and found an "exponential rise." The average in 1915 was slightly more than one; by 1985, the average was more than six. After analyzing the numbers of authors per article in eight journals over the period 1982–92, Richard J. Epstein (1993, 765) reported that "all journals except *Cell* and *Nature* showed a trend towards increasing authorship numbers over the study period." Epstein also reported that journals specializing in clinical research averaged the most authors per article. And Joseph L. Onwude, Anthony Staines, and Richard J. Lilford (1993) confirmed Epstein's report that the trend toward multiple authorship was most striking in medicine.

Some of the increase in multiple authorship in biomedicine may also be the direct result of more complex and costly research equipment, techniques, and protocols, as in physics. Epstein (1993), however, explicitly rejects this hypothesis, as do many others. Indirect causes that are often cited include the increasing pressure in academic medicine to publish, exacerbated by the tendency of some university review committees to evaluate research productivity by sheer quantity of publications rather than by their quality; the pressure to secure ever more competitive grant funding; and the desire to enhance one's reputation and reap whatever benefits might ensue—fame and fortune or their academic equivalents, which include salary increases, promotions, tenure, consultantships, and other markers of prestige and status. Addeane S. Caelleigh (1991, 676), for example, wrote of authorship's having become "currency," just "one more negotiable commodity in the academic marketplace" in an era of "big business/big government/big science."

Despite the unease of journal editors and some scientists about the trend toward multiple authorship, the potential relationship between multiple authorship and misconduct in science did not become clear until two sensational cases of scientific misconduct were exposed in the early 1980s.

Cases of Scientific Misconduct Implicating Co-authors

Fabrication, falsification, and plagiarism have long been identified as the most flagrant examples of misconduct in science. The willingness of researchers to be listed as co-authors on papers reporting work they did not do is wrong also, but the practice attracted no special attention and commentary until coupled with the more blatantly unethical behavior of fabrication and falsification of data. Two notorious cases of scientific misconduct revealed in the early 1980s—those of John R. Darsee and Robert A. Slutsky—brought the practice of unearned authorship into the spotlight (LaFollette 1992, 91–107). Both men fabricated data and submitted fraudulent articles that were accepted for publication in reputable and prestigious biomedical journals. The initial attention in both cases focused on the men's blatant fabrication of data. But in each case, the men had sought as co-authors senior colleagues and experts in their respective fields, or they had listed as co-authors researchers who did not know until after publication that they were so listed. When Darsee and Slutsky were ultimately exposed—in 1981 and 1985, respectively—the co-authors who had been willing to accept credit for work they had not done proved unwilling to share responsibility for the fraudulent papers. Although both cases have been extensively publicized, investigated, and analyzed (Culliton 1983a, 1983b; [Huth] 1983; Knox 1983; Relman 1983; Kastor 1984; Locke 1986; Braunwald 1987; Engler et al. 1987; Stewart and Feder 1987; Powledge 1988; Fye 1990; LaFollette 1992), they deserve discussion here because of their effect on the development of explicit guidelines for scientific authorship.

The Darsee Case

Recommended by his faculty mentors at Emory University as a brilliant researcher and a man of "moral character" (Culliton 1983a, 32), John R. Darsee went to Harvard University when he was 31 years old as a research fellow in the Cardiac Research Laborary of Eugene Braunwald at the Brigham and Women's Hospital. Until May 1981, when he was observed faking lab results of experiments on dogs on two separate occasions (Knox 1983; Culliton 1983a), Darsee seemed to be living up to the promise of his recom-

mendations. He worked hard, published extensively, and gained Braunwald's deep trust and respect. Indeed, when accusations of misconduct
were brought against Darsee, Braunwald at first suspected his accusers of
being motivated by jealousy (Knox 1983). And when Darsee confessed to
falsifying data but insisted that he had done so on only one occasion,
Braunwald believed him, accepting a "single, bizarre act" as an explanation
for Darsee's behavior (Knox 1983, 1803). It was months before Braunwald
was persuaded that Darsee had engaged in a widespread pattern of misconduct, which had begun when he was an undergraduate biology major at
Notre Dame and continued during his years as a cardiology resident and
fellow at Emory. It took years to investigate Darsee's research thoroughly
and to determine how many of his publications were based on fabricated
data. Walter W. Stewart and Ned Feder (1987) published their account of
the flaws in Darsee's publications six years after he was first accused of
research misconduct.

When the dust settled, investigations had revealed that Darsee's nine
Harvard papers, co-authored with Braunwald and Braunwald's research
deputy Robert A. Kloner, were all based on fabricated data and had to be
retracted. These papers had been published in prestigious journals, such as
the *American Journal of Cardiology* and *Proceedings of the National Academy of
Sciences* (Knox 1983, 1803). In addition, most of the ten papers and 45
abstracts that Darsee co-authored with researchers at Emory could not be
validated and had to be retracted (Culliton 1983b). They, too, had been
published in prestigious journals, such as *Annals of Internal Medicine* and
the *New England Journal of Medicine*. Even the two articles Darsee had published as an undergraduate in the *Notre Dame Science Quarterly* were suspect
(Knox 1983).

How did Darsee get away with it for so long? A major contributing
factor, many came to believe (Relman 1983; [Huth] 1983; Kastor 1984;
Stewart and Feder 1987; Powledge 1988; LaFollette 1992), was Darsee's
pattern of seeking co-authors or simply adding co-authors, without their
knowledge, to his papers. Who were these co-authors?

> Of Darsee's 47 co-authors, 24 worked at Emory University School of Medicine
> and 23 at Harvard Medical School. Biographical data were found for 44 of the 47
> co-authors. Thirty-nine were apparently MDs, one was a PhD, and one held
> both qualifications; three apparently had no advanced degree. At the time of
> their involvement with Darsee, about half of the co-authors were 30–40 years
> old and had received their advanced degrees 5–15 years previously. Approx-

imately equal numbers were senior and junior to this group, the latter including technicians, medical students, resident staff at teaching hospitals and junior faculty members. The senior co-authors included professors and department chairmen. (Darsee himself was 33 in 1981.) (Stewart and Feder 1987, 207)

What the co-authors had in common, apparently, was little knowledge of the research Darsee had purportedly done for the paper on which their names appeared. When Stewart and Feder (1987) examined the 109 publications of Darsee and his 47 co-authors, they discovered flaws in the published papers that they believe attentive co-authors (or even extremely vigilant reviewers) should have recognized before the papers were published. That the co-authors did not recognize flaws in the papers is explained in some cases because the co-authors did not know Darsee had listed them as authors until after the papers had been published. In other cases, however, co-authors made statements testifying to their lack of direct involvement in the work reported in papers that bore their names (Stewart and Feder 1987).

In the wake of disclosures about co-authors' lack of involvment in the research and their inattentiveness to details of the papers reporting the work, several journal editors (e.g., Relman 1983; [Huth] 1983; Kastor 1984) and others (Stewart and Feder 1987; LaFollette 1992) wrote about the responsibilities of co-authorship. Arnold S. Relman, editor of the *New England Journal of Medicine* when it published two of Darsee's articles, wrote an editorial titled "Lessons from the Darsee Affair," in which he identified the final lesson as one about the responsibilities of co-authorship:

> Anyone who allows his or her name to appear among the authors of a paper assumes major responsibilities. . . . Coauthors should be able and willing to defend the paper in public, and that means they must be confident about the integrity of the data. Furthermore, coauthorship should never be conferred or accepted as an honor or simply as a reward for providing resources or sponsoring a junior investigator who has done all the work. Coauthorship should denote at least that there has been meaningful participation in the planning, design, and interpretation of the experiments and in the writing of the paper. Multiauthored papers should never be submitted for publication without the concurrence of all authors. Before accepting a multiauthored paper for publication, editors would be well-advised to assure themselves that these conditions have been met, perhaps by having all coauthors sign an appropriate form. (Relman 1983, 1417)

In an unsigned editorial, the editor of *Annals of Internal Medicine,* which had also published two of Darsee's papers, came to a similar conclusion about co-authorship: "The lesson is that if you are a coauthor you take responsibility for the paper on which your name appears, but this responsibility includes what your coauthors have done and written as well" ([Huth] 1983, 267). And John A. Kastor, editor of the *International Journal of Cardiology,* spelled out his journal's position on authorship:

> We hold that authorship should only be assumed by those investigators who have participated in a scientifically fundamental manner from conception of the study through its reporting. Authors devise the protocol, perform the experiments or collect the clinical data, evaluate the information, and write the report. Colleagues who are not primarily involved in these steps but who have contributed useful scientific or editorial advice should be credited in the acknowledgements. Friends, colleagues, bosses, and trainees should not become authors merely because of such relationships. (Kastor 1984, 8)

It is important to understand the lessons of the Darsee case in order to appreciate the statement that the International Committee of Medical Journal Editors (ICMJE) was soon to develop about the criteria for authorship. (Both Relman and Huth were members of the ICMJE at the time.) If not the single instigator of the ICMJE response, the Darsee case was a major influencing factor. Meanwhile, on the other coast, another notorious case of research misconduct was about to unravel.

The Slutsky Case

There are troubling similarities between the case of Darsee and that of Robert A. Slutsky, who also published large numbers of fraudulent articles with many unsuspecting co-authors who knew little about his research. While working as a radiology resident and, simultaneously, as an unsalaried associate clinical professor in the Department of Radiology at the University of California, San Diego (UCSD), Slutsky had been producing approximately one paper every ten days for several years (Locke 1986; Engler et al. 1987; LaFollette 1992). Despite this extraordinary output, which should at least have attracted critical attention to his work, Slutsky's fabrications went undetected until early 1985, when he was being considered for appointment as an associate professor of radiology at UCSD. Then, a member of the departmental committee evaluating Slutsky's work noticed duplicate data in two of Slutsky's articles. Questioned about the duplication, Slutsky abruptly resigned his appointments at UCSD.

In the investigation that followed, a ten-member UCSD faculty committee determined that, of Slutsky's 137 publications, 77 were valid, 48 were questionable, and 12 were fraudulent (Engler et al. 1987). The committee gave as examples of fraud "reporting numerous experiments that were never performed," "reporting procedures that were incorrect or measurements that were never made," and "reporting statistical analyses that were never performed." The committee classified as questionable articles "in which statistical calculation errors were apparent" (Engler et al. 1987, 1383). In answering the question of how Slutsky had been able to get away with his fraud for so long, the committee found, as was true in the Darsee case, that "gift coauthorship was effectively a disguise for an impossible amount of work by one person" (Engler et al. 1987, 1387). The role of such uninvolved co-authors was again called into question:

> The classification of questionable validity or fraud in papers with many authors raises the issue of the responsibility of coauthors. Should the coauthors who were unable at the time of the committee review to vouch for parts of articles have had reason to wonder earlier about the accuracy of the statements made in their names? In multiauthored papers, can one expect, for example, the statistician to know personally how the data were collected? Can a supervisor know what actually went on in the laboratory during every experiment? An unrealistic standard cannot be applied in judging the culpability of coauthors. But the standard should be higher than that of many of Slutsky's coauthors and co-authors of others found guilty of fraud. In the absence of any intent to deceive, many have been careless about verifying the accuracy of publications that carry their names. We believe this to be a culpable degree of carelessness. Acceptance of gift coauthorship (in which no scientific contribution was made) is also a culpable act of deliberate misrepresentation. (Engler et al. 1987, 1384)

As a remedy for abuses of co-authorship, the UCSD committee made several suggestions:

> Integrity regarding criteria for authorship must be as integral a part of scientific publication as is the accuracy of the data, and all coauthors should exercise their responsibility for the quality and accuracy of a scientific publication. At the time of publication each investigator could be asked to specify his or her role in the research and records of their reports could be maintained by each department for review at the time of promotions. Journals could require similar statements to be submitted along with the copyright-transfer form. This practice should clearly identify gift authorship and thereby limit it. Departments could require

the statement of contributors and approval of all submitted papers by all co-authors—a practice that would allow young investigators to voice an opinion concerning their role in research at the departmental level. Senior investigators should not put their names on work unless they actually provided ideas and reviewed data. Coauthorship should reflect scientific involvement and responsibility for the work reported. (Engler et al. 1987, 1387)

The committee's ideas about the basis for authorship were in keeping with those expressed by several journal editors just a couple of years earlier after the Darsee case (Relman 1983; [Huth] 1983; Kastor 1983). Perhaps the most important thing the Slutsky case added was the disturbing awareness that unethical behavior on the part of both senior and junior co-authors was not confined to a single case.

The Responses of Medical Journal Editors: Criteria for Authorship

As already discussed, in the wake of the Darsee case journal editors became much more concerned about the proliferation of multiple authorship. One important result was that the ICMJE, also known as the Vancouver Group (for the city in which they held their first meeting over dinner in January 1978), extended their efforts at establishing uniform guidelines for the format of biomedical articles to include a statement about criteria for their authorship. In his commentary introducing the prospective publication of these criteria, Huth (1986a) linked them explicitly to the Darsee case and to criticisms that standards for authorship had not previously been clearly stated and widely disseminated. The "Uniform Requirements for Manuscripts Submitted to Biomedical Journals," now in its fifth edition (ICMJE 1997), has been adopted in one iteration or another (see chap. 2) by several hundred biomedical journals throughout the world. Thus, these journals have all adopted the ICMJE criteria for authorship.

First published as part of the "Uniform Requirements" in 1985, the ICMJE statement on authorship has become extremely important; it is the best-known and most often adopted guideline for authorship in the biomedical sciences. It rests on the insistence that authors must assume responsibility, as well as accept credit, for publications that bear their names. The first criterion emphasizes the concept of author-as-creator by stressing the necessity for an author to make substantial intellectual contributions to the research being reported. The second and third criteria close the breach that had developed between the act of writing and claims of scientific authorship by requiring that authors must take part in drafting or critically revising the manuscript and that they must approve the final version. Here is the core of the ICMJE statement on authorship:

> All persons designated as authors should qualify for authorship. Each author should have participated sufficiently in the work to take public responsibility for the content.
>
> Authorship credit should be based only on substantial contributions to 1) conception and design, or analysis and interpretation of data; and to 2) drafting the article or revising it critically for important intellectual content; and on 3) final approval of the version to be published. Conditions 1, 2, and 3 must all be met. (ICMJE 1997, 38)

The ICMJE also specifies some of the contributions that do not qualify someone as an author: "Participation solely in the acquisition of funding or the collection of data does not justify authorship. General supervision of the research group is not sufficient for authorship" (ICMJE 1997, 38). It is easy to see underneath these guidelines the concerns about authorship and the suggested remedies that had come to the fore in the Darsee case and been reemphasized by the Slutsky case. In requiring that authors take part in the drafting or revising of the manuscript and that they approve the final version, the ICMJE criteria try to ensure that authors will not only make an intellectual contribution to the research project but also make a contribution to the report of that project and have an opportunity to approve the report before it is published. How else could they be expected to assume responsibility for what the report says?

Persistent Problems of Scientific Authorship

In the first few years after the original publication of the ICMJE criteria for authorship in the "Uniform Requirements" and their appearance in the Instructions to Authors of many biomedical journals, editors may reasonably have believed that they had done what needed to be done: They had established what they considered to be clear guidelines for authorship and disseminated them widely. They had also published editorials and articles to assist in interpreting these guidelines (e.g., Huth 1986b). It is understandable that they expected these guidelines to acquaint researchers with the accepted standards for determining authorship and thereby help prevent the abuses of co-authorship that had been revealed in the Darsee and Slutsky cases. As years have passed, however, evidence mounts that the

ICMJE authorship guidelines in the "Uniform Requirements" have not changed practice as much as was anticipated. One revealing study, for example, shows that patterns of co-authorship among chairs of departments of medicine did not change in the years between 1979 and 1990. That is, results showed that, "among all the chairmen, there was no statistically significant decrease in the average number of articles per year for which the chairmen were last authors, and there was a significant increase in the average number of coauthors per year on published articles." The authors of this study concluded that "changes in the definition of authorship by medical journal editors did not seem to be important influences on the authorship patterns of the chairmen" (Shulkin, Goin, and Rennie 1993, 688).

This conclusion comes as no surprise to those of us who have been teaching in the research ethics course mandated by the National Institutes of Health (NIH) in institutions that have NIH-funded research fellows. We can testify that the ICMJE authorship guidelines are not well known either to postdoctoral fellows and junior faculty members or to some senior faculty members with active research careers who publish frequently. In response to the continued ignorance of authors, some journals, such as the *Journal of the American Medical Association (JAMA)*, have instituted more and more specific requirements with which authors must comply when they submit papers for possible publication. Given these efforts, which require authors to sign statements affirming that they qualify for authorship, it seems unlikely that any author could remain unaware of the ICMJE guidelines for authorship spelled out in the "Uniform Requirements"; yet, if we are to believe what they tell us each year, they do.

Among authors who *are* aware of the ICMJE authorship guidelines, many consider them unrealistic in light of established practice in many departments and research laboratories: including on the author list everyone who has anything to do with a project, no matter how tangential that involvement may be. Mentioned with considerable frequency is the example of the clinician who will not allow researchers access to "his" patients unless he is also listed as a co-author of any publication that ensues. Even researchers who know this is a violation of the guidelines of the journal to which they submit their papers admit that they bow to the pressure and include such clinicians as authors. Another common example is that of international postdoctoral fellows who come to the United States with differing ideas and expectations about authorship. Some come with expectations that they must include mentors from their home country as authors on any publications resulting from the fellows' research in the United States. In sympathy with the plight of these fellows, who are caught between cultures and conflicting value systems, American colleagues sometimes add the name of such a mentor to the authorship list, even though the international mentor has made no contribution to the research or writing and obviously could not fulfill the ICMJE requirements. Other fellows come with expectations that they must publish a certain set number of articles if they are to complete their training in their home country. Thus, they are willing to give authorship credit to colleagues who are willing to reciprocate and give them unearned authorship in return (see chap. 10).

These examples, like the study of authorship patterns of chairs of departments of medicine (Shulkin, Goin, and Rennie 1993), make clear that editors' establishing guidelines for authorship and disseminating them widely may be necessary but are not sufficient to change practice and solve some of the most persistent problems of scientific authorship. Journal editors, as they frequently remind themselves and others, are not police and do not have any means of enforcing the guidelines that they have established; they can expound but not enforce (Powledge 1988).

Thus, despite the best efforts of journal editors to solve problems of authorship, many persist. Among the most persistent problems are guest, gift, or honorary authorship; ghost authorship; denial of authorship; the order of authorship; and credit for those who do not qualify for authorship. Although many of these problems are interrelated, it is important to clarify and discuss each in turn, as well as to identify the interrelationships among them.

Guest, Gift, or Honorary Authorship

Guest, gift, or honorary authorship is authorship that is conferred on someone who clearly does not qualify for authorship (Croll 1984; Jackway and Boyce 1990; Rennie and Flanagin 1994). This is precisely the kind of unearned authorship that received so much attention in the Darsee and Slutsky cases. Statements in the "Uniform Requirements" specifically rule out three common types of guest, gift, or honorary authorship: those conferred on someone for supplying funding, for collecting data, or for general supervision of a research group (ICMJE 1997, 38). Yet in some laboratories and departments, the lab supervisor and department chair expect and may require that their names be listed as authors on every paper written by anyone in their lab or department, whether they are closely enough involved in the research to accept responsibility for it or not. Usually such a name would be added as the last author, the position that some people refer to as senior author. This kind of gift authorship exploits those who have actually done the research by giving credit to some who have not been involved in the work.

Sometimes, however, junior researchers want to confer gift authorship on highly respected researchers in hopes that the name of an illustrious researcher will add luster to the paper at hand, even though the famous one has had nothing to do with the research being reported. In this kind of example, a junior researcher may exploit a more established researcher. A senior researcher may agree to accept authorship, possibly out of altruistic motives of wanting to help a young researcher get published, possibly out of self-serving motives of wanting to extend his or her bibliography with an effortless publication.

Ghost Authorship

Ghost authorship is almost an inversion of guest authorship. In ghost authorship, the person who actually writes the paper is not identified as the author (DeBakey and DeBakey 1975; Rennie and Flanagin 1994; Flanagin and Rennie 1995). Ghost authors may be hired by researchers or clinicians who do not have the time to write a paper, by someone who does not know how to write a paper, or by someone who is not fluent in the language (usually English) in which the paper needs to be written. Sometimes students are expected to draft a paper as part of their educational experience but are not named as authors. Pharmaceutical companies employ large numbers of writers, and it has been reported that these companies pay prominent physicians to allow their names to be placed in authorship of "scholarly reviews about new drugs" that the writers have prepared (Rennie and Flanagin 1994, 470). In ghost authorship, the act of writing is completely severed from the claim to authorship.

Ghost authors are different from author's editors, who are usually hired by individual researchers or by departments to assist researchers in preparing articles for publication. Some institutions maintain an elaborate editing service and require that all publications bearing the institutional affiliation be submitted for editing before being submitted to a journal. Some author's editors cross the line between providing editorial assistance and ghost writing, especially if they are working directly for a single researcher and being paid by that individual. In an effort to expose these ghosts, *JAMA* has recently begun requiring that such assistance be disclosed to journal editors when an article is submitted for review (Rennie and Flanagin 1994).

The Denial of Authorship

Denying authorship to someone who qualifies for it can sometimes be equated with plagiarism: appropriating the work and words of others without giving proper credit and attribution. Examples range from not properly documenting in notes and references the ideas and words of someone else to the flagrant theft of someone else's research. These can be difficult cases to resolve. Often the person who believes that he or she qualifies for authorship but has been denied it is a graduate student or junior researcher. The highly publicized case of Pamela Berge, a former graduate student at the University of Alabama, Birmingham (UAB), falls under this rubric. Research that she undertook as part of her doctoral dissertation was allegedly presented by another UAB graduate student at a professional meeting. Instead of filing charges with the NIH or the Department of Health and Human Services' Office of Research Integrity, Berge filed suit under the False Claims Act because the research ostensibly being conducted by the other graduate student was funded by a federal grant (see chap. 8). In April 1995, the suit was heard by a jury, which awarded Berge $550,000 (Taubes 1995). Although the verdict was later overturned on appeal, the case was notable as the first to invoke the False Claims Act as a possible remedy for denial of authorship.

The Order of Authorship

The order in which authors should be listed on a paper remains one of the least standardized and most troublesome aspects of authorship. The "Uniform Requirements" leaves its determination up to the co-authors:

> The order of authorship should be a joint decision of the coauthors. Because the order is assigned in different ways, its meaning cannot be inferred accurately unless it is stated by the authors. Authors may wish to explain the order of authorship in a footnote. In deciding on the order, authors should be aware that many journals limit the number of authors listed in the table of contents and that the U.S. National Library of Medicine (NLM) lists in MEDLINE only the first 24 plus the last author when there are more than 25 authors. (ICMJE 1997, 38)

The decision of the NLM to list up to 25 authors in MEDLINE is recent and is much more liberal than its previous practice. The special inclusion of the last author reflects what was once an admirable tradition in biomedical publication. At a certain point in a student's development as a budding independent researcher, the student's mentor allowed the student to take first authorship credit for their collaborative research and the mentor took last, sometimes called senior, authorship (Riesenberg and Lundberg 1990; Hulley 1991). When the mentor has participated in the research, last authorship is a position of true honor, one that reflects both generosity and responsibility. Ironically, it is this tradition that has become corrupted by the presumption in some departments and labs that the department chair's or lab supervisor's name will go in last position on every paper that comes out of the department or lab, even if the chair or supervisor has not been involved in the project.

As several studies have shown, only first authorship and last authorship have any generally accepted meaning (Zuckerman 1968; Shapiro, Wenger, and Shapiro 1994). The first author is the person who has taken the initiative and responsibility for a project and carried out most of the work. The final author may be the first author's true research mentor, the senior researcher in a team, or merely a guest author riding on privilege. Beyond these positions, there is no prevailing agreement about what the positions of authors' names on the byline mean, although some fairly detailed and complex schemes have been put forward for determining the order (Ahmed et al. 1997). The most straightforward is one that would have the order of authorship reflect the amount of work on the project. In that scheme, the first author does most work and gets most credit, the second author does the second most work and gets second most credit, and so on. This scheme, however, conflicts with the older tradition of having the most senior and experienced author take last place, the anchor position. In some disciplines, alphabetical listing or occasionally reverse alphabetical listing is considered the fairest way of determining the order of authorship. It avoids the delicate and difficult task, especially when there are many authors, of determining the listing of authors in order of their diminishing efforts on a project. Indeed, some author lists, such as those in high-energy physics, are so long that it would be nearly impossible to determine the relative contributions of authors. In these cases, alphabetical listing seems the only realistic solution.

Because of the different traditions and practices among disciplines, journals, and research teams for deciding on the order of authorship, the advice in the "Uniform Requirements" about explaining in a footnote the rationale for the order is an excellent idea. Without that rationale, readers may make incorrect assumptions about the meaning of the order of authors. This kind of explanation has special importance when someone's publications are being reviewed for tenure and promotion decisions. Otherwise, it is difficult to assess what *intervening authorship (et int.)*—that is, appearing anywhere other than first or last on the authorship list—means (Epstein 1993, 767).

Credit for Those Not Qualifying as Authors

Most of the attacks on the ICMJE definition of authorship have to do with the issue of awarding credit for those involved in a research project who do not qualify for authorship. These may include technicians who carry out experiments, statisticians who do only assigned routine statistical analysis, clinicians who provide access to patients, and those people who are accustomed to receiving guest authorship as a result of their position in the hierarchy. According to ICMJE guidelines, the appropriate way to give credit for contributions to a project that do not qualify someone for authorship is to thank those who made such contributions in the acknowledgments section of an article. No one should be acknowledged, however, without his or her permission. This requirement seems onerous to some, but it is necessary to avoid the implication that someone has endorsed a study when he or she has not.

Proposed Solutions

If the best efforts of the ICMJE could not solve these persistent problems of authorship, how else might they be resolved? Suggested solutions vary widely, from raising awareness and continuing educational efforts within medical schools themselves by developing institutional authorship policies to abandoning the concept of scientific authorship altogether.

The Development of Authorship Policies in American Medical Schools

Medical schools and universities in the United States have gradually developed procedures for responding to allegations of scientific misconduct that involve plagiarism or fabrication or falsification of data (see chap. 9). Less firmly in place, however, are procedures for responding to authorship disputes, which are not infrequent. Among the recommendations of the Commission on Research Integrity (CRI 1995) was that medical schools should develop authorship policies that will make clear to their faculty and students what the institutional standards for authorship include. Even though the report of the commission was not adopted, this suggestion seems well worth considering.

In an effort to discover how many U.S. medical schools have considered or adopted an authorship policy, in mid-December 1996 I sent an Institutional Review Board (IRB)-approved questionnaire to the deans of the 125 U.S. medical schools. By May 1997, after a follow-up letter in March and a final follow-up telephone call in April, I had received 119 responses, for a return rate of 95% (Jones 1997). Of the schools that responded, 25 (21%) have adopted authorship policies. Another 11 schools (9%) reported that they were in the process of trying to develop an authorship policy. And 77 (65%) reported either that they had discussed developing such a policy but had given up any attempts to do so or that they had never discussed such a policy. Six respondents (5%) did not know whether there had been discussions of such a policy on their campuses. Among those who reported having discussed the development of such a policy but having given up the attempt to adopt one, most who made comments said that disciplinary differences made it impossible to develop a policy for the entire school and that such policies would have to be developed within departments or disciplines.

In the statements of the 25 schools that have developed authorship policies, the ICMJE guidelines from the "Uniform Requirements" are often obvious. For example, in the "Guidelines for the Responsible Conduct of Research at Yale University School of Medicine" (1991, 4), the statement on "Authorship of Scientific Papers" has this footnote: "These principles are consistent with the uniform requirements for manuscripts submitted to biomedical journals now endorsed by over 400 biomedical journals." Not surprisingly, then, the Yale guidelines insist on authors' having contributed to the "intellectual content" of a scientific paper, and this intellectual contribution is distinguished from other contributions, such as those "to provide routine technical services, to refer patients for study, to provide a valuable reagent, to assist with data collection and assembly, or to review a completed manuscript for suggestions." The Yale guidelines also insist on authors' writing or revising the manuscript and approving the final version.

The most common variation from the ICMJE (and Yale) guidelines is to expand the first criterion for authorship so that not only intellectual contributions but also "functional" or "practical" contributions to a project may qualify someone for authorship. This variation is highly significant because it opens the way for the inclusion of those who are specifically excluded from authorship by the ICMJE guidelines in the "Uniform Requirements." The statement on authorship from the *Faculty Policies on Integrity in Science* adopted by the Faculty of Medicine of Harvard University

(1996, 5, 7) offers a good example: "The Committee considers the only reasonable criterion to be that the co-author has made a significant intellectual or practical contribution. The concept of 'honorary authorship' is deplorable." For its *Guidelines and Resource Material for the Ethical Conduct and Reporting of Research and Procedures for Handling Allegations of Unethical Research Activities* (1988), the University of Louisville School of Medicine adopted and republished (with permission) the guidelines developed at Harvard University School of Medicine. An interesting addition in the Louisville guidelines is a footnote to the criteria for authorship saying that "Harvard did not intend 'significant practical' to include *routine* technical assistance" (*Guidelines and resource material* 1988, 4n. 4). What Harvard did intend by "significant practical contribution" is not clarified in either the Harvard or the Louisville guidelines, however.

The Harvard and Louisville statements on authorship contain two other deviations from the ICMJE guidelines that are worthy of note. The first is a statement that "criteria for authorship of a manuscript should be determined and announced by each department or research unit" (Faculty of Medicine, Harvard University 1996, 5, 7; *Guidelines and resource material* 1988, 3). The second is a statement placing responsibility for the entire manuscript on the first author. Other authors are expected to review and approve the manuscript "to the extent possible, given individual expertise" (Faculty of Medicine, Harvard University 1996, 5, 7; *Guidelines and resource material* 1988, 4). Thus, co-authors are not responsible for the entire content of an article. This change may have been necessitated by allowing someone to qualify for authorship on the basis of practical rather than intellectual contributions to a paper, but there is no clarification of this point in the guidelines themselves.

The authorship policy of Rush Medical College is adapted from the guidelines of the American Psychological Association (APA) rather than those of the ICMJE. There are striking similarities between them, however. The Rush guidelines also include useful discussion of intellectual versus practical contributions:

> Authorship encompasses not only those who do the actual writing but also those who have made a substantial scientific contribution to a study. Substantial scientific contributions may include formulating the problem or hypothesis, structuring the experimental design, conducting the experiments in a manner that demonstrates independent thought, organizing and conducting the statistical analysis, interpreting the results, or writing a major portion of the paper.

Those who so contribute are listed in the "authorship" byline. Each author listed in the byline of an article should review and approve the entire manuscript before it is submitted.

A technician, research assistant, other employee, research fellow, resident, or student may be a co-author of a publication if, in the opinion of the Principal Investigator, the said individual has made a substantive contribution to the work over and above actually performing required tasks. If the technical staff (support) person has performed the studies prescribed by the PI, but has not made contributions to the experimental design, data analyses, data interpretation, or rationale for the study, then co-authorship is not automatically earned. Likewise, provision of patients, space, and/or research funds do not automatically entitle a collaborator to authorship, though this may be determined to be appropriate after discussion with the PI and co-investigators. Technical assistance may be acknowledged in the "acknowledgment" section of the publication. (*Investigator/authorship guidelines of Rush Medical College* 1996, 8–9)

The *Investigator/Authorship Guidelines of Rush Medical College* (1996, 9) also specifies a process of first appeals for those who think they have been unfairly excluded from authorship or not positioned appropriately on the authorship list: "The PI alone has the primary role in determining co-authorship and the order of co-authors. If any of the individuals involved in the research consider the decision of the PI to be unfair, that individual may appeal to the Department Chairman, or if necessary to the Office of the Dean." This statement points the way toward development of an institutional policy to deal with authorship disputes (see chap. 9).

As these few examples demonstrate, institutional authorship policies raise questions of their own, especially when they allow each department or research division to set its own criteria for authorship. In a time when interdepartmental and interdisciplinary research is being encouraged at many medical schools, an interdepartmental definition of authorship for those participating in such research is clearly desirable. Whatever the limitations of authorship policies, however, the faculty-wide discussion that often goes into their preparation must certainly be helpful, not only to administrators who adjudicate authorship disputes on their campuses (see chap. 9) but also to researchers and their trainees. A written policy is at least a beginning point for education and discussion about criteria for authorship. One potentially troublesome issue rarely addressed is what to do when an institutional authorship policy conflicts with a journal's authorship policy. Presumably, authors would be bound by the more restrictive policy.

Many of the survey responses I received indicated a high level of interest in authorship and authorship policies. Many deans requested a copy of the results of the survey. Some wrote to express their special interest in the topic even though their schools had not as yet discussed developing an authorship policy. Several called to talk about topics ranging from incidents of authorship disputes on their campuses to references they might use in discussing authorship with their faculty members. The interest evoked by the questionnaire reflects willingness on the part of medical school deans to learn more about both practical and ethical aspects of authorship credit (see chap. 11).

National Authorship Policies

Just as the ICMJE guidelines are discernible (even when not explicitly acknowledged) beneath the authorship policies of several American medical schools, they are also the basis for the authorship policies recommended in Australia and Denmark. In Australia, the National Health and Medical Research Council (NHMRC), in conjunction with the Australian Vice-Chancellors' Committee (AVCC), developed guidelines on research practice that include a firm statement about authorship criteria (NHMRC 1997, sec. 3.1):

> Each institution must establish a written policy on the criteria for authorship of a research output. Minimum requirement for authorship should accord with the "Vancouver Protocol". Authorship is substantial participation, where all the following conditions are met: a) conception and design, or analysis and interpretation of data; and b) drafting the article or revising it critically for important intellectual content; and c) final approval of the version to be published. Participation solely in the acquisition of funding or the collection of data does not justify authorship. General supervision of the research group is not sufficient for authorship. Any part of an article critical to its main conclusion must be the responsibility of at least one author. An author's role in a research output must be sufficient for that person to take public responsibility for at least that part of the output in that person's area of expertise. No person who is an author, consistent with this definition, must be excluded as an author without their permission in writing.

The 1995 annual report of the Danish Committee on Scientific Dishonesty (DCSD) reflects concern about the corruption of the ICMJE criteria but responds by reaffirming them: "The only practicable way of solving the problem [of authorship] is undoubtedly to realise the thoughts of the Vancouver Group" (Riis and Anderson 1996). And the DCSD's recently published "Guidelines Concerning Authorship" incorporates the ICMJE requirements for authorship while acknowledging the emerging practice of publishing a *contributor description* to provide more information about each author's contribution to the work. Perhaps the most interesting feature of these DCSD guidelines is the clear and repeated endorsement of the concept of author-as-creator: "Right to authorship is obtained through a creative effort and only through this" (DCSD 1999). Such efforts to establish national guidelines give hope that international guidelines might someday be possible, as, indeed, the ICMJE has attempted to provide.

Abandoning Authorship

At the other end of the spectrum of proposed solutions is that of abandoning scientific authorship entirely. As early as 1984, Fotion and Conrad suggested that traditional authorship should be maintained but an alternative system of credits should be developed to explain exactly what other persons involved in a research project had contributed. By 1997, Drummond Rennie, Veronica Yank, and Linda Emanuel went further and suggested that scientific authorship should be abandoned in favor of a system of contributors and guarantors. In their proposed alternative system, any number of contributors could be listed on a paper, with their respective contributions specified, but there must be at least one guarantor to assume responsibility for the entirety of the research being reported in the paper. In assuming responsibility for the paper, guarantors will function much as traditional authors did—and still do. Contributors, on the other hand, are freed from the responsibilities of authorship: they do not have to make an intellectual contribution to the work, they do not have to engage in writing or revising the manuscript, they do not have to approve the manuscript, and they are not held responsible for the work.

Various objections to this new model include journal editors' concerns that it will take too much space to list all contributors and specify details of their contributions and researchers' fears that such credits will not be understood or valued in an academic setting, thus denying the rewards that accrue to authorship. The alacrity with which the new model was adopted by the *Lancet* (Horton 1997) and the *British Medical Journal* (*BMJ*) (Smith 1997) makes clear that the academic community's review processes will provide a more formidable obstacle than editors' concerns about journal space. The contributor-guarantor model will probably be most attractive to those who cannot qualify for authorship under the ICMJE criteria but who could receive credit as a contributor under the new model. This alternative may help solve the difficulties of awarding credit in large, multicenter trials, for example (see chap. 2). But guarantorship seems so much more important than contributorship that those who are accustomed to being authors will probably aspire to guarantorship. Who, for example, would want to risk grant monies on someone who has been a contributor but who has never assumed the responsibility of a guarantor? Worth passing comment is the fact that Rennie, Yank, and Emanuel (1997) were all identified as co-guarantors of their article proposing this new system.

Conclusions

The criteria for authorship developed in 1985 by the ICMJE powerfully reaffirm traditional values of authorship: they require that an author not only make a substantial intellectual contribution to a research project and accept responsibility for the published report but also either draft the manuscript or revise it critically and then approve the final version. In these specifications, the ICMJE brought together the concepts of author-as-writer and author-as-creator and thereby brought scientific authorship once again into accord with authorship in other academic disciplines. Indeed, how could anyone accept responsibility for a paper that he or she had not had the opportunity to revise and approve?

Those who argue that the ICMJE definition is too strict for contemporary scientists are arguing that scientists should not be expected to make an intellectual contribution to a research project and take part in writing the research report. Those who argue against establishing campus-wide policies of authorship often claim that disciplinary differences make such policies impossible. Yet an intellectual contribution to a project, some involvement in the drafting or revising of the manuscript, and approval of the final manuscript should be minimal requirements for authorship in any discipline. The increasing emphasis on interdisciplinary work, especially in biomedical research, makes such an interdisciplinary definition of authorship not only desirable but necessary. And, as many cases of scientific misconduct have illustrated during the past two decades, traditional values of authorship are inextricably linked with integrity in research. Only if scientific authorship has become irreparably corrupt, as its critics claim (Rennie, Yank, and Emanuel 1997; Horton 1997; Smith 1997), will the contributor-guarantor model become the exclusive way of the future.

References

Ahmed, S. M., C. A. Maurana, J. A. Engle, D. E. Uddin, and K. D. Glaus. 1997. A method for assigning authorship in multiauthored publications. *Family Medicine* 29:42–44.

Alexander, R. S. 1953. Trends in authorship. *Circulation Research* 1:281–83. Reprinted in Roland, C. G. 1970. Good scientific writing. *Archives of Internal Medicine* 125:771–72.

Braunwald, E. 1987. On analysing scientific fraud. *Nature* 325:215–16.

Broad, W. J. 1981. The publishing game: Getting more for less. *Science* 211:1137–39.

———. 1982. Crisis in publishing: Credit or credibility. *Bioscience* 32:645–47.

Burman, K. D. 1982. "Hanging from the masthead": Reflections on authorship. *Annals of Internal Medicine* 97:602–5.

Caelleigh, A. S. 1991. Credit and responsibility in authorship. *Academic Medicine* 66:676–77.

Commission on Research Integrity (CRI), Ryan Commission. 1995. *Integrity and misconduct in research: Report of the Commission on Research Integrity to the Secretary of Health and Human Services, the House Committee on Commerce, and the Senate Committee on Labor and Human Resources.* Washington, D.C.: Department of Health and Human Services, Public Health Service. See also http://www.faseb.org/opar/cri.html. Site accessed 8 April 1999.

Conrad, C. C. 1990. Authorship, acknowledgment, and other credits. In Council of Biology Editors, Editorial Policy Committee, *Ethics and policy in scientific publication,* 184–87. Bethesda, Md.: Council of Biology Editors.

Croll, R. P. 1984. The noncontributing author: An issue of credit and responsibility. *Perspectives in Biology and Medicine* 27:401–7.

Culliton, B. J. 1983a. Coping with fraud: The Darsee case. *Science* 220:31–35.

———. 1983b. Emory reports on Darsee's fraud. *Science* 220:936.

Danish Committee on Scientific Dishonesty (DCSD). 1999. Guidelines concerning authorship. Chap. 6 in *The Danish Committee on Scientific Dishonesty: Guidelines for good scientific practice.* Copenhagen: Danish Research Agency. See also http://www.forskraad.dk/spec-udv/uvvu/guidelines/author.htm. Site accessed 12 July 1999.

DeBakey, L., and S. DeBakey. 1975. Ethics and etiquette in biomedical communication. *Perspectives in Biology and Medicine* 18:522–40.

de Solla Price, D. J. 1963. *Little science, big science.* New York: Columbia University Press.

———. 1964. Ethics of scientific publication. *Science* 144:655–57.

———. 1981. Multiple authorship. *Science* 212:986.

Engler, R. L., J. W. Covell, P. J. Friedman, P. S. Kitcher, and R. M. Peters. 1987. Misrepresentation and responsibility in medical research. *New England Journal of Medicine* 317:1383–89.

Epstein, R. J. 1993. Six authors in search of a citation: Villains or victims of the Van-
    couver convention? *BMJ* 306:765–67.
Faculty of Medicine, Harvard University. 1996. *Faculty policies on integrity in science.*
    Boston: Harvard Medical School. See also http://www.hms.harvard.edu/
    integrity/index/html. Site accessed 8 April 1999.
Flanagin, A., and D. Rennie. 1995. Acknowledging ghosts. *JAMA* 273:73.
Fotion, N., and C. C. Conrad. 1984. Authorship and other credits. *Annals of Internal
    Medicine* 100:592–94.
Fye, W. B. 1990. Medical authorship: Traditions, trends, and tribulations. *Annals of
    Internal Medicine* 113:317–25.
*Guidelines and resource material for the ethical conduct and reporting of research and pro-
    cedures for handling allegations of unethical research activities at the University of
    Louisville School of Medicine.* 1988. Louisville: University of Louisville School of
    Medicine. See also http://www.louisville.edu/research/ethics.htm. Site accessed
    8 April 1999.
"Guidelines for the responsible conduct of research at Yale University School of
    Medicine." 1991. New Haven: Yale University School of Medicine. See also
    http://info.med.yale.edu/sciaffr/grants/guidelin.htm. Site accessed 8 April
    1999.
Hodge, S. E., and D. A. Greenberg. 1981. Publication credit. *Science* 213:950.
Horton, R. 1997. The signature of responsibility. *Lancet* 350:5–6.
Hulley, S. B. 1991. The order of authorship. *JAMA* 265:865.
[Huth, E. J.] 1983. Responsibilities of coauthorship. *Annals of Internal Medicine*
    99:266–67.
Huth, E. J. 1986a. Abuses and uses of authorship. *Annals of Internal Medicine*
    104:266–67.
———. 1986b. Guidelines on authorship of medical papers. *Annals of Internal Medicine*
    104:269–74.
———. 1986c. Irresponsible authorship and wasteful publication. *Annals of Internal
    Medicine* 104:257–59.
———. 1990a. Discussion comment. In Council of Biology Editors, Editorial Policy
    Committee, *Ethics and policy in scientific publication,* 193–94. Bethesda, Md.:
    Council of Biology Editors.
———. 1990b. Editors and the problems of authorship: Rulemakers or gatekeepers? In
    Council of Biology Editors, Editorial Policy Committee, *Ethics and policy in sci-
    entific publications,* 175–80. Bethesda, Md.: Council of Biology Editors.
International Committee of Medical Journal Editors (ICMJE). 1997. Uniform re-
    quirements for manuscripts submitted to biomedical journals. *Annals of Inter-
    nal Medicine* 126:36–47. See also http://www.acponline.org/journals/resource/
    unifreqr.html. Site accessed 8 April 1999.
Investigator/authorship guidelines of Rush Medical College. 1996. Chicago: Rush Medi-
    cal College.

Jackway, P., and R. Boyce. 1990. Gift co-authorships: A tangled web. *Australian Clinical Review* 10:72–75.

Jones, A. H. 1997. Authorship policies in U.S. medical schools: Report of a survey. Paper presented at the 3d International Congress on Biomedical Peer Review and Global Communications, 18 September, Prague. http://www.ama-assn.org/public/peer/ausu.htm. Site accessed 7 April 1999.

Kastor, J. A. 1984. Authorship and the Darsee case. *International Journal of Cardiology* 5:7–11.

Kennedy, D. 1985. *On academic authorship.* Washington, D.C.: American Council of Learned Societies.

Knox, R. 1983. The Harvard fraud case: Where does the problem lie? *JAMA* 249:1797–1807.

LaFollette, M. C. 1992. *Stealing into print: Fraud, plagiarism, and misconduct in scientific publishing.* Berkeley and Los Angeles: University of California Press.

Locke, R. 1986. Another damned by publications. *Nature* 324:401.

Lundberg, G. D. 1998. Publication and promotion: Writing is all. *Lancet* 352:898.

McLellan, M. F. 1995. Authorship in biomedical publication: "How many people can wield one pen?" *American Medical Writers Association Journal* 10:11–13.

National Health and Medical Research Council (NHMRC). 1997. *Joint NHMRC/AVCC statement and guidelines on research in practice.* http://www.health.gov.au/nhmrc/research/nhmrcavc.htm. Site accessed 31 March 1999.

Onwude, J. L., A. Staines, and R. J. Lilford. 1993. Multiple author trend worst in medicine. *BMJ* 306:1345.

Oxford English Dictionary (OED). Compact ed. 1971. s.v. "author."

Powledge, T. M. 1988. *NEJM's* Arnold Relman. *Scientist,* 21 March, 12–13.

Relman, A. S. 1983. Lessons from the Darsee affair. *New England Journal of Medicine* 308:1415–17.

Rennie, D., and A. Flanagin. 1994. Authorship! Authorship! Guests, ghosts, grafters, and the two-sided coin. *JAMA* 271:469–71.

Rennie, D., V. Yank, and L. Emanuel. 1997. When authorship fails: A proposal to make contributors accountable. *JAMA* 278:579–85.

Riesenberg, D., and G. D. Lundberg. 1990. The order of authorship: Who's on first? *JAMA* 264:1857.

Riis, P., and D. Anderson. 1996. Authorship and co-authorship. Chap. 2 in *The Danish Committee on Scientific Dishonesty: Annual report 1995.* Copenhagen: Danish Research Councils. See also http://www.forskraad.dk:80/publ/rap-uk/kap05.html. Site accessed 8 April 1999.

Schwitters, R. F. 1996. The substance and style of "Big Science." *Chronicle of Higher Education,* 16 February, B1–2.

Shapiro, D. W., N. S. Wenger, and M. F. Shapiro. 1994. The contributions of authors to multiauthored biomedical research papers. *JAMA* 271:438–42.

Shulkin, D. J., J. E. Goin, and D. Rennie. 1993. Patterns of authorship among chairmen of departments of medicine. *Academic Medicine* 68:688–92.

Smith R. 1997. Authorship is dying: Long live contributorship. *BMJ* 315:744–48.

Stewart, W. W., and N. Feder. 1987. The integrity of the scientific literature. *Nature* 325:207–14.

Strub, R. L., and F. W. Black. 1976. Multiple authorship. *Lancet* 2:1090–91.

Stumpf, S. H. 1993. Understanding authorship. *Family Medicine* 25:491.

Taubes, G. 1995. Plagiarism suit wins; experts hope it won't set a trend. *Science* 268:1125.

Zook, A., II. 1987. Trend toward multiple authorship: Update and extension. *Journal of Counseling Psychology* 34:77–79.

Zuckerman, H. A. 1968. Patterns of name ordering among authors of scientific papers: A study of social symbolism and its ambiguity. *American Journal of Sociology* 74:276–91.

Richard Horton

The Disquieting Case of Dr. Crohn

The first description of Crohn's disease is attributed to a paper published in 1932 by Crohn, Ginzburg, and Oppenheimer (1932). This apparently straightforward citation hides a story of remarkable relevance to contemporary academic scuffles surrounding the issue of authorship. By 1930, Leon Ginzburg and Gordon Oppenheimer had studied 12 patients who had been operated on by the surgeon A. A. Berg. They wrote these cases up into a paper intended for publication. At the same time, Burrill Crohn had seen two patients with a similar disease process. The common feature was a condition of the terminal ileum characterized by chronic inflammation, mucosal ulceration, luminal stenosis, and fistula formation. Patients presented with "fever, diarrhea, and emaciation, leading eventually to an obstruction of the small intestine" (Crohn, Ginzburg, and Oppenheimer 1932, 1323).

Crohn suggested to Berg that his two cases might be written up and published. Berg demurred, pointing out that a draft manuscript had already been prepared by Ginzburg. Their discussions fell silent until news came that Crohn planned to report all 14 patients at a meeting of the American Medical Association. He had claimed sole authorship, and only Berg's late intervention restored the names of Ginzburg and Oppenheimer. Berg declined the offer of co-authorship because he was unwilling to take credit for a paper he had not written.

Who should take the authorship credit in this instance? Berg saw and operated on all 14 patients. Ginzburg and Oppenheimer saw 12 and wrote the first draft of a paper that was never submitted. Crohn, it seems, attempted to steal credit from his colleagues. Berg was merely acknowledged. The appellation *Crohn's disease* rests on behavior that might at best be described as discourteous; at worst, one might conclude that Crohn's action betrayed scientific misconduct. Whatever lesson one draws from Dr. Crohn's example, it seems difficult to apportion first author (and so eponymous) credit fairly for the discovery of regional enteritis, despite a spate of recent conferences (Horton and Smith 1996a), committees (ICMJE 1997), editorials (Lundberg and Glass 1996), research papers (Eastwood et al. 1996), and guidelines (Goodman 1994) on who constitutes an author and why. The subject of authorship remains an eerie skeleton in the institutional closet.

The Fraudulent Author

The increasing unease about authorship in science is driven largely by a single issue, fraud. One quite astonishing example illustrates how corrosive this phenomenon can be. Francis Collins directs the U.S. National Center for Genome Research at the National Institutes of Health (NIH). His responsibility extends to managing the human genome project (budget, $189 million), an intramural research program (budget, $44 million), and a bioethics initiative (budget, $11 million). Among these hardly trivial affairs, he also runs a research laboratory. One of Collins's interests is leukemia, specifically chromosomal changes found in some patients with the disease. In 15% of people with acute myeloid leukemia, for example, the center of chromosome 16 is turned 180° on its axis. During this rotation, two pieces of normally separated DNA are brought together to form a fusion gene. Collins's team published this observation, including details of the gene's protein product, in 1993 (Liu et al. 1993).

His group went on to study this gene in great detail. One report described the intriguing finding that the gene led to cancerous growth when expressed by mouse fibroblasts. Other workers, however, were unable to confirm these results. There was understandable frustration about this failure, even consternation. Concern came to a head when the editor of *Oncogene,* John Jenkins, invited Collins to respond to a reviewer's question about a Western blot included in a submission to the journal. The reviewer had noted that, if one lane was cut and turned 180°, it appeared to be part of another lane on the same blot—a bizarre and barely believable irony, given the lab's interest in the inverted segment of chromosome 16.

When Collins investigated further, he found an alarming pattern of deceit: control cell lines had been invented and fictional DNA sequences created. Collins immediately contacted the U.S. Office of Research Integrity. In September 1996, he returned to the University of Michigan at Ann Arbor to confront a graduate student in his old lab, whom he now suspected. After hearing three hours of evidence, Amitav Hajra admitted his crime. With Hajra's signed confession in hand, Collins went to Harold Varmus, director of NIH, and together they sent a letter outlining details of the falsified data to a hundred researchers working in Collins's very narrow field. Collins subsequently retracted two papers and part of the data set of a further three.

Although Collins admitted "regret" for what had happened, he clearly did not wish to draw any larger or more troublesome conclusions. As he said, "if [science] is going to be open, if it's going to be creative, if you're going to allow people with talent to explore the unknown, . . . there are going to be people who take advantage" (Marshall 1996, 910). Collins may be correct that overregulation could have damaging consequences for science, but the authorship question—namely, the precise nature of the responsibility that authorship confers—remains elusive and unresolved.

The incoherence of the scientific community's response is revealed in the correspondence published by *Science* after their news report about Collins first appeared (Wooley, de Sa, and Sagar 1996; Gilson 1997; White 1997). De Sa and Sagar argued that co-authors are collectively responsible for their work, but Gilson called this view risky for collaboration, as well as impractical. Gilson's view has a distinguished heritage. In an analysis of the William Summerlin affair, in which a Memorial Sloan-Kettering Cancer Center researcher used a black felt-tip pen to fake a successful skin graft in mice, Peter Medawar (1996b, 139) concluded that "it is not physically possible for the head of an institute of several hundred members to supervise intently the work of each one. Most such directors assume—and as a rule rightly—that young recruits from good schools and with good references will abide by the accepted and well-understood rules of professional behaviour. I write here with the authority of someone who has been the head of a large research institute, and who has himself been once or twice deceived by an impostor." These opposing points of view seem intractable. But both White and Knight offer a solution (White 1997), one I shall explore later—namely, the notion of stating explicitly who was responsible for which particular aspects of the investigation.

For authorship, the celebrated cases of fraud during the past 25 years have pointed relevance not for the individual act of misconduct itself, but for the part played during the investigation by the co-authors. In the cases of John Darsee (Relman 1983), Robert Slutsky (Whitley, Rennie, and Hafner 1994), Malcolm Pearce (Lock 1995), and Thereza Imanishi-Kari (Kevles 1998), for example, the prominence of the co-authors, as with Francis

Collins, drew attention to and damaged the credibility of science, producing two very different reactions.

First, the report of the Commission on Research Integrity (CRI) (1995), chaired by Harvard Professor of Obstetrics Kenneth Ryan, adopted a conciliatory tone toward the issue of authorship. Its message was simple: dialogue, dialogue, and more dialogue. In one short section devoted specifically to authorship, the Ryan report commented that "such conflicts can generally be avoided if researchers have early and frequent discussions on the allocation of authorship and intellectual property" (CRI 1995).

In contrast to this effort to promote awareness, often in the face of strong criticism that any further encroachment into the research process by so-called fraud-busters would be a "scurrilous" and "pernicious" development (Howe 1996, A3), others have indicated an urgent need for a more radical and muscular approach (Lock and Wells 1996). Lock, for example, rates authorship abuse as a more serious breach of conduct than the commission does. After the Pearce case, in which an obstetrician invented data that formed the substance of a clinical trial (Pearce and Hamid 1994) and lied about the supposedly successful transfer of an ectopic pregnancy to the uterus (Pearce, Manyonda, and Chamberlain 1994), Lock (1995, 1548) wrote: "Of all the abuses of scientific research, gift authorship is the most common and the most lightly regarded. . . . Many people accept or confer gift authorship, detection is unlikely, and the rewards are obvious: tenure, promotion, research grants, and fame, especially in a society that measures worth by the weight of papers produced rather than their quality."

In both instances, Pearce had buttressed the face validity of his papers by adding the names of individuals, with their agreement, who had contributed nothing substantive to the research project. In the case of Geoffrey Chamberlain (Pearce, Manyonda, and Chamberlain 1994), co-author status was given on the grounds that he was head of Pearce's department (yet he admitted he had no idea that the operation reported had taken place), editor of the journal in which the report was published (Pearce was a co-editor), and president of the Royal College of Obstetricians and Gynecologists, the body responsible for publishing the journal!

To deal with such abuses, Lock (1995, 1548) concluded that a "central committee would also seem the most suitable pattern for Britain" because of the experience of similar committees in the United States (Office of Research Integrity [ORI]) and Denmark (Danish Committee on Scientific Dishonesty [DCSD]). Simply promoting dialogue seems to represent the "lax approach" criticized by Lock (1995, 1548). Indeed, the failure of the

United Kingdom's medical community to respond to the issues, notably authorship, raised by the Pearce fiasco led him to exclaim: "I feel professionally ashamed and diminished by this sequence of events. The profession here has failed its responsibilities to the community" (Lock 1997, 92). That authorship is central to this discussion is shown by the work of the Danish committee, well over half of whose cases center around authorship disputes (DCSD 1998). The United Kingdom has responded to Lock's critique by establishing a Committee on Publication Ethics (COPE) (1998). Here editors meet to present and discuss ethics problems encountered during the publication process. The group has also found that authorship issues form a considerable part of its work.

If quarrels over authorship constitute the bulk of misconduct cases and if authorship should be taken more seriously as a part of the definition of misconduct, the case for national committees and international guidelines seems difficult to resist. While national policies vary greatly and are the subject of deep disagreement, one set of international rules has commanded at least a measure of support.

The Vancouver Clause

Though unelected and without mandate, the International Committee of Medical Journal Editors (ICMJE, also known as the Vancouver Group), is the self-appointed standard-bearer of good editorial practice. Its guidelines, the "Uniform Requirements for Manuscripts Submitted to Biomedical Journals," have been enormously influential in harmonizing widely divergent editorial policies concerning article format and reference style. Repetitive publication, patients' rights to privacy, conflict of interest, and many other matters of editorial concern are all covered by the group, which includes representatives of ten journals from six countries and three continents.

Authorship has been a central concern of the ICMJE since its first gathering in 1978. Its first statement that went beyond the "Uniform Requirements" was produced in 1985 (Editorial consensus on authorship and other matters 1985, 595):

> Each author should have participated sufficiently in the work to take public responsibility for the content. This participation must include: (a) conception or design, or analysis and interpretation of data, or both; (b) drafting the article or revising it for critically important intellectual content; and (c) final approval of the version to be published. Participation solely in the collection of data does not justify authorship.

All elements of an article (a, b, and c above) critical to its main conclusions must be attributable to at least one author.

In concept, the definition bound *responsibility* to *participation*—that is, whatever an author's degree of participation, that individual must "have participated sufficiently . . . to take public responsibility for the content."

The type of participation these editors had in mind was clearly set out under three broad categories: doing, writing, and approving. Conducting the research meant being involved in the intellectual development of the work, its "conception or design, or analysis and interpretation." Merely collecting data did not justify authorship. This exclusion clause has produced much acrimony and threatens not only the future of the existing definition of authorship but also, as we shall see, the health of collaborative clinical research. In 1985, writing the paper "or revising it for critically important intellectual content" and "final approval" also constituted reasons for claiming authorship (Editorial consensus 1985, 595).

An oddity then appears, one that has also caused a great deal of confusion among researchers and editors alike. The ICMJE indicated that "all" of the elements of doing, writing, and approving should be "attributable to at least one author" of a paper (Editorial consensus 1985, 595). What does this phrase mean? Does it assert that one author and one author only must have participated significantly in all three activities? If not, why use the word "all" when "each" would have been clearer? Or does it simply mean that one author should be able to say that he or she accepts attribution of the doing, or the writing, or the approving, or a combination of any two, or all three? And, in this definition, is attribution synonymous with responsibility? None of these uncertainties is clarified or even acknowledged.

The motivation for the statement, though, does slip out. According to a *Lancet* editorialist, "We hope that the words on authorship will do something to limit the inflationary trend in numbers" (Editorial consensus 1985, 595). Anxiety about the spreading waistline of the authorial corpus has exercised the editorial community for several decades. The "ICMJE effect"—namely, the inducement to limit authorship to six names because any more will invoke the x, y, z, et al. rule for references—has received some preliminary support (Epstein 1993). And editors certainly do use the ICMJE definition to persuade, coax, or bully authors into severing what editors see as unnecessary human appendages. However, most authors view this issue very differently from editors and provide a perspective that editors would do well to heed.

Interpreting these 1985 guidelines is made more difficult by journal inconsistencies in the way the ICMJE definition was published. Although the *Lancet* reported "complete agreement among the editors present" (Editorial consensus 1985, 595), the *British Medical Journal (BMJ)* clearly recalled events very differently. Their representative was the joint founder of the ICMJE, Stephen Lock. He added a further two paragraphs, one drawing attention to the issue of corporate authorship and another making clear the right of an editor to ask authors to justify their claims (ICMJE 1985, 722): "A paper with corporate (collective) authorship must specify the key persons responsible for the article; others contributing to the work should be recognized separately (see Acknowledgments and other information)" and "Editors may require authors to justify the assignment of authorship."

The latest pronouncement by the ICMJE illustrates how this issue has grown in importance in recent years (ICMJE 1997; see chap. 1). The twin issues of responsibility and participation remain the core of the definition. However, it is now made clear that "all" authors must qualify for authorship. Participation continues to be divided into doing, writing, and approving, but this requirement is now qualified by the phrase "substantial contributions to" (ICMJE 1997, 38). No definition of "substantial contribution" is provided. In truth, it is difficult to see how there could be one. The matter must remain at the discretion of the authors, although such discretionary practice may soon be ripe for curtailment.

The ambiguity pointed out in the 1985 definition has now been resolved. To qualify for authorship, an individual must satisfy each condition of doing, writing, and approving. Also, two specific exclusion clauses now exist. First, to the collection of data is now added the acquisition of funding. And second, "general supervision of the research group" (ICMJE 1997, 38) will no longer do. These strictures are at variance with the views of many scientists.

Anxiety about numbers again crops up, this time with the explicit note that the National Library of Medicine (NLM) now imposes its own limits. This citation boundary is hardly repressive; if the total exceeds 25, the NLM will list the first 24 plus the last author. The advent of multicenter collaborative studies, especially in disciplines dependent on molecular techniques, has forced librarians and editors to adopt a more sanguine view of author groups that take on the appearance of shopping lists.

The most significant change to the ICMJE statement is subtle but important. Until recently, the ICMJE highlighted the fact that "Editors may require authors to justify the assignment of authorship" (ICMJE 1993,

2283). This comment appeared in the 1985 *BMJ* statement, but not in that of the *Lancet*. The latest (1997) version now reflects perhaps the more aggressive character of the ICMJE. Editors may not only ask authors to justify their assignment by describing what each contributed, but also publish that information in their journals. This stance was adopted after a conference on authorship at the University of Nottingham in the United Kingdom in June 1996, which was organized by the *BMJ* and the *Lancet* (Horton and Smith 1996b).

Two key issues raised at this meeting led to a noticeable change in mood. First, Drummond Rennie, deputy editor of the *Journal of the American Medical Association (JAMA)*, argued forcefully, as he had done previously (Rennie and Flanagin 1994), that along with credit goes responsibility. Recent instances of scientific fraud (Lock and Wells 1996) had drawn attention to authorial negligence. Authors frequently put their names to papers even though their intellectual contribution, perhaps *any* contribution, had been zero. Thus, publishing the details of authors' contributions received some support. Second, and more controversially, some felt that the ICMJE statement represented a charter designed specifically for senior authors. The only way to identify those who toiled to produce the gruel of research was by citing their material contribution. Thus, an early draft of the new ICMJE codicil read as follows: "Editors may require authors to justify assignment of authorship, and editors may require that each author's contribution, *together with the contribution of other significant parties,* be described. Editors might consider publishing this information somewhere in the article" (my italics). The final version of this sentence, as now published, benefits from being more succinct. But the wish of some editors to widen understanding of both credit and responsibility in scientific authorship was quashed.

Although editors become agitated about gift authorship (an endemic disease, polyauthoritis giftosa, according to Kapoor [1995]), scientists seem to regard it as acceptable (Sharp 1998). Shapiro, Wenger, and Shapiro (1994) examined 20 research articles from each of five science journals and 20 articles from each of five clinical journals. Papers were chosen on the basis of having four or more authors. All first authors were surveyed about the contributions of co-authors to their paper. One-quarter of all authors had contributed either nothing or only to one aspect of the work. In a small survey, Goodman (1994) found that over a third of authors of articles published in one peer-reviewed general medical journal had not made a substantial contribution to the paper.

In the largest survey to date, Susan Eastwood and colleagues (1996) surveyed 1,005 postdoctoral fellows on a wide range of issues relating to publication ethics. One-third responded. The results from questions about authorship are shown in table 2.1. According to the ICMJE, all five of the activities listed under "ICMJE definition" must be satisfied to justify authorship. The percentages of fellows agreeing with each criterion fell far short of 100% in the Eastwood study. More importantly, the specific exclusion criteria cited by the ICMJE—providing funding, collecting data, and being head of the lab—all received substantial support for justifying authorship, especially for those who do the actual laboratory work. This finding provides strong support for the belief that the existing ICMJE definition is elitist in outlook. One-fifth of respondents would include a statistician in their author group. It is difficult, given the sample size, to discover any significant differences between M.D.s and Ph.D.s.

Eastwood et al. (1996, 110) asked a further, revealing question: "If it would make publication of your work more likely or benefit your research career, would you be willing to list someone as an author on your paper, even though he or she did not deserve authorship?" Remarkably, though perhaps not surprisingly given the current academic climate, 32% (103) of the respondents said they would. Interestingly, the replies for women versus men were 36% versus 28% and for M.D.s versus Ph.D.s 37% versus 29%. Are the pressures for women in research and for physicians in a fiercely competitive hierarchy so great as to tempt gift authorship? This hypothesis demands further study. Another perplexing result was that any training in research ethics was significantly associated with a willingness to *offer* gift authorship (39% with training versus 27% without).

A much smaller U.K. study confirmed Eastwood et al.'s findings. Bhopal and colleagues (1997) interviewed 66 researchers in a single medical faculty. Although those questioned supported criteria for authorship, few knew of or used those of the ICMJE. Gift authorship was agreed to be a common practice (66%) but was justified on grounds of pressure to publish, improving chances of publication, repaying favors, encouraging collaboration, and maintaining good working relationships. And Flanagin et al. (1998) showed that gift and ghost authorship are common in papers published by general medical and more specialist journals.

This intensification of debate about authorship has produced extraordinary hand-wringing among editors. Parmley, editor-in-chief of the *Journal of the American College of Cardiology,* called for investigators to take "the high road" by adhering strictly to ICMJE rules. He was explicit: "Certainly,

Table 2.1. The Views of Postdoctoral Fellows on Authorship

Criteria for Authorship	Percentage Agreeing		
	All Fellows	M.D.s	Ph.D.s
ICMJE definition			
Developed hypothesis (all or part)	65.4	71.0	62.0
Designed study (all or part)	91.7	94.0	90.3
Analyzed and interpreted data	84.6	80.0	86.2
Wrote first draft	69.1	72.0	70.3
Revised paper	35.8	45.0	30.8
ICMJE exclusion			
Obtained funding	44.4	37.0	45.6
Performed experiments; collected data	85.8	80.0	87.7
Was head of lab	47.5	49.0	45.6
Miscellaneous contributions			
Completed statistical analysis only	20.1	18.0	19.5
Referred patients; provided material	15.4	26.0	7.2
Commented on paper	2.2	3.0	0.0

Source: Adapted from S. Eastwood, P. A. Derish, E. Leash, and S. B. Ordway, "Ethical Issues in Biomedical Research: Perceptions and Practices of Postdoctoral Research Fellows Responding to a Survey," *Science and Engineering Ethics* 2(1996):89–114. Reprinted with permission.

Note: The question asked was: Please check each item that you believe is a sufficient contribution to warrant authorship of a research paper. Figures are percentages of respondents.

none of the following by themselves constitute grounds for authorship: technical support, providing an assay, director of a laboratory, chief of the division, paying for the study, typing the manuscript, or contributing patients to the study" (Parmley 1997, 702).

Richard Smith, editor of the *BMJ*, invited readers to suggest how to repair the cracks in the ICMJE definition. He resisted the idea of publishing credits in the *BMJ*, but instead encouraged "those who send us papers to experiment" with their authorship attribution (Smith 1997, 922). At the *American Journal of Public Health*, Susser has followed Smith's example (Susser 1997). An editorial in *Nature* agreed that trying to apply general rules would simply "encounter insurmountable obstacles" but concluded that "personal responsibility" was unavoidable (Games people play with authors' names 1997, 831).

As Jane Smith (1994, 1457) argued, "A set of guidelines drawn up by editors will not influence the behaviour of authors." With an ever-increasing number of scientists, greater pressure for individual recognition, and more collaborative research across disciplines and countries, the ICMJE criteria do seem outdated. I, too, reviewed these recent twists and turns (Horton 1997b), and the *Lancet* later jettisoned authors in favor of contributors (Horton 1998d). The *BMJ* followed suit.

At the *Lancet* we have found contributorship a valuable means of assigning proper credit to the particular parts played by individual investigators in a collaborative research process. However, contributorship does not solve all authorship disputes. As evidence summarized in the 1998 and subsequent COPE reports indicates, when conflicts arise within research groups it is hard for editors to get true insight into who did what or who should deserve authorship credit. A policy based on contributors rather than authors may have some place in preventing improper attribution, but it will never be wholly successful.

What Is an Author?

Such is the recent history of attempts to codify the concept of authorship in biomedicine. The main difficulty facing anyone grappling with the question, What is a scientific author? is the lack of available groundwork in mapping out systematically the nature of authorship. From the limited scholarship available, four distinct but interdependent characteristics of a scientific author are identifiable. The *attribution* of a piece of scientific writing reflects the traditional criteria described by the ICMJE (namely, taking public responsibility for the work and participating in the doing, writing, and approving of the paper). This characteristic subsumes both credit and responsibility. However, my notion of attribution differs from that of some editors sitting on the ICMJE. To move toward a more equitable definition of authorship, I favor broadening both credit and responsibility to those individuals who performed the research, including those who "solely" collected the data.

Authorship also implies *authority*. Issues of power and ownership are inextricably tied to the concept of a scientific author. Huth crystallized this least-acknowledged feature vividly (Huth 1985, 276): "The central motive most often, I believe, is to establish oneself as a greater expert among lesser experts, expecting from that gain the benefits likely to follow: the benefits of power, political as well as economic." Eastwood's finding that 48% of postdoctoral researchers would cite the laboratory chief as an author confirms this belief (Eastwood et al. 1996). Attribution and authority are frequently uncoupled, a concern for editors but one seemingly accepted by researchers.

The *animus* of an author combines motivation (incentive) with interpretive intent (purpose); it is the animating spirit underlying authors' words, the reasons why they assert what they do and the meaning of what they do assert. The best way to explain this feature is by showing how animus can rapidly metamorphose into animosity. The Multicentre Acute Stroke Trial–Italy (MAST-I) was published in December 1995 (MAST-I Group 1995). The study began with a seven-member steering committee who, at the conclusion of the trial, sat down to write a final report. A dispute ensued about the meaning of the results (rather fundamentally, whether streptokinase had adverse or beneficial effects in the treatment of stroke), a disagreement that proved irreconcilable. The seven became five when two authors peeled off from the consensus, although the paper was submitted with all seven listed as the writing committee. The paper was reviewed and accepted, and only late in the day was it noticed that two of the seven authors had failed to provide signatures. These were sought but denied. The corresponding author then admitted that these two held views contradictory to the majority. The *Lancet* published a separate interpretation of the study by the two dissenters alongside the full paper (Tognoni and Roncaglioni 1995), together with an editorial explanation (Horton 1995b).

Although all seven "authors" could rightly claim attribution and authority for the work, their animus—motivation and interpretive intent—was a point of intense conflict. The meanings both factions drew from the same work were so at variance with one another that sharing authorship on the same paper proved impossible, although they sought to preserve the collaboration to ease the path to publication. Authorial intentionality is an important but often neglected component of scientific authorship. One wonders how much uncovered and suppressed dissent exists in published research where authorship is shared? More than is admitted, for sure, which makes something of a nonsense of that part of the ICMJE definition calling for public responsibility to be accepted by all authors.

The fourth component in my taxonomy of authorship is *agency*. By this, I wish to ask, Who is the agent of the text? That is, who creates the text? On first reflection, this question seems obvious. It is the writer who creates the text. But this is not so. The creator of the text—the person who creates a meaningful reading or interpretation of the text—is the reader (Horton 1995a, 1997a, 1997d). The author sets out a version of the text, but the reader will never accept that version at face value. Rather, readers will compare the contents of the paper with their own views and knowledge about the subject, creating a unique, interiorized text of their own by combining the two.

The linearity of the scientific paper is formalized by its IMRAD structure (namely, introduction, methods, results, and discussion). The authors' intentions can be set out logically within this structure, and the reader is forced to confront them as such, although the order in which they are confronted is for the reader to determine. Parts of the text, including tables and figures, will be read, other parts skimmed, and some ignored totally. The agent of the text can only ever be the reader.

In the digital environment, this linearity breaks down even further. The path taken by the reader through a text is now far less dependent on the traditional order set by the author. Readers can click themselves to wherever they wish. In this setting, the agency of the text shifts still more to the reader.

These four concepts—attribution, authority, animus, and agency—underlie my understanding of authorship in science. They could provide a useful framework on which to reconstruct a definition of the author. However, we must consider a further challenge faced by authorship in recent years, namely, the clinical trial as a dominant force shaping medical knowledge.

The Clinical Trial: Toward an Impersonal Author

Authorship has, thus far, been amenable to rational investigation and reflection. The clinical trial, however, seems to defeat all attempts at logical analysis from many perspectives.

The Journal

In 1991, Jerome Kassirer and Marcia Angell, editors of the *New England Journal of Medicine,* outlined a new policy on authorship and acknowledgments for larger clinical trials (Kassirer and Angell 1991), essentially banning group authorship. They also insisted on written justification for large author lists and on restricted numbers of acknowledgments. The reaction was devastating. Carbone wrote that "making it harder to receive credit or acknowledgment in journals such as yours is only going to lessen the worth of the clinical investigator" (Carbone 1992, 1084). Hart argued that "your proposed rules will solve your problem, but they make it a little harder for first-rate researchers to work together without academic jealousy on multicenter clinical trials" (Carbone 1992, 1084). Kassirer and Angell immediately revised their rules: "On reflection . . . we are willing to accept so-called corporate authorship" (Carbone 1992, 1085). They also allowed acknowledgments to include some individuals who did not qualify for authorship. They admitted that they were "disappointed" by their readers' responses (Carbone 1992, 1085). The *New England Journal of Medicine*'s authoritarian stance on trial credits has had lasting effects on investigators (Topol 1998).

The Funding Agency

In 1994, Bernard Fisher's contract as chairman of the National Surgical Adjuvant Breast and Bowel Project (NSABP), funded by the U.S. National Cancer Institute (NCI), was abruptly ended after a finding that one physician in a participating center had falsified data about patients included in the trial (Rennie 1994). Fisher was alleged to have failed to act on this information, thereby shirking his public responsibility not only as chairman of the project but also as chief author on published papers that included the falsified data. The editors of the *New England Journal of Medicine* acted quickly to censure Fisher for failing to inform them of the fraud (Angell and Kassirer 1994). As the senior author, he should have contacted the journal immediately. He did not, and the allegation caused the NCI to instruct Fisher's university in Pittsburgh to dismiss him from the NSABP, along with his statistical associate, Carol Redmond. This the university did, although both Fisher and Redmond have since been exonerated.

Like federal funding agencies, the pharmaceutical industry also has huge influence over authors. In 1996, the *Wall Street Journal* (King 1996) reported that a drug company, Boots, had exerted legal pressure on the author of a study it had funded, and which was soon to be published in *JAMA*, to withdraw her paper. The authors' contract with Boots stated that they would not be able to publish "without written consent" from the company (Wadman 1996, 4). This consent had not been given, and it was unlikely to be secured, since the data in question were not favorable to the company's product. Faced with this legal threat, the University of California, San Francisco, withdrew its support from Betty Dong, the senior author (Rennie 1997). Dong's paper was eventually published (Dong et al. 1997) to a hail of criticism from the drug company (Spigelman 1997). Rennie (1997, 1241) argued the obvious point, which Dong and associates had somehow forgotten: "Investigators . . . should never allow sponsors veto power" over publication. This is a fundamental right of an author and lies at the heart of academic freedom. Neither the responsibility of authors nor their independent authority should be taken for granted.

The Institution

Davies and colleagues assessed how multiauthored research was evaluated when Canadian medical faculty were reviewed for tenure and promotion (Davies, Langley, and Speert 1996). Only one dean's office had written guidelines for assessing authorship, and assigning collective authorship to a research group was thought to diminish the credit given to participating researchers. Multicenter versus single-center research was weighted differently by respondents; seven of 15 respondents rated multicenter research more highly, while four thought them to be of equivalent status. Davies, Langley, and Speert concluded that there was no consistency in assigning credit among research collaborators. Given that multicenter research is increasingly common, the need for guidance on evaluating research contributions is of pressing concern.

The Trialist

In June 1996, just after the Nottingham conference on authorship, a widely published U.K. trialist wrote to me. She had participated in a clinical trial published in the *Lancet*, in which she was acknowledged but not listed as an author. This extract is edited to remove any possibility of attribution.

> There is much disquiet [concerning] the vexed question of authorship. I thought it might be interesting for you to have my view of what the "contributors" actually did: [A]—wrote the paper, [B]—did the "hands-on" statistical analyses, [C]—took over as Director of [X] in 1993, [D] is the administrator at [X]. [E]—was formerly director of [X] and retired in 1993, i.e. three years ago. It was significant that this was never discussed [among participants]. As far as the publication itself is concerned, it is ill-informed and poorly discussed. In spite of pointing this out to [A], my comments were ignored. [Our patients] form one tenth of the group that are the body of this publication. As you can see, there are many issues here of responsibility, accountability, and credit. I doubt you can do anything—except use this as a debating example of how authorship in this situation should be anonymous. In our own unit, we have seriously thought of withdrawing our patients from [X].

Options and Objections

There are several possible solutions to questions of authorship in multicenter clinical trials. No consensus exists around any of these, and the ICMJE does not help trialists to reach a practicable solution.

Carbone (1992) proposed the most rational system of authorship to date. In his scheme, used by the U.S. Eastern Cooperative Oncology Group for 20 years, the *first* author is always the primary protocol chairperson. The *second* author is the statistician with involvement in design, randomization, data analysis, and writing of the final paper. In addition, authorship is given to study co-chairpersons (often specialists in particular aspects of the study). Substantial contributions, defined as providing at least 10% of cases in large (more than 100-person) studies or a minimum of ten cases in smaller studies, are also credited with authorship. At least one author from an institution is listed if these criteria are met. Finally, the disease committee chairperson is also included as an author. Carbone, who was group chairperson, never insisted that his name be added merely because of his title.

Oliver (1995, 668) also supported a more careful and systematic approach to trial authorship. His proposal is directed toward more junior collaborators: "The chairperson of the steering committee of a trial [could] provide junior investigators with a certificate of their participation, which could then be used in applications for new posts and during interviews by selection or search committees."

However, if exact guidelines cannot be agreed upon, three further possibilities are available. The trial team can assume *anonymous group authorship*, with all contributors and committees listed and acknowledged but with no individual named as author. The disadvantage of this approach is that the impersonal paper, while a paragon of democracy, may damage rather than help those responsible because it fails to give named credit (Davies, Langley, and Speert 1996). If named contributions are preferred, *bundled authorship* may be agreeable. In this scheme the clinicians associated with the studies are divided equally among the projected publications, and an individual is given major responsibility for preparing each single manuscript. All other contributors would be listed and acknowledged. Finally, a small *writing committee* could assume the authorship of each paper, acting on behalf of a larger trial group, again acknowledging the complete list of contributors.

One danger of providing guidelines about authorship, as with any aspect of publication ethics, is that guidelines tend to become de facto rules. Medical journals have pointed out the risks to clinical research if investigators are overmanaged (Overmanaged medical research 1997). The line between providing the freedom to do creative research (and giving appropriate credit) and giving guidance to make that credit and its attendant

Table 2.2. Authorship Guidelines for Multicenter Collaboration

1. A publication plan should be constructed early on to avoid overlap of contents and ensure fair allocation of authorship. Prior written agreement must be obtained from the principal investigators of all centres whose data are to be used in any paper, and policy on authorship, correspondent, and acknowledgment for each paper should likewise be agreed.

2. Individuals interested in data collected at other sites should circulate their publication proposals to those sites, giving a reasonable specified time period in which to respond.

3. Authorship should reflect relative contributions to the writing of the paper as well as to the analysis, design, and conduct of the study. It may be appropriate for some contributors to be recognized by an acknowledgment.

4. The final draft of any paper must be circulated to all authors, whose written agreement regarding content and target journal must be obtained before each submission for publication. Consent must also be obtained from those whose contribution has been acknowledged.

5. When a public presentation of data is to be made and data are taken from a paper already accepted for publication, collaborating authors must be ackowledged. Where the data for presentation are taken from a paper still in preparation, permission must be obtained from the relevant authors for their findings to be presented and the authors likewise acknowledged. Agreement may be given in advance for certain categories of presentation.

6. All papers which combine data from more than one site should state the affiliation to the wider research collaboration. Papers should be distributed to all members.

Source: This table was first published in the *BMJ* (A. Barker and R. A. Powell, "Guidelines Exist on Ownership of Data and Authorship in Multicentre Collaborations," *BMJ* 314[1997]:1046) and is reproduced by permission of the *BMJ*.

responsibility more equitable is a fine one, but one that should be carefully kept in mind at the earliest stages of the investigation. To this end, the guidelines for multicenter collaboration recently published by Barker and Powell (1997) provide a valuable foundation (table 2.2). These six "rules," which emphasize the importance of a publication plan, deserve wide scrutiny and discussion.

Reconstructing the Author

Despite the ambiguities about definition and quarrels over meaning, the concept of authorship is unlikely to lose its importance in science. Indeed, author inflation is becoming a serious burden to journal editors, reflecting not only increasing interdisciplinary collaboration but also greater competition for credit. The number of papers with large numbers of authors is increasing in many journals (Drenth 1995; Onwude, Staines, and Lilford 1993; Alvarez-Dardet et al. 1985; Sobal and Ferentz 1990; Morgan 1984; Dardik 1977; Mussurakis 1993). Some editors clearly see these shifts as indicating a greed for recognition rather than an evolution in the way science is done, a belief supported by investigators who have given testimony about how they have been treated by senior colleagues more concerned with scientific prestige than academic integrity (Hunt 1991; Horton 1998b, 1998c).

I have outlined three theories of the author: first, the ICMJE view, which binds credit for participation (intellectual rather than actual) to responsibility; second, a scientist-driven perspective, which focuses on writing and collecting data in addition to design, analysis, and interpretation; and third, my preferred separation of authorial characteristics into attribution, authority, animus, and agency. These theories exist in the context of two opposing forces, the increasing pressure to be named as an author for material reasons (such as tenure) and the trend toward greater impersonalization of authorship in clinical trials. Given this complexity any simple solution seems an elusive goal.

Can this confusion be dispersed by a coherent theory of authorship? I think it can, but we need to avoid subsuming too much into the term *authorship*. The word *authorship* signifies a complex concept. The authorship of a scientific paper is neither a single person nor a simple idea linking "work" to "scientific paper." The research enterprise includes two inseparable components: first, the research and, second, the preparation of a manuscript for publication describing that research. These two activities are, of course, related but not necessarily directly so (Medawar 1996a). Research data are generated by an array of individuals from program director to laboratory technician.

Rennie and Flanagin (1994, 471) supported "the idea of encouraging the more formal use of acknowledgments to make clear to the reader who did what." The notion of film credits, where specific and explicit contributions are cited (Moulopoulos, Sideris, and Georgilis 1983), with overall responsibility assumed by one individual, led to the proposal, by Rennie in Nottingham (Rennie, Yank, and Emanuel 1997), to divide authors into guarantors and contributors. In the wake of the fraud exposed by Collins (Marshall 1996), this proposal has received strong support from White and Knight (White 1997). White (1997) explained that

> an alternative means of allocating responsibility for the contents of a paper would simply require the contributions of all authors to be boldly and briefly stated. Such a statement could conveniently be placed in the acknowledgments or in a footnote of a paper giving each author's initials and contribution—for example, "AB, immunohistochemistry, wrote paper; MB, polymerase chain re-

action and Northern blots; EL, physiological recordings; ME, donated antibodies; BS, intellectual contributions, co-authored paper, provided funding and lab space."

If we add a guarantor, which fixes a point of overall responsibility for the research reported in the paper, we have arrived at Rennie's proposal.

Rennie, Yank, and Emanuel proposed that a *contributors list* should appear as a footnote, describing a job-driven identification of contribution. The *byline* is the list of those who "contributed most substantially to the work" (Rennie, Yank, and Emanuel 1997, 583). *Guarantors* are "those people who have contributed substantially, but who also have made added efforts to ensure the integrity of the entire project." They "must be prepared to be accountable for all parts of the completed manuscript, before and after publication" (582). The advantages of this scheme are many. It is precise, it is fair, and it may diminish the risk of fraud. It allows academic promotions committees to discern research contributions. And authorship abuse—gift authorship, ghost authorship (a paper written by a person whose name does not appear on the published article), and the disappearing author (a significant contributor not acknowledged in the author list)—will be lessened. The first six months of the *Lancet*'s experience of contributors have been reviewed by Yank and Rennie (1999).

Questions persist. For example, some editors believe that all authors should be guarantors of the work. Allowing otherwise merely dilutes each author's responsibility. (Not so, since individuals clearly have responsibility for their own portions of the study.) Also, just who is the guarantor? Is it that rare person who can answer all questions about the details of a paper, including the statistical analysis, or is it the senior author, the head of the lab, the principal investigator, the director of the institution, the chairperson of the funding body? In other words, where does final responsibility for the work justifiably end? Can there ever be one guarantor? I suspect not (Horton 1997b). This issue needs further careful thought. The *Lancet* did not introduce the guarantor into its shift toward contributors. And who would enforce these rules? Could a journal's ombudsman have final oversight (Horton 1996, 1998a; Sherwood 1997)?

There is also an issue about how far credit should be apportioned. The list might become, as it seems to have in some films, endless. Furthermore, if a long list of contributors and their contributions appears in the acknowledgments, whose names appear at the front of the paper? It might be too cumbersome to list every contributor. The guarantor/contributor/

Table 2.3. Authorship: Toward a Synthesis of Roles

Role	Film	Scientific Paper	Clinical Trial*
Attribution	Actors	Clinicians and scientists Statistician Data gatherers	Co-chair Major contributors Statisticians
Authority	Producer	Head of laboratory or equivalent	Trial program chairperson
Animus	Director	Principal investigator	Protocol chairperson
Agency	Scriptwriter	Shared	Shared

*After Carbone (1992), although the tendency toward group authorship with detailed acknowledgments is a further way to give reward for taking part. Adapted from data published in P. P. Carbone, "On Authorship and Acknowledgments," *New England Journal of Medicine* 326(1992):1084. Reprinted with permission.

byline route might simply bring us right back to where we started, namely, to the question, What is an author? Is an author only the one who makes a contribution that is so substantial that the individual can claim to be a guarantor?

If we accept a pluralistic definition of the author and the theatrical metaphor, we might be able to identify the key participants who do qualify for credit as authors (table 2.3). It seems ludicrous to exclude the head of a laboratory or the equivalent individual when that person has created and maintained the conditions enabling research to take place but has failed to fulfill precise ICMJE rules. It is also essential to include the statistician in the authorship; his or her intellectual and practical contribution, if the research has been carefully thought out, should equal that of any other participant. That still leaves the question of where one draws a line among participating clinicians and scientists. I believe the bar should be lowered to include those doing the experiment and collecting the data. That would mean more authors for editors to deal with, but the editor's role is to assist the scientific enterprise, not to hinder it. If research projects now include more researchers, then editors cannot alter that fact.

However, the cinematic metaphor, together with the guarantor/contributor/byline proposal, while attractive, clearly possesses its own tensions and inconsistencies. Indeed, on its own, Rennie's proposal is insufficient to deal with the authorship puzzle. He has focused on the research process. But the second part of the research enterprise—writing the manuscript—is less well developed. The byline is a valid journalistic device, but in science it is vulnerable, as the authors listed there are unlikely to have written the paper together in the sense we think of with the word *written*.

Instead, the responsibilities of authorship might better be understood in terms of an intellectual contract or professional covenant between investigator and editor (Horton 1997d). This contract—I emphasize that this is an *intellectual* and not a *legal* or *commercial* contract—is an agreement that binds the parties to it. It is sealed by the respective signatures on the letter of submission and the letter of acceptance. A contract suggests an ethical obligation on both parties. The intellectual contract consists of the offer of a paper by the investigators and its acceptance (one hopes) by the editor. Rather than "authors," the names put on the paper are the *signatories* to the research.

An offer is a proposition (in this case, a scientific paper) put by one person or persons (the investigators) to another (the editor), coupled with an indication that the scientist is willing to be held to that proposition. The offer is made knowing that the editor will decide whether to accept it or not according to the journal's stated procedures (e.g., statistical peer review). The contract must be enforceable, which might be a suitable role for the ombudsman when disputes arise. The duties of each party are clear. Investigators agree that the findings reported are honestly arrived at and that they will defend them if criticized. The editor agrees to be prompt in decision making, securing good reviews, and moving efficiently to publication.

An intellectual contract has several advantages. First, it dispenses with the widely perceived authoritarian status of the editor and places a more formal obligation on editors to honor their obligations toward investigators. That is, a contractual model imposes equity between researcher and editor. Second, it acknowledges that investigators and editors act, in the main, according to their own interests. Editors want to publish the best research they receive; investigators want their work published in the best and most appropriate journal. Third, the intellectual or professional nature of this contract implies a higher obligation than is provided for in a single legal agreement. The relationship between investigator and editor is close. They may come from the same specialist community, and they are certainly likely to have a relationship beyond the life of the paper in question. Therefore, although self-interest governs the relationship, each party should act well above this imperative, given the professional nature of the contract.

I would like to see this approach, and the concepts of contributors and signatories underlying it, replace the ICMJE definition. It is more practical, is more in tune with the wishes of scientists (Hopfield 1997), and provides a means of resolving several thorny editorial difficulties. A few issues do remain, especially those related to promotion and tenure practices. Efforts to use multiple indicators in the assessment of an individual's research record are under investigation (Lewison, Anderson, and Jack 1995). Editors also need ways to allow genuine interpretive disagreement among authors to be reflected in their final published paper (Horton 1995b). One solution might be, as with judicial opinions, to include separately authored statements within the discussion.

Finally, a question about the need for research police (Jacobsen 1997) still hangs over science. The DCSD (1998) deals mainly with authorship issues, as does the United Kingdom's COPE. It may be useful for individual countries to create a similar forum. However, it is important to recognize, first, that the range of scientific misconduct is broad (Horton 1995c; Stewart and Feder 1987) and, second, that no single committee can reasonably be expected to handle authorship disputes and full-blown accusations of fraud. Nevertheless, the matter is pressing (Nylenna et al. 1999; Horton 1999), since authorship disputes are becoming more common. For example, Linda Wilcox (1998) reported that the proportion of complaints to her Harvard Ombuds Office rose from 2.3% in 1996 to 10.7% in 1997. Future efforts should probably be directed toward educating scientists to appreciate the importance of their responsibility as co-authors (Relman 1984), both as contributors and signatories. This task will not be easy. In a study of the Robert Slutsky affair, Friedman (1990) concluded that journal editors resisted publication of retractions when co-authors lived in "psychological denial" of proven fraud. And Wendela Hoen, H. C. Walvoort, and A. J. P. M. Overbeke (1998) recently showed that many published authors in one Dutch medical journal were unfamiliar with the ICMJE criteria.

Coda

The cultural importance of the author in science is unassailable. The author exists as a source of interpretive authority for the reader. The meaning of a piece of published research is heavily, though not totally, influenced by the way in which the author "performs"—that is, the rhetorical intentions driving the authors, which lie behind the apparently formal presentation of the data (Horton 1995d). The "performance of science" was carefully discussed by Dorothy Nelkin (1998, 893), who noted that "the credit practices in scientific journals have not kept [pace] with the changes in the production of knowledge. Acknowledgement of these changes, however, is not just a simple matter of listing credits, but the dispersal of control and responsibility in the scientific community."

Three further forces are likely to shape our views of authorship during coming years. First, the advent of systematic reviews, especially the quantitative meta-analysis, raises several new concerns. Huston and Moher (1996) described how, in their review of the medical literature for trials on the antipsychotic drug risperidone, authorship seemed to have become a random game of musical chairs while the same data set was reported in different journals at different times. Such variable authorship, on a background of apparent multiple publication, will surely complicate the meta-analytic process. Agreement about authorship (as well as rules on repetitive publication) is essential to promote valid reviews into clinical effectiveness.

Second, the increasing influence of industry as a funding source for research presents several difficulties, some of which relate to authorship (Horton 1997c). Industry representatives may assist investigators with the conduct of their work, especially a clinical trial. They can help with data gathering and data analysis, in particular. How they do so might materially affect the outcome and interpretation of the study. For example, a company might suggest an analytic technique that favors its product or, as a major contributor to the research, it might have wider say on the slant of the paper's final conclusion than is wise.

To identify and describe these influences over data handling and interpretation, editors need to ask the signatories to the paper to report in the methods section how the company was involved. This idea was first applied to *Annals of Internal Medicine* by its editor, Frank Davidoff (1997). The implication is that it is not the company in the abstract that has been involved with a trial, but an individual—and this person should be cited as a contributor and/or signatory.

Third, the rapid developments in electronic publishing are likely to further loosen the bonds between author and text (Horton 1997b; McConnell and Horton 1999). The power of the author is also likely to be compromised. For instance, the systematic reviews produced by members of the Cochrane Collaboration (a movement to collate and combine data about clinical interventions) are made freely available without copyright under the Cochrane imprint. These studies tend to be discussed under the Cochrane label; the authors have become vestigial accompaniments.

The electronic text, set as it is in hypertext-mark-up language, allows the reader to assume the role of author. A reader can create a text, written by many individuals or impersonal groups of authors, which is unique for that reader. The author as a center of interpretive authority now begins to dissolve; attribution becomes blurred; the animating spirit behind the text and so its agency now shifts to the reader.

The author as a presence separate from the reader is now tacit rather than real. If constructing rules for what we now imagine to be authors is a trying task, the entrance of the tacit author is likely to be totally defeating. Yet this shift from the imagined or impersonal author to an implied authorship is likely to be the characterizing, perhaps even stigmatizing, change in scientific communication in the digital era.

Huth (1985, 280) foresaw this threat over a decade ago: "But will electronic publishing be as attractive to authors as today's books and journals? In electronic formats authors will not be as visible as they are on paper. Do not sell short the value of that visibility: referrals, consultations, political self-promotion, academic advancement, tenure. Remember that publishing means to make one's paper—a paper in the sense of a coherent intellectual package of question, data, and answer—visible for readers today and in the future."

The difficulty we face is simply that we have come to rely too heavily on the author as our interpretive *source* (Anderson 1992). Rather, we should see the author's text as a *site* for interpretation. Or, as Luca Toschi (1996, 204) put it, a "territory for experimentation." A theory of authorship is a thin cover for a theory of interpretation. Wolfgang Iser (1978, 20) had much to say on this misreading: "So long as the focal point of interest was the author's intention, or the contemporary, psychological, social, or historical meaning of the text, or the way in which it was constructed, it scarcely seemed to occur to critics that the text could only have meaning when it was read." Only when we come to understand that, from the point of view of a text's meaning, the most important author is the reader will we truly begin to appreciate the limitations of our conventional notions of authorship.

References

Alvarez-Dardet, C., E. Gascon, P. Mur, and A. Nolasco. 1985. Ten-year trends in the *Journal*'s publications. *New England Journal of Medicine* 312:1521–22.

Anderson, C. 1992. Authorship: Writer's cramp. *Nature* 355:101.

Angell, M., and J. P. Kassirer. 1994. Setting the record straight in breast-cancer trials. *New England Journal of Medicine* 330:1448–50.

Barker, A., and R. A. Powell. 1997. Guidelines exist on ownership of data and authorship in multicentre collaborations. *BMJ* 314:1046.

Bhopal, R. J., J. M. Rankin, E. McColl, L. H. Thomas, E. F. Kaner, R. Stacy, P. H. Pearson, B. G. Vernon, and H. Rodgers. 1997. The vexed question of authorship: Views of researchers in a British medical faculty. *BMJ* 314:1009–12.

Carbone, P. P. 1992. On authorship and acknowledgments. *New England Journal of Medicine* 326:1084 (Discussion by R. G. Hart, A. J. Pinching, D. Canter, M. F. Fathalla, P. F. A. Van Look, J. P. Kassirer, and M. Angell, pp. 1084–85).

Commission on Research Integrity (CRI), Ryan Commission. 1995. *Integrity and misconduct in research: Report of the Commission on Research Integrity to the Secretary of Health and Human Services, the House Committee on Commerce, and the Senate Committee on Labor and Human Resources.* Washington, D.C.: Department of Health and Human Services, Public Health Service. See also http://www.faseb.org/opar/cri.html. Site accessed 17 February 1999.

Committee on Publication Ethics (COPE). 1998. *The COPE report, 1998.* London: BMJ Books.

Crohn, B. B., L. Ginzburg, and G. D. Oppenheimer. 1932. Regional ileitis: A pathologic and clinical entity. *Journal of the American Medical Association* 99:1323–29.

Danish Committee on Scientific Dishonesty (DCSD). 1998. *The Danish Committee on Scientific Dishonesty: Annual report 1997.* Copenhagen: Danish Research Councils. See also http://www.forskraad.dk/spec-udv/uvvu/ann-report97/index.htm. Site accessed 31 March 1999.

Dardik, H. 1977. Multiple authorship. *Surgery, Gynecology and Obstetrics* 145:418.

Davidoff, F. 1997. Where's the bias? *Annals of Internal Medicine* 126:986–88.

Davies, H. D., J. M. Langley, and D. P. Speert. 1996. Rating authors' contributions to collaborative research: The PICNIC survey of university departments of pediatrics. Pediatric Investigators' Collaborative Network on Infections in Canada. *Canadian Medical Association Journal* 155:877–82.

Dong, B. J., W. W. Hauck, J. G. Gambertoglio, L. Gee, J. R. White, J. L. Bubp, and F. S. Greenspan. 1997. Bioequivalence of generic and brand-name levothyroxine products in the treatment of hypothyroidism. *JAMA* 227:1205–13.

Drenth, J. P. 1995. Authorship inflation: A trend reversed. *Lancet* 345:1242–43.

Eastwood, S., P. A. Derish, E. Leash, and S. B. Ordway. 1996. Ethical issues in biomedical research: Perceptions and practices of postdoctoral research fellows responding to a survey. *Science and Engineering Ethics* 2:89–114.

Editorial consensus on authorship and other matters. 1985. *Lancet* 2:595.

Epstein, R. J. 1993. Six authors in search of a citation: Villains or victims of the Vancouver convention? *BMJ* 306:765–67.

Flanagin, A., L. A. Carey, P. B. Fontanarosa, S. G. Phillips, B. P. Pace, G. D. Lundberg, and D. Rennie. 1998. Prevalence of articles with honorary authors and ghost authors in peer-reviewed medical journals. *JAMA* 280:222–24.

Friedman, P. J. 1990. Correcting the literature following fraudulent publication. *JAMA* 263:1416–19.

Games people play with authors' names. 1997. *Nature* 387:831.

Gilson, M. K. 1997. Responsibility of co-authors. *Science* 275:14. (See related commentary by T. I. Baskin, J. M. Pasachoff, and C. Loehle, p. 14.)

Goodman, N. W. 1994. Survey of fulfillment of criteria for authorship in published medical research. *BMJ* 309:1482.

Hoen, W. P., H. C. Walvoort, and A. J. P. M. Overbeke. 1998. What are the factors determining authorship and the order of the authors' names? *JAMA* 280:217–18.

Hopfield, J. J. 1997. Authorship: Truth in labeling. *Science* 275:1403.

Horton, R. 1995a. The interpretive turn. *Lancet* 346:3.

———. 1995b. MAST-I: Agreeing to disagree. *Lancet* 346:1504.

———. 1995c. Revising the research record. *Lancet* 346:1610–11.

———. 1995d. The rhetoric of research. *BMJ* 310:985–87.

———. 1996. The *Lancet*'s ombudsman. *Lancet* 348:6.

———. 1997a. Prague: The birth of the reader. *Lancet* 350:898–99.

———. 1997b. The signature of responsibility. *Lancet* 350:5–6.

———. 1997c. Sponsorship, authorship, and a tale of two media. *Lancet* 349:1411–12.

———. 1997d. The unstable medical research paper. *Journal of Clinical Epidemiology* 50:981–86.

———. 1998a. The journal ombudsperson: A step toward scientific press oversight. *JAMA* 280:298–99.

———. 1998b. Publication and promotion: A fair reward. *Lancet* 352:892.

———. 1998c. The unmasked carnival of science. *Lancet* 351:688–89.

———. 1998d. Who should be an author? In *How to write a paper,* ed. G. W. Hall. London: BMJ Books.

———. 1999. Scientific misconduct: Exaggerated fear but still real and requiring a proportionate response. *Lancet* 354:7–8.

Horton, R., and R. Smith. 1996a. Signing up for authorship. *Lancet* 347:780.

———. 1996b. Time to redefine authorship. *BMJ* 312:723.

Howe, P. J. 1996. Exonerated MIT Nobel laureate lashes out. *Boston Globe,* 29 October, A3.

Hunt, R. 1991. Trying an authorship index. *Nature* 352:187.

Huston, P., and D. Moher. 1996. Redundancy, disaggregation, and the integrity of medical research. *Lancet* 347:1024–26.

Huth, E. 1985. The physician as author of medical information. *Bulletin of the New York Academy of Medicine* 61:275–82.

International Committee of Medical Journal Editors (ICMJE). 1985. Guidelines on authorship. *British Medical Journal* 291:722.

———. 1993. Uniform requirements for manuscripts submitted to biomedical journals. *JAMA* 269:2282–86.

———. 1997. Uniform requirements for manuscripts submitted to biomedical journals. *Annals of Internal Medicine* 126:36-47. See also http://www.acponline.org/journals/resource/unifreqr.htm. Site accessed 8 March 1999.

Iser, W. 1978. *The act of reading.* Baltimore: Johns Hopkins University Press.

Jacobsen, G. 1997. Do we need a research police? *Journal of the Royal College of Physicians of London* 31:8–9.

Kapoor, V. K. 1995. Polyauthoritis giftosa. *Lancet* 346:1039.

Kassirer, J. P., and M. Angell. 1991. On authorship and acknowledgments. *New England Journal of Medicine* 325:1510–12.

Kevles, D. J. 1998. *The Baltimore case.* New York: Norton.

King, R. T. 1996. Bitter pill: How a drug company paid for university study, then undermined it. *Wall Street Journal,* 25 April, 1, 33.

Lewison, G., J. Anderson, and J. Jack. 1995. Assessing track records. *Nature* 377:671.

Liu, P., S. A. Tarle, A. Hajra, D. F. Claxton, P. Marlton, M. Freedman, M. J. Siciliano, and F. S. Collins. 1993. Fusion between transcription factor CBF beta/PEBP2 beta and a myosin heavy chain in acute myeloid leukemia. *Science* 261:1041–44.

Lock, S. 1995. Lessons from the Pearce affair: Handling scientific fraud. *BMJ* 310:1547–48.

———. 1997. Fraud in medical research. *Journal of the Royal College of Physicians of London* 31:90–94.

Lock, S., and F. Wells, eds. 1996. *Fraud and misconduct in medical research.* 2d ed. London: BMJ Publishing Group.

Lundberg, G. D., and R. M. Glass. 1996. What does authorship mean in a peer-reviewed medical journal? *JAMA* 276:75.

Marshall, E. 1996. Fraud strikes top genome lab. *Science* 274:908–10.

MAST-I Group. 1995. Randomised controlled trial of streptokinase, aspirin, and combination of both in treatment of acute ischaemic stroke. *Lancet* 346:1509–14.

McConnell, J., and R. Horton. 1999. *Lancet* electronic research archive and international health eprint server. *Lancet* 354:2–3.

Medawar, P. 1996a. Is the scientific paper a fraud? In *The strange case of the spotted mice and other classic essays on science,* 33–39. Oxford: Oxford University Press.

———. 1996b. The strange case of the spotted mice. In *The strange case of the spotted mice and other classic essays on science,* 132–43. Oxford: Oxford University Press.

Morgan, P. P. 1984. How many authors can dance on the head of an article? *Canadian Medical Association Journal* 130:842.

Moulopoulos, S. D., D. A. Sideris, and K. A. Georgilis. 1983. Individual contributions to multiauthor papers. *British Medical Journal* 287:1608–10.

Mussurakis, S. 1993. Coauthorship trends in the leading radiological journals. *Acta Radiologica* 34:316–20.

Nelkin, D. 1998. Publication and promotion: The performance of science. *Lancet* 352:893.

Nylenna, M., D. Andersen, G. Dahlquist, M. Sarvas, and A. Aakvaag. 1999. Handling of scientific dishonesty in the Nordic countries. *Lancet* 354:57–61.

Oliver, M. F. 1995. AI, or the anonymity of authorship. *Lancet* 345:668.

Onwude, J. L., A. Staines, and R. J. Lilford. 1993. Multiple author trend worst in medicine. *BMJ* 306:1345.

Overmanaged medical research. 1997. *Lancet* 349:145.

Parmley, W. W. 1997. Authorship: Taking the high road. *Journal of the American College of Cardiology* 29:702.

Pearce, J. M., and R. I. Hamid. 1994. Randomised controlled trial of the use of human chorionic gonadotrophin in recurrent miscarriage associated with polycystic ovaries. *British Journal of Obstetrics and Gynaecology* 101:685–88.

Pearce, J. M., I. T. Manyonda, and G. V. Chamberlain. 1994. Term delivery after intrauterine relocation of an ectopic pregnancy. *British Journal of Obstetrics and Gynaecology* 101:716–17.

Relman, A. S. 1983. Lessons from the Darsee affair. *New England Journal of Medicine* 308:1415–17.

———. 1984. Responsibilities of authorship: Where does the buck stop? *New England Journal of Medicine* 310:1048–49.

Rennie, D. 1994. Breast cancer: How to mishandle misconduct. *JAMA* 271:1205–7.

———. 1997. Thyroid storm. *JAMA* 277:1238–43.

Rennie, D., and A. Flanagin. 1994. Authorship! Authorship! Guests, ghosts, grafters, and the two-sided coin. *JAMA* 271:469–71.

Rennie, D., V. Yank, and L. Emanuel. 1997. When authorship fails: A proposal to make contributors accountable. *JAMA* 278:579–85.

Shapiro, D. W., N. S. Wenger, and M. F. Shapiro. 1994. The contributions of authors to multiauthored biomedical research papers. *JAMA* 271:438–42.

Sharp, D. 1998. A ghostly crew. *Lancet* 351:1076.

Sherwood, T. 1997. *Lancet* ombudsman's first report. *Lancet* 350:4–5.

Smith, J. 1994. Gift authorship: A poisoned chalice? *BMJ* 309:1456–57.

Smith, R. 1997. Authorship: Time for a paradigm shift? *BMJ* 314:992.

Sobal, J., and K. S. Ferentz. 1990. Abstract creep and author inflation. *New England Journal of Medicine* 323:488–89.

Spigelman, M. K. 1997. Bioequivalence of levothyroxine preparations for treatment of hypothyroidism. *JAMA* 277:1199.

Stewart, W. W., and N. Feder. 1987. The integrity of the scientific literature. *Nature* 325:207–14.

Susser, M. 1997. Authors and authorship: Reform or abolition? *American Journal of Public Health* 87:1091–92.

Tognoni, G., and M. C. Roncaglioni. 1995. Dissent: An alternative interpretation of MAST-I. *Lancet* 346:1515.

Topol, E. J. 1998. Drafter and draftees. *Lancet* 352:897–98.

Toschi, L. 1996. Hypertext and authorship. In *The future of the book,* ed. G. Nunberg, 169–207. Berkeley and Los Angeles: University of California Press.

Wadman, M. 1996. Drug company "suppressed" publication of research. *Nature* 381:4.

White, B. 1997. Multiple authorship. *Science* 275:461 (see also related commentary by J. Knight, p. 461).

Whitley, W. P., D. Rennie, and A. W. Hafner. 1994. The scientific community's response to evidence of fraudulent publication: The Robert Slutsky case. *JAMA* 272:170–73.

Wilcox, L. J. 1998. Authorship: The coin of the realm, the source of complaints. *JAMA* 280:216–17.

Wooley, C. F., P. de Sa, and A. Sagar. 1996. "Struck" by fraud. *Science* 274:1593.

Yank, V., and D. Rennie. 1999. Disclosure of researcher contributions: A study of original research articles in *The Lancet*. *Annals of Internal Medicine* 130:661–70.

Fiona Godlee

Biomedical journals exist to publish accurate and useful information for scientists and clinicians. Editorial peer review—by which journal editors and their external advisors decide which manuscripts should be published and in what form—is a means to that end. It represents an attempt on the part of the scientific community to ensure that decisions about what is published are valid rather than arbitrary or partial. Success in this attempt would mean that all work ending up in print was relevant to the journal's audience, important, original, and methodologically and ethically sound. It would also mean that no work that met these criteria was overlooked. Few of those involved in the peer-review process—whether authors, reviewers, editors, or readers—could claim it has succeeded.

Decisions about what to publish have a clear ethical dimension. First, it is unethical to publish bad science, just as it is to practice bad science. Whatever one's definition of bad science (irrelevant, inaccurate, sloppy, incomplete, fraudulent), its publication compounds the initial waste of research effort by misleading those who cannot distinguish it from good science and alienating those who can. It clogs up a system already overburdened with information, leaving less room for better work. And vitally in the biomedical sciences, it reduces the likelihood of patients receiving appropriate, high-quality care. Second, it is unethical to fail to publish good and important science. Journals should facilitate rather than obstruct the dissemination of innovative research that could extend our understanding or improve the way in which patients are managed. And third, it is unethical to give credit to the wrong people. Since publication is the currency of success in science, it should be awarded fairly, based on the quality of the work, and not for reasons of prestige, prejudice, or personal gain.

Current expectations of peer review are high, and perhaps as a result its critics are many. It is viewed both as one answer to science's problems and as its Achilles heel. At its worst, peer review is seen as expensive, slow, biased, open to abuse, patchy at detecting scientific flaws, and almost useless at detecting fraud or misconduct. This chapter will take as its starting point two questions posed a quarter of a century ago by the then-editor of the *New England Journal of Medicine,* Franz Ingelfinger (1974): Does peer review ensure that journals make good decisions about what to publish? And is it worth the price?

Does Peer Review Ensure That Journals Make Good Decisions?

Editorial peer review in its current form is a relatively new concept. Although peer review was a feature of the very earliest scientific journals dating back to the seventeenth century (Lock 1992), until the middle of this century most editors made their own decisions on what to publish in their journals. Over the past 50 years, as science has become more complex and competitive, more and more journals have formed to serve specialties and subspecialties, and peer review has developed into a vast industry. Lock (1992) estimated that about three-quarters of scientific journals now use peer review to assess research articles for publication.

The term *peer review* covers a multitude of different systems of evaluation. Because of this, while editors, researchers, and the public tend to see the term as a certificate of excellence, the National Library of Medicine does not require peer review for a journal to be selected for *Index Medicus* or MEDLINE (Colaianni 1994). In the context of biomedical journals, the term should be reserved for systems of decision making that involve editors seeking advice from independent external experts. According to the International Committee of Medical Journal Editors (ICMJE), a peer-reviewed journal is "one that has submitted most of its published articles for review by experts who are not part of the editorial staff" (ICMJE 1997, 43). Even this definition leaves scope for wide variation. Smaller journals with part-time editors tend to rely on their external advisers to decide the fate of a manuscript. If two reviewers disagree, a third may be asked to adjudicate. Editors of larger journals, on the other hand, use reviewers for advice only and may have additional systems, such as a weekly panel meeting of editors and external expert advisers, to help them decide on publication. Some journals obtain statistical peer review on all manuscripts before publication; others do not. A few journals pay their reviewers; most do not. Whatever the type of system, the peer-review process involves the combined input of journal editors and external reviewers. In addition, it involves not only the decision to accept or reject an article for one particular journal but also decisions on how accepted articles should be revised before publication.

The Aims and Failings of Peer Review

The aims of peer review are twofold: first, to help editors decide which articles to accept and, second, to improve accepted manuscripts before publication. The first of these aims is the one in which peer review meets most criticism, perhaps because the all-or-nothing nature of publication leaves many disgruntled authors understandably questioning the validity of the process by which their articles were rejected. This question of whether peer review leads journals to make good decisions can only be approached with a clear recognition of the large subjective element within peer review. According to Jacob Bronowski (1965, 63–64) in *Science and Human Values*, "Those who think that science is ethically neutral confuse the findings of science, which are, with the activity of science, which is not." If this is true, we should not expect peer review to be ethically neutral either, since it is part of the activity of science.

Editorial peer review is about making choices. To pretend otherwise is to deny the very function of journals. Journals add value to the scientific enterprise by selecting this paper and not that, by asking authors to emphasize these data and omit those, by shortening here and expanding there. These choices reflect the values of the journal. The criteria on which they are based should, of course, be made explicit and should be justifiable in terms of their contribution to the advancement of biomedical science and the improvement of patient care. But within these criteria, there is a general sense that making good decisions should mean that bad science is excluded and good and important science included, that reviewers of the same paper broadly agree about its strengths and weaknesses, and that their recommendations and editors' decisions are the same when confronted with the same paper a second time.

The evidence that peer review has, on occasion, failed on all these counts is overwhelming. Several of the more celebrated pieces of fraudulent research have passed through the peer-review process unnoticed (Lock 1993). Secondary review of manuscripts after they have been published has shown that errors are rife. Nor does peer review reliably identify lack of originality or the extremes of this—plagiarism and repetitive publication. In their study of institutional bias in peer review, Peters and Ceci (1982) resubmitted slightly altered versions of published papers to the journals that had originally published them. The journals identified only three of the 12 articles as resubmissions, and only one of the remaining nine articles was reaccepted.

Reviewers of the same paper do not agree much more than would be expected by chance, either in the nature of their comments or in their final recommendations (Oxman et al. 1991). The level of consensus varies according to the discipline. Complete agreement between two reviewers on whether to publish or reject an article has been reported in two-fifths (Ingelfinger 1974) to three-quarters (Zuckerman and Merton 1971) of cases, tending to be lower in biomedical journals than pure science journals and higher when a paper is of poor quality. Studies that involved sending the same manuscript to large numbers of reviewers have found similar rates of agreement (Godlee, Gale, and Martyn 1998).

However, these failings of peer review must be put into perspective. In examining the cognitive tasks involved in manuscript assessment, Kassirer and Campion (1994) drew an analogy between a reviewer's recommendation and a diagnostic test. They suggested that manuscript assessment, like even the most sophisticated diagnostic tests, has a certain sensitivity and specificity and must therefore lead to a certain number of false-positive and false-negative results, even in the hands of the most objective reviewers. Erroneous recommendations are, therefore, an inevitable and unavoidable aspect of the review process.

Does Peer Review Recognize Important New Research?

Quality control is an important function of peer review, but it is not the only or even the main function. Horrobin (1990, 1438) argued that

> the fundamental purpose of peer review in the biomedical sciences must be consistent with that of medicine itself, to cure sometimes, to relieve often, to comfort always. Peer review must therefore aim to facilitate the introduction into medicine of improved ways of curing, relieving, and comforting patients. The fulfillment of this aim requires both quality control and the encouragement of innovation. If an appropriate balance between the two is lost, then peer review will fail to fulfill its purpose.

Horrobin's fear was that quality control has been emphasized to the detriment of creative innovation. He suggested that, while the overall accuracy and reliability of medical articles have improved substantially over the past 60 years, there has been a relative failure of innovation. Part of the responsibility for this he laid at the door of journal editors and peer reviewers. Citing Cade's discovery of the effects of lithium in mania, he suggested that these crude experimental results would never have satisfied today's reviewers. He also cited examples of innovations, now known to be important, that were repeatedly rejected by peer-reviewed journals.

It would be difficult to establish the extent to which innovations are suppressed or the role played in this suppression by journals: increasingly, it is funding agencies that decide what gets investigated and therefore what eventually reaches journals. Even so, Horrobin asked that editors be alert to the rare possibility of a highly innovative article crossing their desk. If they suspect one, he suggested that they should take extra care in choosing a careful, open-minded, and unbiased reviewer and should not accept negative reviewers' comments without careful examination of the article themselves.

However, editors have a clear responsibility to ensure that published work is methodologically sound. Where doubts exist about the methodological rigor of an article, one option is to publish it as a "hypothesis promotor," with its status made clear to readers in an accompanying commentary or editorial note. General medical journals, which exist largely to publish work that is directly applicable to clinical medicine, may redirect startling but unproved innovative research to more specialist journals, where it can be examined by those who are in a position to take the ideas forward, but where it will be less likely to get picked up by the press.

Is Peer Review a Filter or a Traffic Policeman?

Directing research to the appropriate journal is an important function of peer review that has often been undervalued and misinterpreted. The finding that most papers rejected by high-impact journals are eventually published elsewhere (Wilson 1978; Relman 1978; Lock 1991; Chew 1991; Abby et al. 1994) has been interpreted as showing that, if authors persist long enough, they will get their work published. But Lock framed the issue in more helpful terms. He asked whether peer review acts as a filter, removing from circulation those papers that are below certain standards, or as a traffic policeman, directing research away from one journal to another (Lock 1991, 128). The evidence suggests that it performs both functions.

Studies in the 1970s found that 85% of articles rejected from the *Journal of Clinical Investigation* and the *New England Journal of Medicine* (Wilson 1978; Relman 1978) and 73% rejected from the *British Medical Journal (BMJ)* (Lock 1991) were subsequently published elsewhere. All three journals have high impact factors (based on the rates at which their articles are cited in the *Science Citation Index*) and high rejection rates. This means that they will tend to reject many submitted articles for editorial reasons (because they are not sufficiently original or relevant to the journal's readership, for example), rather than because of methodological weaknesses. The fact that manuscripts rejected from such journals are published elsewhere does not mean that peer review has failed. Only 11% of the articles rejected from the *BMJ* were subsequently published in other journals with high impact factors (Lock 1991), and a more recent study at the *American Journal of Surgery* found that only 38% of rejected articles were published in journals indexed in MEDLINE within three years of rejection (Abby et al. 1994). The authors concluded that peer review is an effective filter, keeping most of the papers it rejects out of the core medical literature.

Does Peer Review Improve the Published Article?

Despite the importance of this question in assessing the value of peer review, few studies have examined it adequately. One that has is a study by Goodman et al. (1994). Peer reviewers were asked to assess the quality of two versions of 111 consecutive manuscripts that had been accepted for publication by *Annals of Internal Medicine*. The first version was the manuscript as originally submitted to the journal; the second version was the manuscript as revised after peer review and editing. The two versions were prepared in the same format, and the reviewers were unaware of which version of the manuscript they were reviewing. They were asked to judge the quality of the manuscript on 34 points of written presentation, focusing on clarity, completeness, and balance of interpretation in all sections of the manuscript.

The study found that the peer-reviewed and edited versions of the manuscripts were judged to be of higher quality than the initial submissions, especially if the initial submission was very weak. Of the 34 elements, 33 were rated higher in the peer-reviewed and edited manuscripts. Nine of the first versions were judged to be of low quality (less than half of the items rated acceptable), compared with only one of the second versions. The improvements were not huge, but the manuscripts were already highly selected for quality, being those that had passed through the journal's peer-review process. Another study also showed that peer review and editing improve the readability of published articles (Roberts, Fletcher, and Fletcher 1994).

Several other studies, not directly intended to assess the effects of peer review, also suggest that proper peer review improves the quality of publications. Rochon et al. (1994) found that trials published in journal supplements were generally of lower quality than trials published in the parent journal. They concluded that this difference in quality probably results from the fact that, as shown in two previous studies (Bero, Galbraith, and Rennie 1992; Massie and Rothenberg 1993), articles in supplements are not subjected to the same rigorous peer review as articles in the parent journal.

Peer review may improve manuscripts, but it does not make them perfect. Many studies attest to the flaws in published articles revealed by secondary peer review. And in the study by Goodman et al. (1994), none of the peer-reviewed and edited manuscripts received perfect grades from the reviewers.

With all its flaws, however, the peer-review system lives on. This may be because the vested interests of editors, in whom much of the power currently resides, tend toward maintaining the status quo or because the system has intrinsic worth. Peer review will never be a perfect guard against fraud, inaccuracy, or unoriginality, nor, according to Kassirer and Campion (1994), should we expect it to be. This does not by any means justify complacency. But it does help to put the performance of peer review in perspective. Even given the documented poor standards of review (Godlee, Gale, and Martyn 1998), there is little doubt that the combined efforts of peer reviewers and editors result in the publication of better reports of better science. Let us, then, examine the price.

Is Peer Review Worth the Price?

It has been argued that peer review is inherently threatened by corruption (Judson 1994). Four interrelated aspects of peer review as it currently exists justify such a statement. First, science is a competitive enterprise, increasingly so as funds become limited. Second, peer review controls the currency of success—publication—from which flows funding, position, recognition, and power in science. Third, in sending manuscripts for review by experts in the same field, journals are putting them in the hands of the very people most likely to be in direct competition with the authors. Fourth, most journals preserve the anonymity of their reviewers by removing their names from the comments that are sent on to the authors. Such anonymity has been considered necessary to obtain uninhibited comment, but it has the effect of giving reviewers power without responsibility. Where ethical standards are lacking, this system, which grew up partly from a desire for greater accuracy and fairness in assessing people's work,

can become an opportunity to misappropriate data, breach the confidential relationship between author, editor, and reviewer, and make partial
judgments, whether consciously or unconsciously, to the detriment of
rivals or the benefit of friends.

In November 1978, a physician at the National Institutes of Health
(NIH) submitted a paper, with two co-authors, to the *New England Journal of
Medicine*. After two and a half months the paper was rejected with conflicting reports from peer reviewers. Within days of receiving the news, the
author, Helena Wachslicht-Rodbard, was asked by the head of her department to give her opinion on a paper on the same subject, which he had been
asked to review for another journal. To her amazement the paper, from a
group at Yale, contained not only data similar to her data but also verbatim
passages from her paper. Guessing correctly that the authors, Vijay Soman
and Philip Felig, had written the negative review that had contributed
to the rejection of her paper by the *New England Journal of Medicine*,
Wachslicht-Rodbard fired off an angry letter to the editor accusing Soman
and Felig of plagiarism and clear conflict of interest as reviewers of her work.

From the investigation that followed, as described in *Science* (Broad
1980), several important facts emerged. The *New England Journal of Medicine* had sent Wachslicht-Rodbard's paper to Felig, then a well-respected
professor at Yale and vice-chairman of the Department of Medicine. He had
passed it on to his junior colleague, Soman, for additional comments. Soman, an assistant professor, was also well respected in his field. In 1976 he
had received approval from the institutional review board at Yale to study
insulin binding in patients with anorexia nervosa. However, he had made
little progress with the work by the time that the Wachslicht-Rodbard paper, reporting findings from a study of insulin binding in patients with
anorexia nervosa, arrived on his desk two years later. Soman gave Felig a
negative report of the work, photocopied the manuscript without telling
Felig, and set to work on his own paper. Lacking sufficient numbers of
patients, he fabricated data on at least one case. Felig advised the *New
England Journal of Medicine* to reject Wachslicht-Rodbard's paper but made
no mention of the fact that his junior colleague was working on an identical study. Within a month, he and Soman submitted their paper to the
American Journal of Medicine, of which Felig was an associate editor.

Soman's fraud was subsequently found to extend to at least ten other
papers, for nine of which he was unable to produce the raw data. He
was asked to resign, and the fraudulent papers were eventually retracted.
Wachslicht-Rodbard's paper was published in the *New England Journal of*

Medicine but shortly afterward she quit the NIH for clinical work. It had taken her two years to convince people of any wrongdoing. Although Felig was apparently unaware of Soman's fraud, he was considered culpable in failing to declare a conflict of interest with regard to Wachslicht-Rodbard's paper, accepting authorship on a paper about which he could claim no direct knowledge, and inadequately supervising a junior colleague. He, too, was eventually forced to resign. Such extreme scientific misconduct is rare. But individual elements of the story—breach of confidentiality, misappropriation of data, and conflict of interest—may be less rare.

Confidentiality

A manuscript submitted for publication is and remains the intellectual property of the authors and is submitted to the journal on the understanding that it will be treated as a confidential document by editors and reviewers. The unwritten contract between editor and author should be as sacred as that between physician and patient. Editors should not show manuscripts to or discuss them with anyone outside the office except reviewers. Moreover, they should not even acknowledge to anyone, other than the authors and reviewers, that a particular manuscript is under consideration. If, as often happens, a member of the press asks for information about a manuscript that they have been told by the author is due for publication soon, the editors should decline to comment, however unhelpful this may seem.

Reviewers should follow the same code of practice. While some journals allow reviewers to seek advice from colleagues, most require them to ask the journal's permission to do this and to let them know whom they are consulting. Such consultation, if well supervised, is an important means of training junior colleagues in the art of peer review. But the colleagues should either sign the review or be acknowledged in the main reviewer's covering letter. In this way, journals can keep track of who has seen the paper during the review process. Reviewers should not make copies of the paper and should destroy or return it once the review has been written. Editors are well aware that such scrupulous conduct is by no means universal. But most reviewers are also current or prospective authors, who therefore have an interest in maintaining ethical standards of peer review.

The Misuse of Data

Improper use of a manuscript's contents is a subset of breach of confidentiality, and it can be a gray area. Clearly, wholesale plagiarism is wrong, as is the conscious theft of an idea. The ICMJE (1997, 44) says that "reviewers should not use knowledge of the work, before its publication, to further their own interests." But it would be inhuman to expect researchers not to take into account a convincing report suggesting, for example, that the technique they are using to study a problem may be inadequate or flawed. To continue to use the technique under such circumstances might even be considered foolish. Some societies, such as the Society for Neuroscience, state that it is ethical to use information contained in a manuscript under review to discontinue a line of research (Society for Neuroscience 1998, 14). Even the most scrupulous of us may find it difficult to remember where we read about a new finding, whether in a published report or when reviewing an unpublished manuscript. Papers that spend a long time in the review process or do the rounds of several journals before publication are especially at risk of misuse.

Editors have a clear obligation to protect authors' work from being misappropriated. They should make sure that reviewers know that the manuscript is confidential, that it should not be photocopied, and that it should be destroyed or returned once the review has been written. They should ensure that reviewers complete their evaluations speedily, and they should make their own decisions promptly. Editors should destroy rejected manuscripts and keep a record of who has seen the paper and when, in case authors subsequently raise concerns.

Conflict of Interest

Fraud may be considered rare in science, breaches of confidentiality and misuse of data less so, but conflict of interest is almost universal. According to the ICMJE (1997, 44), there is conflict of interest "when a participant in the peer review and publication process—author, reviewer, and editor—has ties to activities that could inappropriately influence his or her judgment, whether or not judgment is in fact affected." This distinction is important. Conflicts of interest are not best judged by those who have the conflicts, and therefore it is the possibility of such influence, rather than its actually being felt, that must be considered.

The ICMJE (1997, 44) suggests four main causes of conflict of interest: financial relationships, personal relationships, academic competition, and intellectual passion. Financial relationships are usually thought to be the most important, though this may be partly because, of all possible causes of conflict of interest, they are the easiest to articulate. Examples of financial conflicts of interest include working for or owning stock in companies providing services or products. When trials of a thrombolytic agent were under review at a cardiology journal, the editor was much criticized for having a financial interest in the company that manufactured the agent (O'Donnell 1991).

Personal relationships and academic competition can influence reviewers and editors alike. Reviewers may be more likely to give favorable reviews of papers written by friends and colleagues, and editors may be more likely to accept them. Enemies and competitors may be given unfairly critical review or unwarranted rejection, as in the Soman case. Such conflicts of interest are especially likely among reviewers and editors of small subspecialty journals, who will know many of the authors submitting manuscripts for review. Ensuring impartiality under such circumstances requires particular care and vigilance.

Intellectual passion is perhaps the most difficult form of conflict of interest to guard against. Reviewers and editors may have strongly held beliefs and opinions, which they may have spent the best part of their careers developing and expounding in print and on which their reputations now depend. Such people are not best placed to give a fair hearing to research that supports an opposite view. For Franz Ingelfinger, a former editor of the *New England Journal of Medicine,*

> the ideal reviewer should be totally objective, in other words, supernatural. Since author and reviewer usually are by selection engaged in similar endeavors, they are almost unavoidably either competitors or teammates. Even the most conscientious reviewer will find it difficult to wax enthusiastic about an account that undermines his tenets or to disparage a report supporting his work. If a reviewer is less conscientious, the reviewing system will falter grievously. (Ingelfinger 1974, 688)

Recent evidence has shown the influence of conflicts of interest on the views espoused by authors of review articles. Three studies found that authors with financial links to drug companies or the tobacco industry were more likely to draw favorable conclusions about a drug or to discount the effects of passive smoking than were those without such links (Stelfox et al. 1998; Barnes and Bero 1998). However, there is no direct evidence showing that the peer-review process is affected by conflicts of interest. Until such evidence is found, attempts to minimize the influence of conflict of interest in the peer-review process are based on the assumption that peer reviewers and editors are just as likely to be influenced as are authors.

It would be foolish to try to eliminate conflict of interest. The only way to do this would be to send papers to reviewers who had no interest in the area of research under review. This would largely defeat the object of peer review. Nor should there be any suggestion that conflict of interest is a crime. Some degree of conflict of interest is almost inevitable. The aim of any intervention should be to heighten awareness of the possibility of conflict of interest among editors and reviewers, to encourage disclosure of any recognized sources of conflict of interest with regard to a particular paper, and to take steps to minimize conflicts in the future. As the ICMJE (1997, 44) states, "Public trust in the peer review process and the credibility of published articles depend in part on how well conflict of interest is handled."

To heighten awareness and encourage full disclosure, many journals now ask reviewers to sign a statement, at the time they are asked to review each paper, either saying that they have no conflicts of interest or detailing any of which they are aware. Reviewers can then choose to disqualify themselves from the review of a particular paper or, having informed the editors, to act on their advice. The editor may feel that the declared conflict is not sufficiently serious to interfere with the reviewer's judgment and ask him or her to go ahead with the review. Asking reviewers to sign such a form does not at all guarantee that existing sources of conflict of interest will be disclosed. Reviewers may choose not to declare conflicts or may be unaware, especially in the case of intellectual passion, that any such conflict exists. It is therefore up to the editor to select reviewers who will be as far as possible free from such influences. For research that challenges a commonly held belief, editors may need to seek several different reviews and to be alert to the influences at work.

Journals are looking at ways of making it more likely that reviewers will declare any conflicts. The *BMJ* has decided to focus on a narrower definition of conflict of interest, involving only financial conflicts rather than the whole gamut of personal, professional, and political conflicts. And several journals are moving away from the pejorative term *conflict* in favor of more neutral terminology. The *BMJ*, for example, now uses the term *competing interests*. More open peer-review processes may encourage peer reviewers to declare conflicts, in the knowledge that the authors and possibly the readers will be told who they are and may know of existing conflicts. But at journals where peer reviewers remain anonymous, editors must be the authors' advocates. This they can be only if they are themselves aware that a conflict of interest exists. Peer reviewers should therefore be asked to declare all relevant conflicts of interest. It could also be argued that authors of letters that comment on published work are putting themselves in the role of peer reviewers and should therefore be required to declare conflicts of interest.

Editors can do a great deal to minimize the potential for conflicts of interest in their own dealings with papers. First, editors who make final decisions about papers should have no financial interest in the areas of research under review. Several journals, including the *New England Journal of Medicine* and the *BMJ*, have made it a rule that editors should not receive payments from or own stock in medically related companies. Second, where possible, editors should disqualify themselves from making final decisions on papers by authors with whom they have close personal or academic relationships or where they think the strength of their own beliefs or intellectual opinions might inappropriately influence their judgment. In such cases, they should seek advice from their editorial board or advisory committee.

Finally, because peer review costs money, the process itself introduces an important source of conflict of interest for editors: the need to raise revenue through pharmaceutical advertising (Fletcher and Fletcher 1992). The cost of peer review varies across journals. Larger journals have full-time editors who may spend more than half their time reading papers, selecting reviewers, assessing reviews, asking authors to revise papers, and assessing revisions, all of which constitutes peer review. Also, some journals pay their reviewers, either in cash or in subscriptions to the journal. While some journals raise revenue through subscriptions, most, including the major general medical journals and membership association journals, rely largely on advertising, most of which comes from the pharmaceutical industry. Editors can thus find themselves under pressure from their publishers to attract advertisers as well as subscribers. Systems should be in place to prevent such pressure from influencing editorial decisions. Most major journals have systems that prevent their advertising departments from knowing what is being published and when.

Bias on the Part of Reviewers and Editors

Bias in peer review occurs when decisions about publication are influenced by factors other than a paper's methodological quality or relevance to the journal's readers. The scope of bias is seemingly endless. A student of human nature could perhaps predict the main types of bias to which editors and peer reviewers, whether consciously or unconsciously, might fall prey—a preference for statistically significant results, for example, or for papers from prestigious authors or institutions. The existence of some of these biases has now been well documented, while some expected biases have been looked for but not found. The fundamentally subjective nature of peer review makes some degree of bias inevitable, but it is important to understand the sources of bias if we are to minimize their effect.

It has long been assumed that peer review favors well-known authors or those from prestigious institutions. However, proving this is not easy. Authors who are well known may be justly so, because of the high quality of their work, and may therefore be more likely to have their work published in the future. In addition, authors working in prestigious institutions have already been selected, one hopes, on the basis of merit and have all the added benefits that prestigious institutions can offer: the stimulation of other high-powered academic researchers, good laboratory facilities, and a competitive atmosphere. To provide convincing evidence of author or institutional bias, studies need to take into account these other factors that may legitimately influence decisions about publication.

In a celebrated study, Peters and Ceci (1982) resubmitted slightly altered versions of 12 articles to the psychology journals that had already published them. They chose articles from prestigious institutions, made minor changes to the titles, abstracts, and introductions, changed the authors' names, and changed the names of the institutions to unprestigious-sounding fictitious ones (such as the Tri-Valley Center for Human Potential). Three journals recognized the articles as resubmissions of previous work. Of the other nine articles, only one was accepted. The eight rejections were on grounds of poor study design, inadequate statistical analysis, or poor quality, not lack of originality. The authors concluded that the study showed bias against papers coming from unknown institutions. Despite much criticism (Lock 1991, 34–38), this study was widely quoted as proving that peer review was biased in favor of authors from prestigious institutions. But other studies failed to confirm such a bias (Mahoney 1977; Garfunkel et al. 1994), at least on the part of referees, or concluded that any difference could be explained by the quality of the papers themselves (Perlman 1982).

Peters and Ceci were researching in the 1970s. Since then, science has become less clubby and more competitive. Recent research suggests that any bias now existing may be in favor of less prestigious authors. In a study by Fisher, Friedman, and Strauss (1994), 57 consecutive manuscripts submitted to the *Journal of Developmental and Behavioral Pediatrics* were independently assessed, using a five-point scale, by two reviewers who were told the identity of the authors (unblinded reviewers) and two who were not told their identity (blinded reviewers). The study used the number of previous publications on the authors' curriculum vitae as a measure of how well known the authors were. All assessors gave higher grades to authors with more previous publications, but, surprisingly, the positive correlation between high grade and high numbers of publications was statistically significant only for blinded reviewers. Nonblinded reviewers, who were aware of the authors' identities, judged well-known authors more harshly than did the blinded reviewers, who had only the quality of the manuscript to go on. Fisher, Friedman, and Strauss (1994) suggested that this harsher treatment of better-known authors might be explained by professional jealousy and competition. An alternative explanation is that reviewers expect more from authors with strong publication records.

If less well-known authors can have more confidence in reviewers as a result of this research, they may still have justifiable concerns about bias among editors. Evidence suggests that editors may be susceptible to the pull of prestige. Zuckerman and Merton (1971) looked at the effect of the authors' status on how papers were treated at the major physics journal, *Physical Review.* The researchers graded authors according to their awards and membership in professional societies. They found that reviewers' recommendations regarding publication were not affected by the status of the authors; despite this, however, the papers of higher-ranking authors were more likely to be accepted and were dealt with more quickly. Zuckerman and Merton suggested that this might partly be explained by another of their findings—if a paper had higher-ranking authors, editors were more likely to come to a decision without sending it out for peer review.

As with reviewers, editors' characteristics and behavior may have changed with time. Lock (1991) quoted a paper from the 1960s, in which Crane (1967) analyzed characteristics of authors and editors of three American journals, *American Sociological Review, American Economic Review,* and *Sociometry.* The authors whose papers were accepted for publication were similar in professional age and academic background to the editors. In the first period of the study, editors were largely from prestigious universities, and authors from prestigious universities were more likely to be offered publication. In the second period of the study, both the successful authors and the editors were more academically diverse. This could, of course, reflect a secular trend within science and scientific journals.

The conclusion seems to be that peer review is susceptible to biases relating to certain characteristics of authors and their institutions, but that, as one might expect, the direction of those biases depends on the prevailing culture. The evidence of editorial bias seems rather to puncture the confident pronouncement by Arnold Relman and Marcia Angell (1989, 829), of the *New England Journal of Medicine*, that "the best guarantee of an unbiased review system is a fair and conscientious editor." Editors' assumptions, based on their experience that research from prestigious institutions is likely to be of higher quality, may be justifiable. But it might be preferable to know that decisions had been made without the benefit of this additional information. So what can be done to minimize the effects of bias?

Multiple Review

Belshaw (1982) suggested that sending a paper to multiple reviewers (as many as 15) would reduce the effect of each reviewer's individual biases. While this might seem plausible in theory, the practical problems of obtaining and collating up to 15 separate sets of comments would be enormous, not to mention the influence such a practice would have on the academic community's workload if every journal adopted it.

Blinding

The arguments for and against blinded peer review have raged for years, mainly without the benefit of evidence for or against its effectiveness. Those in favor of blinding have argued that it would reduce bias. Those against have suggested that the process of blinding rarely succeeds in removing all signs of the authors' identities and that removing authors' names may remove information that could be useful to reviewers in assessing the paper, such as knowledge of the authors' previous work. Some journals, about 20% of medical journals (Cleary and Alexander 1988), have adopted blinded peer review. Others introduced blinded review but then reverted to nonblinded review because blinding was time consuming and often unsuccessful, in that reviewers were able to identify authors (Morgan 1984; Squires 1990). The past decade has seen a much clearer understanding of the need for evidence to guide decisions about the peer-review process in general and blinding in particular. We now have at least some evidence with which to address two key questions: Is blinding possible, and does it reduce bias?

Rates of successful blinding, as judged by reviewers' success in identifying the authors and institutions of blinded papers, range in different studies from 50% to 76% (van Rooyen et al. 1998; Godlee, Gale, and Martyn 1998; Fisher, Friedman, and Strauss 1994; McNutt et al. 1990). The rate of success will depend on the rigor with which any mention of the authors and their work in the text and references is removed and to some extent on the size of the scientific field, since the smaller the field the more likely reviewers and authors are to know one another. Asking authors to submit blinded copies of manuscripts reduces the workload within the journal office, but manuscripts would still need to be carefully checked for clues to the authors' identities. Cho et al. (1998) found that more experienced reviewers were less likely to be successfully blinded to the authors' identities.

What of the effect of blinding on the behavior of peer reviewers? In a randomized trial, McNutt et al. (1990) found that blinded review was associated with a small, statistically significant improvement in the quality of reviewers' reports as judged by the editors. Other studies also found that blinding made reviewers more critical (Blank 1991). Fisher, Friedman, and Strauss (1994) found that blinded reviewers were less critical of papers from well-known authors than were nonblinded reviewers and concluded that blinding reduces bias, in this case caused by academic competition or high expectations. Three more recent randomized trials also looked at the influence of blinding on peer reviewers' comments. One found no difference in quality of comments but found that blinded reviewers were less likely to recommend rejection (Godlee, Gale, and Martyn 1998). The other two found that blinding made no significant difference to either the quality of comments or reviewers' recommendations regarding publication (van Rooyen et al. 1998; Justice et al. 1998).

Because the success and effects of blinding are likely to differ in different journals and disciplines, journals trying to decide whether or not to adopt blinding should base their decision on research at their own or similar journals. Blinding reviewers would not, of course, have any influence on the biases of editors.

Open Review

Traditionally, peer reviewers' comments have remained anonymous. Journals have justified this practice on various grounds. The main arguments are that reviewers would be unwilling to sign their reviews, making it difficult for editors to recruit good reviewers; that there would be more animosity and resentment within science; that acceptance rates would increase; and that reviewers might tone down their comments, especially if the reviewer were junior and the author eminent and politically powerful. But anonymity is increasingly out of favor in biomedical publishing—editorials, for example, are now rarely anonymous—and society in general is less tolerant of what it sees as power without responsibility. The need for and advantages of anonymous peer review are increasingly questioned.

For a start, anonymity can spread confusion. Authors may wrongly identify the reviewer and harbor unjustified resentment against innocent colleagues for criticism and rejection. Authors submitting manuscripts to *Psychological Medicine* were asked if they knew who the reviewers were: 5.9% identified the reviewer correctly, 14.3% incorrectly, and 79.7% had no idea (Wessely et al. 1996).

Studies have shown that some and, increasingly, most reviewers are willing to sign their reviews. McNutt et al. (1990) invited reviewers to sign their reviews for the *Journal of General Internal Medicine*. Forty-three percent did so. In two pilot studies at the *BMJ* in 1994, 42–44% of reviewers declined to be identified to the authors of the paper and 12–22% declined to be identified to a co-reviewer. But in two subsequent randomized controlled trials at the same journal, performed in 1997 and 1998, only 8% refused to have their identity revealed to their co-reviewer (van Rooyen et al. 1998), and a similar percentage refused to be identified to the author (van Rooyen et al. 1999). In the trial of electronic peer review at the *Medical Journal of Australia* (1996–97), almost all reviewers signed their comments (Bingham et al. 1998). From these data, it seems that fears about reviewers' willingness to sign their comments are increasingly misplaced.

Concern that reviewers might change the nature of what they say if they are asked to sign their comments may be less misplaced. In the study by McNutt et al. (1990), authors found the signed reviews fairer and editors found them more constructive and courteous than unsigned reviews, but reviewers who signed their comments gave less critical reviews and recommended publication more often. No such differences were found in three randomized trials in which reviewers were asked to sign their reports (Godlee, Gale, and Martyn 1998; van Rooyen et al. 1998, 1999).

Fabiato (1994, 1135) rehearsed the arguments for open peer review, in which reviewers sign their comments. First, open review would discourage reviewers from indulging in "an exaltation of ego behind the protection of anonymity" and from emphasizing "this judgmental role at the expense of the other role of the reviewer, which is to help the authors . . . and thereby the progress and diffusion of science." Second, the credentials of the reviewer would add credibility to the comments. Fabiato suggested that reviewers' comments would be less likely to be ignored, as they often are (Wilson 1978; Lock 1991), if the authors knew that they came from a respected source. Third, open review renders reviewers more accountable, forcing them to support their opinions with facts. Fourth, open review should eliminate abuses of the system, such as reviewers delaying or even preventing the publication of data. Fifth, open review may lead to useful discussion between author and reviewer to solve specific problems. Editors have tended to discourage such contact, even when both parties are willing. But this squeamishness is lessening, and, as a first step, reviewers are now often asked to write editorial comments to accompany the publication of papers they have reviewed. Sixth, open review would make the reviewing process more courteous. This is borne out by the gentler tone of reviewers' comments noted by McNutt et al. (1990). Fabiato (1994) ended with perhaps the most convincing argument for introducing open review—that electronic publishing, with comments on open-access Web sites, will soon render it a necessity.

In a commentary following Fabiato's review (1994), Rennie (1994) stated his belief that the only ethically justifiable systems of peer review are either completely closed (with no one but an editorial assistant knowing the identity of the authors and only the editor knowing the identity of the reviewer) or completely open. He then gave a clear call for open review: "We have an ample history to tell us that justice is ill served by secrecy. And so it is with peer review. Two or three hundred years ago, scientific papers and letters were often anonymous. We now regard that as quaint and primitive. I hope that in 20 years, that's exactly how we will look on our present system of peer review" (Rennie 1994, 1143). Whatever individual journals decide to do in the short term (before societal and technological changes make anonymity a thing of the past), any changes to the reviewing system should be made explicit, so that reviewers know what they are committing themselves to and prospective authors know by what process their paper will be judged.

Publication Bias

Blinding and open review will have little influence on another ethically important source of bias in biomedical publication. *Publication bias* refers to the bias in favor of studies with positive (or statistically significant) findings (Dickersin 1990). Early evidence of its existence came from Mahoney (1977), who sent out different versions of the same paper, which the reviewers were told was intended for publication in a symposium on "Current Issues in Behavioral Modification." The different versions had identical introductions, methods, and references, but the results and discussion sections were altered to reflect either positive, negative, or mixed findings.

In addition, some versions of the paper had no results or discussion, as if these were in preparation. The 67 reviewers who responded did not differ significantly in their views of the relevance of the topic. But those reviewing positive versions of the paper judged the methods, the results, and the overall scientific contribution of the paper to be greater than those reviewing negative versions. In his comments on this study, Lock (1991, 33) questioned whether the findings would apply to medicine, where data tend to be more absolute and less open to interpretation. But other research has found clear evidence of the existence of publication bias in biomedical publishing (Dickersin, Min, and Meinert 1992). The bias also extends beyond publication to citations: trials that support a beneficial effect are cited more often than are unsupportive trials (Gotzsche 1987; Ravnskov 1992).

What has publication bias to do with ethics? The answer is that it gives only part of the picture and so distorts our views on what is the best treatment for patients. Negative studies are just as important to scientific understanding, if less exciting for researchers and editors, as positive studies: "If one believes that judgments about medical treatment should be made using all good, available evidence, then one should insist that all evidence be made available" (Dickersin 1990, 1385).

The need for the whole picture has become more apparent since the development of meta-analysis, which allows the results from more than one study to be combined. Combining studies means having larger numbers of subjects; provided that the individual trials are of sufficient quality, it should also mean being able to have more confidence in the final result. But if the studies represent a biased sample (those with positive results) of all the relevant studies (positive and negative), the meta-analysis will simply magnify this bias. Publication bias is the most likely explanation for the discrepancies that have recently been found between large, randomized, controlled trials and meta-analyses addressing the same question (Egger and Smith 1995).

So what can be done? Authors, reviewers, and editors all seem to contribute to publication bias. Authors may lose interest in writing up studies that find nonsignificant results, believing, perhaps with some justification, that journals will be less interested in publishing them (Scherer, Dickersin, and Langenberg 1994); pharmaceutical companies may suppress results that do not favor their own products (Lauritsen et al. 1987); and reviewers and editors may favor positive studies (Mahoney 1977).

As one solution to publication bias, Maxwell (1981) suggested a journal of negative results. A more serious solution is already in train, the setting up of a register of trials by the Cochrane Collaboration (Scherer, Dickersin, and Langenberg 1994). This should help to ensure that all trials are listed, whether or not they are eventually published. Duplication of effort should thus be avoided, and all trials of sufficient quality can more easily be cited and included in meta-analyses. In the hope of encouraging authors who have failed to publish or write up their results, a large group of journals announced an amnesty on unpublished trials from September 1997 (Horton 1997a). The *Lancet* has taken the lead in another initiative to reduce publication bias by introducing a system for review of study protocols and provisional commitment, before the results of the study are known, to publish those that meet certain standards (Horton 1997b).

How Can We Improve the Quality of Peer Review?

Many of the perceived problems of the peer-review process come down to the poor quality of the reviews themselves. Journals can improve review quality by helping to improve the reviewers they use, by selecting different reviewers, and by changing their system of peer review.

Training and Support

Reviewers are usually unpaid and overworked. Informal inquiries suggest that some reviewers may have as many as six articles for review from different journals at any one time. Overburdened reviewers may pass the task on to junior colleagues with no proper supervision. Few reviewers are trained in scientific methodology or the critical appraisal of research reports. Journals should have systems to reward good reviewers and to prevent some reviewers from receiving too many manuscripts. They should also encourage training in critical appraisal for editors and reviewers. This training, along with the provision of clear guidelines and checklists, provides a framework for assessing the quality of manuscripts and should reduce the arbitrary element in peer review.

Selection

Several studies have looked at which reviewers produce the best reviews. In their study at the *Journal of General Internal Medicine*, Evans et al. (1993) found that the best reviews came from reviewers under the age of 40, those who were affiliated with an academic institution, those with training in epidemiology, and those who were known to the editors. Other studies confirmed some of these findings (Black et al. 1998) and tended to encourage journals to select younger reviewers with relevant training.

Changes to the System

I have outlined various changes that might improve ethical standards in peer review, such as blinded and open review. These might equally be considered for their influence on the quality of peer reviewers' comments. McNutt et al. (1990) found a small but statistically significant improvement in blinded reviews as judged by editors and in signed reviews as judged by authors. Laband and Piette (1994) found that articles in economics journals that used blinded review were of higher quality than those in journals not using blinded review, after adjusting for other differences in the articles and the journals.

Conclusions

Ingelfinger (1974) acknowledged the failings of peer review but concluded that it did ensure the validity of published science. Since then, research has revealed more and more holes in peer review's woodwork, and 25 years on, Lock's answer to the same question was, No, peer review does not ensure validity (Lock 1991, 128). That, he said, is the role of time. Most editors would agree. Publication is but one step in a wider process of peer review. After publication, peer review and validation continue in the journal's letters columns, in attempts by other researchers to replicate studies, and ultimately in the decisions of medical practitioners to adopt or not to adopt medical interventions in the care of their patients. Peer review is essentially a subjective process and is prone to error or, as Kassirer and Campion (1994) suggested, to the variation expected of any diagnostic test. But this does not mean that editorial peer review is useless. Alongside the evidence of its failings, there is evidence that it contributes to maintaining standards in published science, both by ensuring that lower-quality research does not appear in the higher-impact journals and by improving the quality of accepted articles before publication.

Much can be done to improve the ethical standards of peer review, through training and guidance of editors and reviewers, through further research into sources of bias and corruption, and through the development of an ethical code for biomedical publishing. Important changes, in particular a move toward more open peer review, will inevitably follow from societal and technological changes. These changes journals would do well to welcome and even encourage, rather than resist. As Judson (1994) pointed out, the current system of peer review is a social construct, not a law of nature. While working to improve the existing system, the scientific community should remain open to the possibility of other ways of achieving quality control in biomedical publishing.

References

Abby, M., M. D. Massey, S. Galanduik, and H. C. Polk Jr. 1994. Peer review is an effective screening process to evaluate medical manuscripts. *JAMA* 272:105–7.

Barnes, D. E., and L. A. Bero. 1998. Why review articles on the health effects of passive smoking reach different conclusions. *JAMA* 279:1566–70.

Belshaw, C. 1982. Peer review and the *Current Anthropology* experience. *Behavioral and Brain Sciences* 5:200–201.

Bero, L. A., A. Galbraith, and D. Rennie. 1992. The publication of sponsored symposiums in medical journals. *New England Journal of Medicine* 327:1135–40.

Bingham, C. M., G. Higgins, R. Coleman, and M. B. Van Der Weyden. 1998. The *Medical Journal of Australia* Internet peer-review study. *Lancet* 352:441–45.

Black, N., S. van Rooyen, F. Godlee, R. Smith, and S. Evans. 1998. What makes a good reviewer and a good review for a general medical journal? *JAMA* 280:231–33.

Blank, R. M. 1991. The effects of double blind versus single blind reviewing: Experimental evidence from the *American Economic Review*. *American Economic Review* 81:1041–67.

Broad, W. J. 1980. Imbroglio at Yale (1): Emergence of a fraud. *Science* 210:38–41.

Bronowski, J. 1965. *Science and human values*. Rev. ed. New York: Harper & Row.

Chew, F. S. 1991. Fate of manuscripts rejected for publication in the *AJR*. *AJR American Journal of Roentgenology* 156:627–32.

Cho, M. K., A. C. Justice, M. A. Winker, J. A. Berlin, J. F. Waeckerle, M. O. Callaham, and D. Rennie. 1998. Masking author identity in peer review: What factors influence success? *JAMA* 280:243–45.

Cleary, J. D., and B. Alexander. 1988. Blind versus nonblind review: Survey of selected medical journals. *Drug Intelligence and Clinical Pharmacology* 22:601–2.

Colaianni, L. A. 1994. Peer review in journals indexed in *Index Medicus*. http://www .ama-assn.org/public/peer/7_13_94/pv3107x.htm. Site accessed 13 July 1999.

Crane, D. 1967. The gatekeepers of science: Some factors affecting the selection of articles for scientific journals. *American Sociologist* 2:195–201. Cited in S. Lock. 1991. *A difficult balance: Editorial peer review in medicine*, 31. London: BMJ Publishing.

Dickersin, K. 1990. The existence of publication bias and risk factors for its occurrence. *JAMA* 263:1385–89.

Dickersin, K., Y.-I. Min, and C. L. Meinert. 1992. Factors influencing publication of research results: Follow-up of applications submitted to two institutional review boards. *JAMA* 267:374–78.

Egger, M., and G. D. Smith. 1995. Misleading meta-analysis. *BMJ* 310:752–54.

Evans, A. T., R. A. McNutt, S. W. Fletcher, and R. H. Fletcher. 1993. The characteristics of peer reviewers who produce good-quality reviews. *Journal of General Internal Medicine* 8:422–28.

Fabiato, A. 1994. Anonymity of reviewers. *Cardiovascular Research* 28:1134–39.

Fisher, M., S. B. Friedman, and B. Strauss. 1994. The effects of blinding on acceptance of research papers by peer review. *JAMA* 272:143–46.

Fletcher, R. H., and S. W. Fletcher. 1992. Medical journals and society: Threats and responsibilities. *Journal of Internal Medicine* 232:215–21.

Garfunkel, J. M., M. H. Ulshen, H. J. Hamrick, and E. E. Lawson. 1994. Effect of institutional prestige on reviewers' recommendations and editorial decisions. *JAMA* 272:137–38.

Godlee, F., C. R. Gale, and C. N. Martyn. 1998. Effect on the quality of peer review of blinding reviewers and asking them to sign their reports: A randomized controlled trial. *JAMA* 280:237–40.

Goodman, S. N., J. Berlin, S. W. Fletcher, and R. H. Fletcher. 1994. Manuscript quality before and after peer review and editing at *Annals of Internal Medicine*. *Annals of Internal Medicine* 121:11–21.

Gotzsche, P. C. 1987. Reference bias in reports of drug trials. *British Medical Journal* 295:654–56.

Horrobin, D. F. 1990. The philosophical basis of peer review and the suppression of innovation. *JAMA* 263:1438–41.

Horton, R. 1997a. Medical editors trial amnesty. *Lancet* 350:756.

———. 1997b. Pardonable revisions and protocol reviews. *Lancet* 349:6.

Ingelfinger, F. J. 1974. Peer review in biomedical publication. *American Journal of Medicine* 56:686–92.

International Committee of Medical Journal Editors (ICMJE). 1997. Uniform requirements for manuscripts submitted to biomedical journals. *Annals of Internal Medicine* 126:36–47. See also http://www.acponline.org journals/resource/unifreqr.htm. Site accessed 5 February 1999.

Judson, H. F. 1994. Structural transformations of the sciences and the end of peer review. *JAMA* 272:92–94.

Justice, A. C., M. K. Cho, M. A. Winker, J. A. Berlin, and D. Rennie. 1998. Does masking author identity improve peer review quality? A randomized controlled trial. *JAMA* 280:240–42.

Kassirer, J. P., and E. W. Campion. 1994. Peer review: Crude and understudied, but indispensable. *JAMA* 272:96–97.

Laband, D. N., and M. J. Piette. 1994. A citation analysis of the impact of blinded peer review. *JAMA* 272:147–49.

Lauritsen, K., T. Havelund, L. S. Laursen, and J. Rask-Madsen. 1987. Withholding unfavourable results in drug company sponsored clinical trials. *Lancet* 1:1091.

Lock, S. 1991. *A difficult balance: Editorial peer review in medicine.* London: BMJ Publishing.

——. 1992. Journalology: Evolution of medical journals and some current problems. *Journal of Internal Medicine* 232:199–205.

——. 1993. Research misconduct: A resume of recent events. In *Fraud and misconduct in medical research,* ed. S. Lock and F. Wells, 14–39. London: BMJ Publishing Group.

Mahoney, M. J. 1977. Publication prejudices: An experimental study of confirmatory bias in the peer review system. *Cognitive Therapy and Research* 1:161–75.

Massie, B. M., and D. Rothenberg. 1993. Publication of sponsored symposiums in medical journals. *New England Journal of Medicine* 328:1196–97.

Maxwell, C. 1981. Clinical trials, reviews, and the journal of negative results. *British Journal of Clinical Pharmacology* 1:15–18.

McNutt, R. A., A. T. Evans, R. H. Fletcher, and S. W. Fletcher. 1990. The effects of blinding on the quality of peer review: A randomized trial. *JAMA* 263:1371–76.

Morgan, P. P. 1984. Anonymity in medical journals. *Canadian Medical Association Journal* 131:1007–8.

O'Donnell, M. 1991. Battle of the clotbusters. *BMJ* 302:1259–61.

Oxman, A. D., G. H. Guyatt, J. Singer, C. H. Goldsmith, B. G. Hutchison, R. A. Milner, and D. L. Streiner. 1991. Agreement among reviewers of review articles. *Journal of Clinical Epidemiology* 44:91–98.

Perlman, D. 1982. Reviewer "bias": Do Peters and Ceci protest too much? *Behavioral and Brain Sciences* 5:231–32.

Peters, D. P., and S. J. Ceci. 1982. Peer-review practices of psychological journals: The fate of published articles, submitted again. *Behavioral and Brain Sciences* 5:187–95.

Ravnskov, U. 1992. Cholesterol lowering trials in coronary heart disease: Frequency of citation and outcome. *BMJ* 305:15–19.

Relman, A. S. 1978. Are journals really quality filters? In *Coping with the biomedical literature explosion: A qualitative approach,* ed. W. Goffman, J. T. Bruer, and K. S. Warren, 54–60. New York: Rockefeller Foundation.

Relman, A. S., and M. A. Angell. 1989. How good is peer review? *New England Journal of Medicine* 321:827–29.

Rennie, D. 1994. Commentary on: Fabiato A. Anonymity of reviewers. *Cardiovascular Research* 28:1142–43.

Roberts, J. C., R. H. Fletcher, and S. W. Fletcher. 1994. Effects of peer review and editing on the readability of articles published in *Annals of Internal Medicine. JAMA* 272:119–21.

Rochon, P. A., J. H. Gurwitz, C. M. Cheung, J. A. Hayes, and T. C. Chalmers. 1994.

Evaluating the quality of articles published in journal supplements compared with the quality of those published in the parent journal. *JAMA* 272:108–13.

Scherer, R. W., K. Dickersin, and P. Langenberg. 1994. Full publication of results initially presented in abstracts: A meta-analysis. *JAMA* 272:158–62.

Society for Neuroscience. 1998. Responsible conduct regarding scientific communication: Guidelines prepared by the Ad Hoc Committee on Responsibility in Publishing. Version 7.7. http://www.sfn.org/guidelines/guidelines-v7-7.doc. Site accessed 13 July 1999.

Squires, B. P. 1990. Editor's page: Blinding the reviewers. *Canadian Medical Association Journal* 142:279.

Stelfox, H. T., G. Chua, K. O'Rourke, and A. S. Detsky. 1998. Conflict of interest in the debate over calcium-channel antagonists. *New England Journal of Medicine* 338:101–6.

van Rooyen, S., F. Godlee, S. Evans, R. Smith, and N. Black. 1998. Effect of blinding and unmasking on the quality of peer review: A randomized trial. *JAMA* 280:234–37.

van Rooyen, S., F. Godlee, S. Evans, N. Black, and R. Smith. 1999. Effect of open peer review on quality of reviews and on reviewers' recommendations: A randomised trial. *BMJ* 318:23–27.

Wessely, S., T. Brugha, P. Cowen, L. Smith, and E. Paykel. 1996. Do authors know who refereed their paper? A questionnaire survey. *BMJ* 313:1185.

Wilson, J. D. 1978. Peer review and publication. *Journal of Clinical Investigation* 61:1697–1701.

Zuckerman, H., and R. K. Merton. 1971. Patterns of evaluation in science: Institutionalisation, structure and functions of the referee system. *Minerva* 9:66–100.

Peer Review and the Ethics of Internet Publishing

4

Craig Bingham

Peer review has evolved from an occasional aid to editorial decision making to become the chief guarantee of a learned journal's scientific validity. The proper conduct of peer review therefore has a central place in publication ethics. Although peer review is generally well supported by editors, authors, and readers of biomedical research, some longstanding criticisms have been reinforced by the perception that the Internet now provides alternative methods of communicating research. Some see peer review as thwarting the flow of knowledge and would prefer to do without it (Ginsparg 1996; LaPorte et al. 1995; Odlyzko 1994). They point to a future after "the death of biomedical journals" (LaPorte et al. 1995, 1387), in which all scientific information is published on the Internet by the authors themselves, with readers selecting from this unbounded research literature with the aid of new (thus far largely undeveloped) electronic systems. Others admire the speed and economy of electronic publishing, but still see value in the quality control and filtering of information imposed by peer review (Harnad 1995a).

At the *Medical Journal of Australia* (*MJA*), we are experimenting with using the Internet to open and extend our peer-review processes. In March 1996, we began the *eMJA* Online Peer Review Trial, in which articles accepted for publication after the usual process of peer review were published on the Internet together with the peer-review comments, and readers were invited to submit further comments, which were passed on to the authors and peer reviewers as feedback (Bingham et al. 1998). Authors could reply to comments on the Web site or revise their articles in response before the articles were edited and printed in the journal.

Participation in the study was voluntary, but we quickly discovered that more than 80% of authors and peer reviewers wanted to participate. We concluded that the Internet has made possible a fairer, more open model of peer review, closely integrated with a rapid system of electronic publication (Bingham et al. 1998). But the study also suggested that (at least for medical research publishing) many virtues of traditional peer review should be retained. We are now engaged in a second study, in which the entire reviewing process takes place online.

In the previous chapter, Fiona Godlee reviews the ethical dilemmas raised by traditional peer review. In this chapter, I suggest that the Internet has not created an academic environment in which we can do without peer review, but that it may offer solutions to some longstanding problems.

The Ethics of Internet Publication of Research

Given that medical research has the potential to save lives and ameliorate suffering, it is an ethical duty of the publication system that it be as rapid and effective as possible. There is some conflict between these two aims: To be effective, the publication system must include some means of establishing the priority of important communications and it must avoid promoting errors, but the quality-control procedures this requires will reduce the speed of publication.

One of the great virtues that the Internet promises to medicine is the possibility of more rapid communication; one of the great questions is whether this can be achieved with safety. There have been objections to the open electronic publication of biomedical research (which was a feature of the *eMJA* study and of some other proposals for biomedical research publication on the Internet) because of the possibility of harm being done to unqualified readers (Kassirer and Angell 1995). For example, some might cease or avoid necessary treatment based on something they had read about a rare side effect; they might pester their doctors for access to an unproven therapy; they might worry needlessly about their condition or the possibility of succumbing to some new condition. Research articles are not written for the general public and so can be misinterpreted; one way of preventing this danger would be to keep them out of public view.

The extent of the risk needs to be put in proportion. Research articles have always been available to anyone who was willing to go to a medical library and read them. Putting articles on the Internet *might* make them easier to find but does not reduce the primary reasons for inaccessibility, which are the narrow focus of most research articles, the level of assumed medical knowledge, the use of jargon, and the high reading level. These features mean that research articles on the Internet are not nearly as accessible to nonmedical readers as several less authoritative and potentially much more dangerous sources of health information from television, newspapers, magazines, alternative therapists, and Web sites specifically tailored to the interests of the general public. These represent the real risk of misinformation, to which the research literature (difficult as it may be) may represent an antidote.

The developing ethical response within medicine toward overcoming patient ignorance or misapprehension has been patient education, with fuller disclosure of information and an acknowledgment that the patient has autonomy and that doctor and patient must share decisions on the direction of treatment (Deber 1994; Pemberton and Goldblatt 1998). In medical research it is mandatory that any patients involved should be fully informed and give their consent; this being so, it is appropriate that patients have access to the published results of the research, for how else are they to check that the research methods and outcomes as published are consonant with the research endeavor in which they agreed to participate?

In general, it is ethically wrong to withhold information from patients because of the theoretical possibility that some may misinterpret it. On the contrary, it would be ethically responsible for medical publishers to make information available not only to the doctors who might apply it, but also to the patients to whom it might be applied. Such a process is difficult in the printed literature, but it may be simpler on the Internet. Sites can be structured so that nonmedical readers are given extra information and cautionary advice, specialist articles can be linked to a more general commentary, and research sites can provide links to reliable public information sites. These are strategies built on open access to information and the promotion of appropriate levels of information for different people.

Just as it is no longer seen as appropriate for a doctor to withhold information from a patient and make decisions on the patient's behalf, no longer should the research literature be seen as private for doctors: Ethicists, other health-care workers, consumer advocates, and patients themselves are entitled to see the literature and contribute to the research debate. This is an essential component of a health-care system that respects patient autonomy.

Purposes of Peer Review That Might Be Differently Achieved via the Internet
Fair Assessment

Peer review originated in the practice of editors seeking an expert opinion on the value of a paper that was beyond their expertise. It is obviously fairer to authors if their work is assessed by someone who fully understands it. It also seems fairer if the editor's decision to accept or reject an article is guided by more than one opinion, hence the common use of more than one reviewer per article or the use of an extra reviewer in the case of a dispute.

Quality Control

Peer review corrects or rejects bad work (Pierie, Walvoort, and Overbeke 1996; Lock 1991, 56–70). Expert reviewers can detect errors of reasoning or fact and point to ways in which the article might be improved. Their familiarity with the subject and the literature means that they may detect fraud, plagiarism, and duplicate publication.

Education of Editors and Authors

Peer review's education of editors and authors is not so often discussed. Editors rely on peer reviewers to extend their knowledge of specialist subjects, to identify new trends, to suggest priorities for publication, and to guide the preparation of the article. Authors may be introduced to new insights into their subject, alerted to misconceptions, driven to further research, and so on.

Criticisms of Peer Review

I summarize only the weaknesses of peer review for which Internet-based review methods may provide some solutions.

Delay

Delay results from the editorial and administrative procedures required to secure peer review, the time taken by reviewers, and the time taken by authors to revise papers in response to reviewers' comments. The amount and proportions of these times vary from journal to journal; at the *MJA*, the first takes up to four weeks (about half of which would be required even if no peer review was intended), reviewers take up to six weeks, and author revision takes a highly variable period, most often about two months. Thus, the longest part of this delay is usually while the article is in the authors' hands. Certainly, the whole delay is much less than the time spent conducting the research and writing the paper.

Failures of Quality Control

Most articles are eventually published somewhere, suggesting that peer review does not prevent the publication of bad work (Lock 1991, 39–41). It does, however, tend to move bad papers down the journal hierarchy, re-ducing the chances that they will be read or cited as evidence. An often-lamented failure of quality control is that peer review sometimes produces the same outcome for good papers, especially if they are truly original or controversial (Horrobin 1990). Peer review also seems to have a limited ability to detect fraud, plagiarism, and duplicate publication (Lock 1991, 44–49, 51–55) or even factual errors in articles (Nylenna, Riis, and Karlsson 1994; Godlee, Gale, and Martyn 1998).

Unfairness

Peer review may be unfair in many ways, beginning with the editor's arbitrary control of the process. The editor can accept or reject a paper without having it reviewed. (I do not know whether this counts as an unfair aspect of peer review, but it is a fact of life in peer-reviewed journals.) An editor could make a bad or biased choice of reviewers. (A bad choice is picking an incompetent reviewer; a biased choice is picking a reviewer with a view to obtaining a certain kind of response.) Editors can make a bad or biased selection from the reviewers' advice (choosing to ignore some rec-ommendations or passing on a misleading selection of the reviewers' ad-vice to the authors). And editors can ignore the reviewers' advice and elect to accept, reject, or recommend revisions of a paper contrary to the balance of reviewer opinion.

The editor of a journal must have the final say over editorial content, and it is only practical that the editor must be able to overrule the peer reviewers, who may give conflicting advice and who, despite their expert knowledge, may not represent the interests of the journal or its readers. The ethical issue is not that editors have these powers, but how they ex-ercise them. Editors make their decisions in private, reveal only as much of the documents as they wish, do not have to record the details of their decisions, and answer to no higher authority. Arguably, there is a lack of *procedural fairness* in editorial decision making.

Of course, editors do not have an obligation to publish or authors an affirmative right to publication in the journal of their choice, so a strictly legal requirement of procedural fairness does not exist. Yet an expectation of procedural fairness arises from the way journals and journal editors represent themselves to readers and authors. Journals advertise their com-mitment to quality and to peer review as the means of selecting quality. Readers are invited to expect that the journal publishes the best papers at its disposal; this leads authors to expect that, if they submit a good paper within a particular journal's terms of reference, it will be accepted (or at least will receive fair consideration). The journal system could not thrive without these expectations, and journal editors generally strive to improve the fairness and accuracy of their decision-making processes because they perceive that this will tend to improve the quality and success of their journals. Procedural fairness, therefore, should be an important objective even if it is not a legal obligation.

That there is not a greater disaffection with peer review in the scientific community than presently exists points to the diligence with which most journal editors exercise their powers. Nonetheless, the procedural arrangement lends itself to abuse, and actual examples of "abuse of editorial power" have been reported (Altman, Chalmers, and Herxheimer 1994, 166). The *Lancet* has addressed this issue by appointing an ombudsman who will hear appeals from authors who feel that they have been unfairly treated (Horton 1996). While this is commendable, it is limited. Neither authors nor reviewers are in a position to detect most of the potential editorial abuses of peer review. A reviewer may feel that his advice has been ignored, but he does not know what contradictory advice other reviewers may have given. An author who is sent peer-review comments does not know who made them or whether that was really all they had to say. To a large extent editors can do as they please, while still presenting the final outcome as a product of independent peer review.

Normally, journal editors have little reason to interfere with the publication recommendations that follow peer review. But they may feel that the readership demands something other than what the experts recommend, they could be influenced by commercial or political pressures (advertisers, boards of directors, lobby groups, professional associations), they may have personal biases, and they can make mistakes. The closed nature of peer review means that the possibility of unfairness through the editor's control cannot be discounted.

The reviewer can do a poor job of reviewing the paper, give a biased review of a paper, steal ideas from a paper, or attempt to delay competitive work by negatively reviewing a paper. Again, the closed nature of peer review does much to prevent any abuses being discovered. The authors do not know the identity of the reviewer, and it has been suggested that this puts them at a psychological disadvantage in case of a dispute (the "Oz-behind-the-curtain effect") (Abate 1995). The masked authority of the reviewer may, for instance, make authors feel that they must accommodate criticisms that they consider trivial or vexatious simply to achieve publication. Reviewer anonymity also makes it more difficult for authors to trace plagiarism by reviewers or to recognize that they are being obstructed by a competitor. Editors are also limited in their assessment of reviewer performance: They may not have the specialized subject knowledge to identify a poor job of reviewing or a biased review, and although they will have a good idea of what is published in their own journals, they may not identify plagiarism or competing publications by reviewers when they are published elsewhere.

Taken together, potential unfairness at the hands of the editor or the peer reviewer forms the strongest ethical objection to our current peer-review system and one that asks for a systemic reform. Although the education of peer reviewers and editors or the introduction of formal policies for the conduct of peer review and the hearing of authors' objections can reduce the chances of inadvertent unfairness, they do not address the fundamental problem, which is the lack of openness in the decision-making process.

Proposed Solutions to Problems with Peer Review

The blinding of reviewers to the identity of authors, the audits of reviewer performance, and the use of guidelines and checklists to standardize reviewing procedures have all been proposed and sometimes implemented in response to criticisms of peer review. These attempts at improvement within the current framework (see chap. 3) do not directly address the closed and restricted nature of peer review, which lies at the root of the criticisms of its fairness. And while these criticisms carried little weight with editors and authors when there seemed to be no alternative, the rise of electronic publishing on the Internet has inspired several proposals for reform. Each of these may have advantages and difficulties (including new problems that arise from having a more open system).

Proposal 1. Abolish Peer Review

This proposal is usually put in the form, "abolish the learned journals," with the faults of peer review being one of the main reasons for abolition (Ginsparg 1996; LaPorte et al. 1995; Odlyzko 1994). The prototype for a system to replace the learned journals is Paul Ginsparg's electronic preprint server in high-energy physics, which has virtually superseded journals as the main mode of research communication for several physics specialties. The preprint server replaces the paper preprints that physicists used to send each other in the months before their articles appeared in the journals with an electronic preprint (an *e-print*). The server (a computer archive of articles accessible via the Internet) gives researchers a central location where they can publish articles as soon as they are ready; the service is free to authors and readers and fully automated.

Ginsparg (1996) suggested that peer review is of little value, especially when "the author and reader communities (and consequently as well the referee community) essentially coincide." This is the friendly situation in his own specialized field of physics and might also be said to apply in the subspecialties of medicine. Ginsparg acknowledged that the situation may be different when the reader community is much wider than the author/ reviewer community, as is the case in much biomedical publishing, especially the general medical journals. He also listed several other special characteristics of the physics research community that do not apply to medicine (or many other scientific disciplines): "a well-defined and highly interactive community of voracious readers with a pre-existing hard-copy preprint habit, with a standardized word processor and a generally high degree of computer literacy, with a rational means of assigning intellectual priority (i.e. at the point of dissemination rather than only after peer-review), and with little concern about patentable content" (Ginsparg 1996). Differences between medicine and physics in this regard are important.

- Medical researchers, particularly those who are also practicing clinicians, are perhaps less likely to be "voracious readers" of research.
- The boundaries of specialization and subspecialization may be less tightly defined within medicine than in theoretical physics; in other words, there may be a requirement to scan a wider literature in medicine and less certainty about what is relevant.
- There is no general acceptance of preprints or e-prints in the medical sciences. An online discussion forum conducted by the *British Medical Journal (BMJ)* indicated that many doctors among those who use the Internet are opposed to unreviewed e-prints, seeing them as potentially dangerous to the uninformed and time-wasting for the practicing professional (Delamothe 1996). The *New England Journal of Medicine* published an editorial aimed at discouraging researchers from publishing e-prints (Kassirer and Angell 1995).
- Whereas physicists have developed a uniform system of word processing and electronic communication to cope with the textual demands of their specialty, communication methods in medicine are more diverse, and the spread of technological competence is much wider.

- Intellectual priority is established in medical publishing as the date of acceptance of a paper by a peer-reviewed journal, and nothing has yet moved to change that.
- Concern with patentable content is, if anything, growing in medical research (Patent craze and academia 1993; Loughlan 1995).

Furthermore, peer review never functioned in quite the same way in physics as in medicine. Evidence cited by Lock (1991, 17) suggests that physics journals had low rejection rates (about 24%), while "the more humanistically orientated the journal, the higher the rate of rejecting manuscripts for publication." Rejection rates in medical journals are commonly higher than 50% and are up to 90% in major international journals. Thus, when physicists gave up peer review, they were not committing themselves to reading nearly as much extra material as medical readers would face without the filtering it provides.

There have been proposals for an e-print server in biomedical sciences and even a couple of attempts to start such a thing. For example, LaPorte and others (1995) founded the Global Health Network (http://www.ghn.com) in 1995 with this as one objective, although the site did not subsequently develop in that direction, perhaps because of a lack of submissions from authors. Another effort was the World Journal Association (http://www.journalclub.com), which in 1996 provided a system for biomedical authors to publish online and for readers to score the articles (a crude system of postpublication peer review). After several months of inactivity, the World Journal Association listed dozens of articles (mostly laboratory studies in biosciences), but the scoring system went unused, suggesting a lack of reader interest. At some time in 1997, the site vanished from the Web.

In April 1999 Harold Varmus of the National Institutes of Health published a proposal for an e-print server to be called E-biomed (Varmus 1999). This proposal is both complex in its structure and vague in its detail, and it seems destined to be the subject of much argument. In June the *BMJ* responded by announcing its intention to establish an e-print server in cooperation with Stanford University (Delamothe and Smith 1999). This e-print server may be operating by the end of the century, and then we will see whether medical writers and readers are willing to leap the cultural divide. But what of the ethical arguments? Neither Varmus nor Delamothe and Smith see the e-print server as threatening the peer-reviewed journals, but let us for the moment assume, like LaPorte (LaPorte et al. 1995, 1388), that a "global health information server" will eventually replace the current hierarchy of journals. How does it address the tasks of the present system?

Fair Assessment?

The health information server bypasses this issue by making publication equally accessible to all, but this only postpones the inevitable. Medical readers cannot double or quadruple the amount of time they spend reading and selecting for reading; some assessment system to guide reading choices must be introduced to replace the filtering previously provided by peer review. Otherwise, junk would have the same prominence and accessibility as useful research. For medical information with the potential to affect people's health, this is not an ethical option.

LaPorte et al. (1995, 1388) suggested a postpublication scoring system: "Individuals . . . could comment or ask for comments from the author or the other readers. When pulling up the abstract or the title so as to decide whether to read the paper, the reader could also pull up the average 'priority score' as well as the comments. The selection could be based on reviewers who are researching that topic or are otherwise concerned with the content—for example, statisticians."

Critics of this proposal have objected to the concept that scores provided by self-selected readers could be an accurate guide to the scientific worth of an article (Kassirer and Angell 1995). In an automated and unpoliced system, there can be no guarantee that the opinion of the best qualified has been given or that spurious opinions have not been given undue weight. This objection applies even more strongly to the simpler proposal, also made by LaPorte et al., that articles be rated by access scores. It does not follow automatically that a widely read article is the best article on the subject or that a little-read article is of poor quality. What about the idea that ratings could be based on the scores given by "reviewers who are researching that topic" (LaPorte et al. 1995, 1388)? In this automated system, such people are self-identified. This may be satisfactory in certain fields of medical research; it is likely to be inadequate in others.

It is easy to see the potential for unfairness in the current system, but it takes a leap of faith to believe that an automated numerical system for assessment of articles will work better and more fairly. What would be the mechanisms for detecting biased assessments (achieved, e.g., by vote stuffing) or inadequate assessments (resulting, e.g., from the lack of appreciative readers of a good article from a little-known worker)? Some potential biases under the current system may actually be worse in such a publication environment. For example, peer reviewers may be inclined to give favorable treatment to articles from well-known institutions, but readers may be even more likely to do this if they are faced with an undifferentiated literature.

Quality Control?

The *eMJA* study results suggest that readers' comments via the Internet are an inadequate substitute for commissioned peer reviews as a means of assessing and promoting quality. Fewer than 2% of accesses to articles in the *eMJA* study led to a comment being made. This suggests that systems depending solely on unsolicited comment and democratic assessment may be underused and therefore unrepresentative. Few readers' comments attempted anything like a comprehensive review of the article, and even these were not as comprehensive as most commissioned reviews. Most comments addressed one or two points in the article, usually with a specific criticism or piece of additional information. In this respect, the comments were more like the letters to the editor that often follow the publication of an article than like peer reviews. Such comments were often valuable, but they did not add up to an assessment of the merit of an article.

There is an apparent difference between the critical attitude and methods of a commissioned peer reviewer and those of a self-directed reader. Perhaps peer reviewers are conscious of discharging a responsibility for and on behalf of their peers; perhaps they are more "ego-involved" because their opinions were actively sought; perhaps they are well guided by the instructions of the commissioning journal. Readers who are engaged primarily because of their own need for information are less likely to offer comments or criticism and are much less likely to make the conscientious effort required for thorough evaluation of an article. These observations are now supported by the experience of other journals that have initiated discussion forums on their Web sites to encourage postpublication comment on articles (e.g., *Lancet, BMJ, American Journal of Ophthalmology*). Many articles receive no comment, very few readers comment, and the comments are generally specific to a particular aspect of the article.

Authors often responded differently to unsolicited comments received after publication than they did to commissioned reviews before publication. Most authors did respond to Internet comments, but a large minority did not or responded in a cursory fashion. Perhaps this represents the important psychological difference between debating when a key issue is still open (whether the article will be published) and debating when the issue is closed (the article is assured of publication or already published). Thus, several improvements to articles that take place before publication under traditional peer review might never take place after publication in the health information server model: first, because the level of commentary may be less conscientious and comprehensive; second, because the authors may be less motivated to respond conscientiously.

In a discipline such as medicine, which involves not only hard quantitative science but also a large amount of fuzzy data about human behavior, an intelligently directed and deliberate attempt at quality assessment is likely to be more effective than an automated system for comment collecting and counting. The traditional human system engages the *conscience* of reviewers and authors more effectively than the computer system does: This psychological difference has an ethical outcome.

Educating Editors and Authors?

In the health information server model, editors are defunct and we need not trouble ourselves about their education. But what about the authors? The *eMJA* study suggests that traditional peer review gives a level of advice to authors that is not matched by unsolicited comments and often forces authors to consider ideas and respond to queries about their work in a way that will not be required if peer review is removed.

The Ethics of the Global Health Information Server

Sidestepping the ethical problems of peer review is not the same as solving them. Allowing publication to all initially avoids the unfairness, delay, and conservatism that may mar peer review, but these issues reappear as soon as the practicalities of selecting a usable and high-quality literature are addressed. The idea is primarily attractive to researchers seeking immediate communications within their exact specialty (who are confident that they can identify meaningful articles). Without the quality-control system of peer review, however, the global health information server would not serve the wider readership of medical journals.

An ethical argument for the global health information server is that it will make medical information available to doctors in the developing world at a cost much less than that of subscribing to a raft of print journals, but this purpose is not advanced if a drought of information is turned into a shapeless deluge. The *BMJ* Web site was inaugurated with the stated policy of publishing freely and in full those articles most likely to be of use in the developing world (Editor's choice 1995); such a policy, applied consistently by the major international journals, would do much to guarantee a better flow of useful information to those in need.

There is no reason that a global health information server could not include effective processes of peer review—except, perhaps, that peer review is expensive, and the proponents of this idea dream of a publication system that is cheap, so that information is virtually free. The Internet certainly presents the possibility of reducing the costs of access to peer-reviewed information, mainly by reducing reliance on print and physical distribution. But the costs of editing and peer review themselves are not greatly altered.

Proposal 2. Create Opportunity for Papers to Circulate before Peer Review

What about combining e-prints with the continued existence of peer-reviewed journals (LaPorte and Hibbits 1996)? Allowing the circulation of e-prints before peer review might answer criticisms of the delay and conservatism inherent in peer review, while maintaining a successful quality-control and selection process for the archival literature. Such an outcome is envisaged by the *BMJ* editors who have proposed an e-print server: "The server will, we hope, be useful to researchers. We do not expect it to be much use to doctors who are not researchers, and nor would E-biomed be of much use to them. They are likely to continue to want to receive pre-digested, well presented accounts of research that matters for their practice. This is a role that journals are likely to continue to have" (Delamothe and Smith 1999, 1638). But would e-prints tend to replace peer-reviewed articles as the important unit of research communication, introducing a trend toward abolishing peer review? Such a possibility is apparently envisaged by the *New England Journal of Medicine,* which has set its face against e-prints (Kassirer and Angell 1995).

The arguments of the *New England Journal of Medicine* editorial merit consideration, as they are likely to be influential throughout medical publishing.

A study found to be badly flawed during peer review may be completely revised or never published. Publishing preprints electronically sidesteps peer review and increases the risk that the data and interpretations of a study will be biased or even wrong. Investigators cannot be expected to judge their own work dispassionately. They are usually enthusiastic about their hypotheses and may be unaware of flaws in the design of their experiments or of the insufficiency of their data to support their conclusions. They need independent experts to evaluate their data. (Kassirer and Angell 1995, 1709)

These objections imply two assumptions: (1) that (potentially unreliable) e-prints may find a wide medical readership and (2) that authors who publish e-prints are seeking to avoid the criticism of their peers. Both assumptions may be false.

Because of their unreviewed and uncertain status, e-prints are unlikely to be read or relied upon by general medical readers, most of whom display a conservative and skeptical approach to new information. There is no general demand for e-prints in preference to peer-reviewed articles. The exception is that researchers in a specialized field are known to seek data ahead of journal publication from other researchers in the same field. These members of the so-called invisible colleges (i.e., the informal communities of specialists with a common expertise and research interest) already use "letters, assessing articles for publication, conversations, workshops, discussions at meetings, and preliminary presentations at conferences" (de Solla Price 1981, cited in Lock 1991, 12) to communicate results, and e-prints would be a useful addition to the list.

Authors who publish e-prints may well be seeking the critical attention of the invisible college, the readers who are most likely to have an urgent use for the data and ideas they contain and also most likely to be able to identify their worth and faults. These researcher-readers include those most likely to be called on to do the peer reviewing if and when the article is submitted for journal publication. They have least to gain from a journal's peer-review process, which they may well see as narrow and partial compared with the open process of discussion among peers that can center on an e-print, and they are the group most likely to be irritated by the delays engendered by formal journal publication. In short, publishing a preprint may well be a path to open and extensive peer review.

Possibly e-prints and traditional peer review could coexist, the first fulfilling the needs of specialized readers, the second those of the wider medical community and the archival literature. However, such a system might involve a certain amount of wasted peer-review effort. If journal editors are outside the discussions of the invisible college, they will be unaware of the extent of peer review and revision that an article underwent as an e-print and will initiate formally (and perhaps repetitiously) a process that might already be well advanced.

To continue their control of the medical literature, journals could themselves publish e-prints in an unreviewed section of their Web sites. Editors could then monitor and evaluate the discussion generated by an e-print, perhaps using this information as part of the formal peer-review process. The *Australian Electronic Journal of Nursing Education* has been divided into reviewed and unreviewed sections since its inception in 1996, and the *BMJ* introduced a highly selective scheme for preprinting and openly reviewing some articles in October 1998 (Help us peer review an article on line 1998). However, journal e-prints entail some interesting problems.

- Will editors select articles that they are willing to e-print? If so, is selection without peer review any advance over selection with peer review? Presumably editors will e-print the articles they would be prepared to accept if peer review subsequently turned out to be favorable, but the editorial decisions at this level might simply become the new frontier for arguments about fairness.
- How would the journal ensure that the proper distinction between its peer-reviewed pages and its unreviewed pages was observed? Would it seek to prevent the citation of e-prints, and how could that be managed? The *BMJ* has asked people not to cite its e-prints (Help us peer review 1998), while acknowledging that an e-print is a publication—an illogical position. In fact, there is no way that people can be prevented from citing a publication, although it may be desirable that e-prints be cited as "unreviewed publication."
- What would happen to the e-print version of an article if and when it passed through peer review and were accepted as a reviewed publication?
- More difficult, what would happen to the e-print if the article were rejected after review?
- What if the article were accepted for publication by another journal?
- What should an editor do if offered an article that had been e-printed by another journal?

Although answers to all these questions can be found, it is no wonder that most journal editors would simply prefer authors not to consider e-prints. At bottom, the issue is whether the literature should accommodate two standards of publication, reviewed and unreviewed. As the reviewed medical literature already encompasses the randomized controlled trial, the hypothesis-generating speculation, the case report, and the cohort study (publications representing widely differing standards of evidence and argument), it is arguable that there is room for unreviewed publications (representing another standard of evidence). The ethical requirements are that unreviewed publications should be clearly labeled and cited as such.

Finally, let's not forget that there have always been unreviewed medical publications. Their status and evidential value are low.

Proposal 3. Continue Peer Review as It Now Is but Improve Other Publication Processes by Using the Internet

Journals need only to break free of the habit of the print issue cycle to achieve substantial improvements in the speed with which they deliver peer-reviewed articles. Although this involves no actual improvement to peer review, it might silence some critics of peer-reviewed journals by reducing the overall amount of delay in the system, and it would address the ethical responsibilities to do good and prevent harm by making the findings of research available as rapidly as possible. However, thus far most print journals that have begun the migration to the Internet have made little use of its virtues. Most print journals are organizing their Web sites by issue and tying publication to the print issue cycle, ignoring the possibility of publishing articles more quickly and of organizing and disseminating them more effectively.

Proposal 4. Augment Peer Review with Improved Peer Commentary after Publication

Stevan Harnad (1991) is a lyrical supporter of the power of the Internet to speed up the process of research communication. He calls the process *skywriting:* "Skywriting promises to restore the speed of scholarly communication to a rate much closer to the speed of thought, while adding to it a global scope and an interactive dimension that are without precedent in human communication, all conducted through the discipline of the written medium, monitored by peer review, and permanently archived for future reference." The hyperbolic claim that Internet publishing approaches the speed of thought means simply that written intellectual debates on the Internet can be conducted within days, without the weeks or months of delay that intervene between proposition and response in print journals.

Harnad's important innovations in electronic publishing have centered on the peer-reviewed e-journal *Psycoloquy.* They are

- the demonstration that a peer-reviewed journal can be produced electronically from within the resources of an academic department and distributed freely to readers all over the world (certainly not possible in print);
- the use of the Internet to promote and accelerate the process of postpublication commentary on articles, creating a more immediate debate between the authors and their peers than is possible in print;
- the use of a peer-reviewed journal to publish articles at an earlier stage of investigation, deliberately seeking peer commentary on hypotheses and preliminary findings before pushing the work to its conclusion.

Harnad (1995b) is in favor of maintaining traditional peer review, seeing the rigor that it brings to scholarly publishing as an essential antidote to the growing amount of "dross." His term for unreviewed self-publication is *vanity publishing*—which puts him in opposition to the enthusiasm of LaPorte for self-publishing—yet he is similarly critical of the print-based journal publishers and their control over the intellectual property of researchers (Harnad 1995b, 1991).

Harnad has relatively little to say about the criticisms of peer review. He described the editor as the weak link in the review system and suggested that using the Internet may allow a wider choice of reviewers. Another problem he acknowledged is delay, and again he suggested that using the Internet might help, by spreading the workload around more reviewers and speeding up the communication of reports (Harnad 1995b). But he is emphatic that peer commentary is no substitute for peer review and that scholarly skywriting can only really take off after traditional peer review is complete. Much of what Harnad has said and demonstrated about the value of open peer commentary can be carried over successfully to the reform of peer review, which itself would benefit from being conducted as a more open and immediate discussion between the various participants.

Proposal 5. Use the Internet to Open and Extend Peer Review Processes: The *eMJA* Study

The possibility that the Internet could be used to open and extend peer review processes has been foreshadowed by other writers, particularly (in relation to biomedical publishing) by Horace Judson (1994). Thus far, there has been little practical experimentation to flesh out the concept. A published survey of scientific, medical, and technical e-journals up to 1995 reported none with an online peer-review process (Hitchcock, Carr, and Hall 1996).

The first *eMJA* study ran from March 1996 to June 1997 (Bingham et al. 1998). As articles in the study had received standard treatment until being accepted for publication, the study preserved the virtues of traditional peer review, but the online review period that followed served to address several criticisms.

- The process that led to the acceptance of the article was opened to scrutiny, increasing the chance that any deficiencies would be revealed. This is peer review for peer review, an important reform toward procedural fairness in editorial decision making.
- Expanding the number of reviewers by open review meant that authors received additional comments that they sometimes found valuable. For 12% of articles, comments led to further changes.
- Nearly two-thirds of the reviewers in the study volunteered to sign their reviews. In addition, most comments received via the Internet were signed. Identification of reviewers provides a check on potential abuses, such as undeclared conflict of interest, plagiarism, lack of qualification to comment on a particular issue, or competitive bias.
- By publishing peer reviews and opening a peer-review debate, the *eMJA* study widened the educational function of peer review for editors and authors and extended it to interested readers for the first time.
- Although the peer-review process was extended, by electronically publishing articles as soon as they were accepted, the *eMJA* was able to shorten publication delays.

In summary, the new model of peer review tested in the *eMJA* study made improvements to peer review in all three of its key functions (fair assessment, quality control, and education of editors and authors), and it added educating readers to the list. To quote Ginsparg (1996): "One of the foremost problems at present is the large amount of information lost in the conventional peer review process, with the end result only a single one-time all-or-nothing binary decision. Although this may somehow be adequate for the purpose of validating research for job and grant allocation, it clearly provides little benefit to the average reader." The *eMJA* received positive feedback from readers about the usefulness of being able to read the peer reviewers' and editors' comments, both for the perspective they provided on the content of the article and for the insight into the editorial process. Reviewers, too, were given better insight into how their colleagues undertook the task of reviewing and how the editor dealt with reviews.

Of course, not everybody wants to read the peer reviews. Only about one in four readers who accessed articles went on to access the reviewers' reports. Yet 25% is a significant minority. Similarly, only a very few readers offered comments, yet this was a valuable contribution, and the study empowered these readers to make it. The Internet makes this extra exchange of information possible and affordable for those who desire it, without inflicting it upon those who do not. The *eMJA* study is a successful demonstration of the power of the Internet to provide faster publication with an improved peer-review process, but it exposed some potential problems.

Articles were published without copyediting. Articles presented in the study (like e-prints) had not been copyedited. No readers complained about this, although copyediting usually shortens articles, improves readability and presentation, and corrects minor (and sometimes not so minor) errors. For example, one article in the study contained information with the potential to identify patients (an ethical breach) that would normally be removed during copyediting.

What about the rejects? The study did not provide any means for scrutinizing the peer review of articles that were not accepted for publication. As some of the greatest failures of peer review may be expressed in the rejection of deserving articles, this is a serious limitation.

Open review occurred after the critical decision. One *MJA* reviewer suggested that there was little motivation to review an article when the decision to publish had already been made. He suggested that an open review process that preceded decision making would attract a higher level of interest from qualified peers. But can this be done without publishing articles that are to be rejected after peer review?

An Advanced Model of Internet Peer Review

The *MJA* is now experimenting with an advanced model of open peer review (similar to a model first described in 1996 by Sumner and Shum and used for the *Journal of Interactive Media in Education*). Here is the procedure:

1. *Submitted articles are assessed by the editor for prima facie suitability.* If suitable:
2. *Articles are posted to a secure site on the Internet, accessible only by the authors, editor, reviewers, and a small consultant panel.* The authors promise not to offer the article for publication elsewhere while it is under

review. Copyright remains with the authors until an agreement is made at the time of accepting the article for publication.

3. *Reviews and comments from the consultant panel are added to a discussion list linked to the article as they are received.* The participants are directed to an online guide to the etiquette and purposes of the review discussion (Protocol for Internet peer review study II 1998) and advised of the rules for participation (see table 4.1). The editor can edit the list when necessary (e.g., to remove abuses, irrelevancies, or computer-generated errors). The reviewers are asked to perform their traditional task, but they can interact with each other and the authors as well as with the editor. The consultant panel provides a means of continuous independent audit of the actions of editors, authors, and reviewers, and it provides a wider range of expertise for the consideration of articles. The consultant panel members are given a different brief than that of the reviewers; they are invited to comment but not expected to provide comprehensive reviews. (Indeed, they are advised that they need do no more than observe the review discussion.) In ethical terms their importance is as witnesses of fair play. Members of the consultant panel in this model are representatives of the journal's "virtual college": the journal's community of peer reviewers and highly motivated readers (those who actively follow and contribute to the literature in a particular subject area). As a general medical journal, the *MJA*'s virtual college includes practicing clinicians as well as researchers, statisticians, ethicists, and other experts with useful external perspectives. For a specialist journal, the virtual college may be consubstantial with the invisible college of researchers working in that particular specialty, and it would be possible for such a journal to include the entire virtual college within the consultant panel for an article. In effect, this would turn the peer-review process into an e-print service for the invisible college.

4. *The authors contribute responses or offer revisions of their article to meet criticisms.* The authors are in a better position in relation to this form of peer review, able if they wish to respond to comments as they are received or to wait until the discussion has played itself out before acting on the editor's summary advice. Authors can answer queries and propose revisions on the fly or submit an entire revision of their article at any stage of the discussion.

5. *The editor, who moderates the discussion, indicates a decision (reject, return for revision, or accept for publication).* The controlling role of the editor is abundantly clear in this system. What is new is that the editor is per-

Table 4.1. *eMJA* Rules for Participation in Internet Peer Review

1. The purposes of peer review are to advise the editor on the suitability of the article for publication and to advise the authors on ways that they may be able to improve their article. All contributions to the review process should serve these purposes.
2. The editor reserves the right to make a publication decision based on his/her own assessment of the best interests of the journal and its readers.
3. The article under review is a confidential document not yet accepted for publication. It should not be shown to or discussed with colleagues, cited as a reference, or used in your own work.
4. The editor will chair the review discussion. Contributors should follow any instructions from the editor given during the discussion.
5. Contributions to the review discussion should be as brief as possible. Contributors should not reiterate points that others have already made, although it is acceptable to send a note of agreement.
6. References to the article under review should quote the relevant paragraph number. [Paragraphs are numbered to facilitate cross-references to the discussion list.]
7. Assertions of fact should be backed with appropriate references.
8. All contributors should conduct themselves with professional courtesy. Remarks that may be construed as insulting or defamatory will be removed from the record.
9. Contributors who breach the required standards of the review process will be barred from further participation by the editor.

Source: "Protocol for Internet Peer Review Study II," *Medical Journal of Australia* (1998). Reprinted with permission.

forming these functions in a forum of peers. If the article is rejected, the discussion is closed and remains confidential. There is the possibility for appeals to be considered in the same forum or for new participants to be added for a reconsideration. If the article is returned for revision, the discussion list lies dormant until the article is resubmitted. If the article is accepted, it moves to the next stage.

6. *The article is edited for publication, and the edited version is reviewed online and published (i.e., made publicly available on the Web) when the authors' approval is received.* Traditionally, copyediting takes place after peer review, and the reviewers are not consulted about its effect. However, at the *MJA* (and some other journals), copyediting can be quite extensive, involving significant revisions to the order of material and sometimes shortening by as much as 20%. Although these changes are never made without the approval of the authors, it is true that they are under pressure to acquiesce in order to finalize their article and achieve publication. The new review procedure provides stronger oversight of the results of copyediting (or, to put this in positive terms, it provides better feedback to manuscript editors on the effectiveness of their work). The review discussion list and earlier versions of the article are published as well, linked to the article and forming a historical record.

7. *The process of open review and discussion continues after publication.* The peer-review process up to this point can be presented in full or edited for brevity and clarity. We are not yet sure how much of the review history should be retained. In theory, a fully accountable system would retain the whole record (including the superseded versions of articles); this is also the easiest option in administrative terms. On the other hand, an edited version of the review process may be more useful and may even be shaped to present the article in a broad context of commentary and additional information. Revision or editing of the article can continue until the final version is defined for publication in print (i.e., for a few weeks).

Some Open Questions Arising from New Models of Peer Review

How will journal editors adapt to the new openness? Journal editors who chair the review discussion are entering into a new relationship with their authors and reviewers. Their decisions are on view, more open to criticism and response from a variety of sources. Will editors respond by keeping a low profile in discussions, letting authors and reviewers bat it out until it seems clear that a decision can be announced? Or will the best policy be an active one, in which editors comment on articles themselves and indicate to authors which reviewers' comments they think are important and which are safe to ignore?

What is the place for anonymous peer review? There are arguments for allowing anonymous reviews in some instances (some critics may fear reprisals or may be prevented from commenting if they must expose their affiliations), but does this compromise the scrutiny of peer review or allow reviewers to behave unfairly under the cover of anonymity? Drummond Rennie (1998) has argued strongly against anonymous reviewing in this context; in our study we are allowing it to see how many reviewers opt for anonymity and to observe what effects this seems to have.

How do you punctuate the new publication continuum? When is a paper "finished"? What version(s) and how much of the surrounding discussion should be archived? Fortunately, Web servers can provide detailed statistics on what is being accessed, and this information will help to guide decisions over time.

What is the new role for manuscript editors in all this? When should we edit? How should we edit? The emphasis shifts from the effort to be "right first time" to a more interactive process of responding to demonstrated reader needs.

Can we afford a peer-review system that is extended through the Internet to encompass a wider circle of peers? The exact effects on journal economics are uncertain. Is electronic peer review more or less expensive than the paper-based version? What new revenues may journals expect from the development of electronic services? Most journals would save vast amounts of money if they could move subscribers from print to electronic delivery. What are the chances of this saving being made? In 1997 the *BMJ* extended free Web access to include the entire content of the journal, with the editors stating that this experiment would continue for at least a year and that they hoped it would be effectively subsidized by increased print subscriptions (and, I wonder, advertising revenues?). This experiment will soon yield some answers to these questions, but the circumstances of a major international journal are different from those of a national journal or a specialty journal.

Possible Faults of the New Advanced Model

The exclusion of those not "Internet capable." This is a serious but rapidly declining problem. Authors, reviewers, or readers who cannot use the Internet can be specially served by providing printouts of the online process and by converting their contributions to electronic form at the editorial office.

The herd effect. If the first reviews to appear with an article are by senior figures of powerful position and high reputation, others may be reluctant to make comments in disagreement, or there may even be a tendency to produce an unthoughtful chorus of agreement. I doubt that this will be a frequent problem in practice because medical researchers are a fairly independently minded group. I would expect that, more often, prominent figures would see their opinions challenged in review discussions by newcomers who wished to make their mark (and this, if it did occur, seems less of a problem to me).

Chaos. An article may provoke a hail of comment indicating wildly divergent assessments of its value. This could occur with articles that report work at the edge of controversial areas of medical science. How much of a problem it is will depend on the attitude of the editor. Arguably, any article that excites major disagreement among qualified peers should be published and debated fully.

More heat than light. If a discussion group is deeply split on intellectual lines or if it contains prominent antagonists who cannot resist the opportunity to do battle, an editor may find that open peer review is turned into an arena for contests that have little to do with assessing the merits of an article. The control of this problem is within the editor's hands. The editor can end the debate on an article at any time, reject certain comments and excise them from the debate, enter the debate to urge moderation and observation of etiquette, or remove disruptive reviewers from participation.

Information overload. The discussion group may generate too much discussion of an article, leaving the author and editor with an impossible task of sifting and evaluating the comments. In conversations with editors about this model of peer review, this is often the first and loudest objection, but the evidence we have thus far suggests that it is not a problem in practice.

Increased pressure on editors. Open peer review puts the opinions and the decisions of the editor under much stronger scrutiny. Some editors may feel that they cannot work that way. They may, at times, feel that they are drawn into debates about their decisions which they do not have the time or the inclination to enter. Editors will have to remember (and remind others) that when they adopted open peer review they did not give away their power to decide the content of their journals. If editors do feel increased pressure, in some cases it may be because their decisions do not withstand scrutiny. As controllers of peer review, it is editors who have the greatest opportunity to act mistakenly, unfairly, or with bias. In the future, however, when some editors adopt open peer review and others do not, who will be in the best position to justify their decisions? The open-peer-review editor will be able to say, "You may not agree with all my decisions, but at least you can see how I reached them, and I have nothing to hide." Most of the time, the open process will lend support to rational editorial decisions and arm the editor against the unreasonable objections of authors and reviewers.

Difficulties in submitting rejected articles to other journals. If an article is rejected after open review by a large discussion group, the authors may find that their submission to another journal is rejected simply on the grounds that the article has already been published. This is not a problem in our study, where the discussion groups are small, but could be a problem if a journal opened peer review to its entire virtual college. The editor of the second journal might take the view that distribution of the article to the virtual college was effectively publication. There is some evidence that the *New England Journal of Medicine* would take this view. Then again, seldom would the *New England Journal of Medicine* be an author's *second* choice of journal; other journals lower in the hierarchy of journal prestige may well take a more friendly attitude to secondary submissions. The ethical question for the editor to ask (rather than the question of commercial advantage) is simple: Does the article merit publication because it is useful and the journal can carry it to the readers who could use it?

Nothing definitive can be asserted about these or any other potential problems of the new model. Our study is still in its early days. It will be necessary for other journals with different readerships to try these procedures before we have adequate data.

The Advantages of the New Model

The advanced model of open peer review calls for articles to be reviewed in an open discussion among peers, followed by an open period of publication and review before the article is finalized. In this model, comments by the reviewers, responses of the author, and the interventions and decisions of the editor(s) are all open to criticism and review. The model is as free and fair as a strict quality-control and selection system could be. It would be reasonable to expect better outcomes and a better appreciation of the outcomes by all parties under such a system. This makes it (or something like it) the ethical choice for peer review in an age of electronic communications.

References

Abate, T. 1995. What's the verdict on peer review? *21st C* 1(1). http://www.columbia.edu/cu/21stC/issue-1.1/peer.htm. Site accessed 19 March 1999.

Altman, D. G., I. Chalmers, and A. Herxheimer. 1994. Is there a case for an international medical scientific press council? *JAMA* 272:166–67.

Bingham, C. M., G. Higgins, R. Coleman, and M. B. Van Der Weyden. 1998. The *Medical Journal of Australia* Internet peer-review study. *Lancet* 352:441–45.

Deber, R. B. 1994. Physicians in health care management: 7. The patient-physician relationship: Changing roles and the desire for information. *Canadian Medical Association Journal* 151:171–76.

Delamothe, T. 1996. Preprint debate. *BMJ* Web site. http://www.bmj.com/preprint.htm. Site accessed 19 March 1999.

Delamothe, T., and R. Smith. 1999. Moving beyond journals: The future arrives with a crash. *BMJ* 318:1637–39. See also http://www.bmj.com/cgi/content/full/318/7199/1637. Site accessed 29 June 1999.

de Solla Price, D. 1981. The development and structure of the biomedical literature. In *Coping with the biomedical literature: A primer for the scientist and clinician,* ed. K. S. Warren, 3–16. New York: Praeger. Cited in Lock, S. 1991. *A difficult balance: Editorial peer review in medicine,* 12. London: BMJ Publishing.

Editor's choice: Come with us into cyberspace. 1995. *BMJ* 310:n.p. See also Delamothe, T. *BMJ* on the Internet. http://www.bmj.com/archive/6991e-1.shtml. Site accessed 19 March 1999.

Ginsparg, P. 1996. Winners and losers in the global research village. http://xxx .lanl.gov/blurb/pg96unesco.html. Site accessed 19 March 1999.

Godlee, F., C. R. Gale, and C. N. Martyn. 1998. Effect on the quality of peer review of blinding reviewers and asking them to sign their reports: A randomized controlled trial. *JAMA* 280:237–40.

Harnad, S. 1991. Post-Gutenberg galaxy: The fourth revolution in the means of production of knowledge. *Public-Access Computer Systems Review* 2:39–53. See also ftp://cogsci.ecs.soton.ac.uk/pub/harnad/harnad91.postgutenberg. Site accessed 19 March 1999.

——. 1995a. Implementing peer review on the Net: Scientific quality control in scholarly electronic journals. In *Electronic publishing confronts academia: The agenda for the year 2000,* ed. R. Peek and G. Newby, 103–18. Cambridge: MIT Press. See also ftp://cogsci.ecs.soton.ac.uk/pub/harnad/harnad95.peer.review. Site accessed 19 March 1999.

——. 1995b. Re: Peer commentary vs. peer review. http://cogsci.ecs.soton.ac.uk/ ~harnad/Hypermail/Theschat/0007.html. Site accessed 19 March 1999.

Help us peer review an article on line. 1998. *eBMJ.* http://www.bmj.com/misc/ peer/index.shtml. Site accessed 19 March 1999.

Hitchcock, S., L. Carr, and W. Hall. 1996. A survey of STM online journals 1990–95: The calm before the storm. In *Directory of electronic journals, newsletters and academic discussion lists,* 6th ed., ed. D. Moggee, 7–32. Washington, D.C.: Association of Research Libraries. See also http://journals.ecs.soton.ac.uk/survey/ survey.html. Site accessed 19 March 1999.

Horrobin, D. F. 1990. The philosophical basis of peer review and the suppression of innovation. *JAMA* 263:1438–41.

Horton, R. 1996. *The Lancet's* ombudsman. *Lancet* 348:6.

Judson, H. F. 1994. Structural transformations of the sciences and the end of peer review. *JAMA* 272:92–94.

Kassirer, J. P., and M. Angell. 1995. The Internet and the *Journal. New England Journal of Medicine* 332:1709–10.

LaPorte, R. E., and B. Hibbitts. 1996. Rights, wrongs and journals in the age of cyberspace: "We all want to change the world." *BMJ* 313:1609–10. See also http://www.bmj.com/archive/7072fd2.htm. Site accessed 19 March 1999.

LaPorte, R. E., E. Marler, S. Akazawa, F. Sauer, C. Gamboa, C. Shenton, C. Glosser, A. Villasenor, and M. Maclure. 1995. The death of biomedical journals. *BMJ* 310:1387–90.

Lock, S. 1991. *A difficult balance: Editorial peer review in medicine.* London: BMJ Publishing.

Loughlan, P. L. 1995. The patenting of medical treatment. *Medical Journal of Australia* 162:376–80.

Nylenna, M., P. Riis, and Y. Karlsson. 1994. Multiple blinded reviews of the same two manuscripts: Effects of referee characteristics and publication language. *JAMA* 272:149–51.

Odlyzko, A. M. 1994. Tragic loss or good riddance? The impending demise of traditional scholarly journals. http://www.-mathdoc.ujf-grenoble.fr/textes/Odlyzko/amo94/amo94.html. Site accessed 25 March 1999.

The patent craze and academia. 1993. *Lancet* 342:1435–36.

Pemberton, P. J., and J. Goldblatt. 1998. The Internet and the changing role of doctors, patients and families. *Medical Journal of Australia* 169:594–95.

Pierie, J. P., H. C. Walvoort, and A. J. Overbeke. 1996. Readers' evaluation of effect of peer review and editing on quality of articles in the *Nederlands Tijdschrift voor Geneeskunde. Lancet* 348:1480–83.

Protocol for Internet peer review study II. 1998. *Medical Journal of Australia.* http://www.mja.com.au/public/information/iprs2doc.html#rules. Site accessed 19 March 1999.

Rennie, D. 1998. Freedom and responsibility in medical publication. *JAMA* 280:300–302.

Sumner, T., and S. B. Shum. 1996. Open peer review and argumentation: Loosening the paper chains on journals. http://www.ariadne.ac.uk/issue5/jime/. Site accessed 19 March 1999.

Varmus, H. 1999. E-BIOMED: A proposal for electronic publications in the biomedical sciences. http://www.nih.gov/welcome/director/ebiomed/ebi.htm. Site accessed 29 June 1999.

Edward J. Huth

Journals involve everyone in scientific communities. Authors value publication of their papers for benefits: audiences for their work, useful feedback from readers, and professional gains that can follow, like promotion and tenure. Readers apply information from journals in enhancing their reputations as being well informed and in solving their problems in research or practice. Editors apply peer review and personal judgments in support of the value of the information they publish.

But these three parties can have conflicting interests. Authors wishing for as large an audience as possible may seek to report a single definable body of research in more than one paper, in repeated reports of the same work, in fractional reports, or in reports in more than one language. Editors who need to use their resources economically do not wish to publish information that has already been or will be published elsewhere; such repetitive or divided publication can damage their journals' reputations for publishing new information and can waste resources. Readers do not wish to be confused by ambiguities about what is new information or a repetition of what they have already read. Can standards of conduct for controlling repetitive and divided publication be established that will maximize values of publication for all three parties while minimizing damage to scientific literature from conflicting interests?

Definitions

Various terms have been used to describe publication of the same information in more than a single paper. The largest cluster of terms turned up in an editorial by Susser and Yankauer (1993): *prior, duplicate, repetitive, fragmented,* and *redundant publication.* Other terms have been used: *dual publication* (Hanke et al. 1990) and *double publication* (Hammerschmidt 1992).

Duplicate publication (or *duplicative publication*) has probably been the term most widely used to describe republication of the same information, either as an entire paper or as information of smaller dimensions than a complete paper. This term strikes me as inadequate as a generic term. *Duplicate* and cognate terms derive from *duplicare,* "to double." There are instances in which the same information appears in print more than twice ("duplicated"), although most cases of repetitive publication probably represent only a second appearance. The wide use of *duplicate publication* may stem from a policy the National Library of Medicine (NLM) (1998) installed in 1989 of indexing journals' notices of duplicate publication for its MED-LINE bibliographic file and connecting its references to such notices to the papers indicated by them as "duplicate."

The term *redundant publication* is also unsatisfactory, despite its use in some authoritative documents (e.g., a Council of Biology Editors [CBE] paper [1996]). *Redundant* in this context reflects the dictionary definition of *redundant,* as "superfluous . . . unnecessary" (*New Shorter Oxford English Dictionary on Historical Principles* 1993). The reader of the redundant paper concludes, "I don't think this publication of this information is needed; once was enough"; sometimes redundancy can be justified, as in publication of the same information in two languages.

Repetitive publication seems to represent objectively and more accurately the appearance of the same information two, or more than two, times. The term readily covers the republication of an entire paper or a closely similar version representing the same body of research. Identity of text among or between the texts is not required in this definition; scientific information such as data or descriptions can be readily presented in variations of text. A second species of repetitive publication is *partial repetitive publication.* This term seems appropriate for a fragment of information already published within another paper in a different context but not identified in the later paper as to its original source.

A third useful term is *divided publication* for a phenomenon related to repetitive publication. The information from a single research study is divided for publication into two or more papers. An example is a research study of the effects in humans of a new drug reported in three papers, one reporting on cardiovascular effects, another on pulmonary-function effects, and a third on systemic effects. This practice has been called "salami science" (Huth 1986) because it represents, in effect, the slicing up of a single study into several pieces ("least publishable unit" [Broad 1981, 1137]) for publication. Here the repetition is not rereporting of data but rereporting of study design and perhaps other information, such as the background to the research. This phenomenon can be termed *topically divided publication.*

Another variety of divided publication, *fractionally divided publication,* is the reporting in a single paper of only a fraction of the data that have been or will be reported in their entirety in another paper. This phenomenon was well illustrated by Huston and Moher (1996). After a literature search for reports of primary research on risperidone, an antipsychotic drug, and examination of the papers identified, they concluded that 20 articles and a few unpublished reports actually represented only two major and seven smaller trials. What is especially important for the interests of readers is that these disaggregations were "far from obvious, because of the chronology of publications, changing authorship, lack of transparency in reporting, and the frequent citation of abstracts and unpublished reports" (Huston and Moher 1996, 1024).

Should publication in a formal paper of data already published in an abstract be considered republication? In a literal sense, yes. If one assumes, however, that critical readers, such as meta-analysts, would not accept data as reliable information when they are reported in an abstract without the support, as in a formal paper, of a full description of the research design and methods and a statistical analysis, then such "republication" is not true republication as defined and discussed here.

Is publication in a formal paper of data reported previously in an informal format (such as a medical newsmagazine) republication? Such *prior publication* may render subsequent formal publication unacceptable to some journals. This is the policy of the *New England Journal of Medicine* as it was set forth by Franz Ingelfinger in the 1960s, a policy since known as "the Ingelfinger rule."[1] If the data were originally published in some informal format (newsmagazine, newspaper), their subsequent republication in a formal and complete format should not be considered republication if one applies the same analysis and criteria as for abstracts.

Another related question is whether the publication of data in an electronic online format is to be regarded by journals receiving a second version of the data as prior publication (Flanagin, Glass, and Lundberg 1992). My view is that an analysis of this question ought to follow the lines indicated above for abstracts and publication in the news media: If the preceding publication carried insufficient content bearing on the scientific rigor of the study (such as the lack of a full description of methods, analyses, and other kinds of evidence), the prior publication need not be considered as disqualifying a full subsequent scientific report from formal publication. An editor may not wish to publish the full report because it lacks news value, but that is not the same judgment as equating an incomplete, informal report with a full formal report and considering the second report as repetitive. My view here is, perhaps, a minority view, one likely to be rejected by editors who believe that the reappearance of data constitutes repetitive publication, even if they first appeared in an informal and scientifically inadequate format. If, however, the electronic version was a formal scientific report, the second version does represent repetitive publication (which may be desirable for readers not able to access electronic sources).

Some types of repetitive publication may be considered legitimate and not a species of undesirable scientific conduct. Brief descriptions of these types will reduce any ambiguity about the meaning of *repetitive publication* in this chapter. There are two critical requirements for accepting these types of repetitive publication as desirable. First, both parties to the repetitive publication—authors and editors—must be aware that it is taking place and assent to it. Second, all versions of such repetitive papers must carry complete, unequivocal bibliographic identifiers of the related papers so that readers know exactly what they are seeing and where else it has appeared or will appear.

The first acceptable type is repeated publication of such papers as policy statements of medical associations, expert-written guidelines, documents, and other similar position papers that serve primarily didactic or enlightening functions in two or more fields of medicine. For example, guidelines on proper immunization practice in infants could be published in the Centers for Disease Control and Prevention's *Morbidity and Mortality Weekly Report* for the public-health audience and also in a pediatrics journal for practicing pediatricians.

The second acceptable type is publication of the same paper in two different languages.[2] For example, an initial report by Norwegian investigators could be published in English in the *New England Journal of Medicine* and followed by a version of the paper in Norwegian in a Norwegian national journal. The second version would cite the English-language version as the primary publication, and the English-language version would call attention to the scheduled publication of the Norwegian version.

A third type, arguably not acceptable, is the publication of two or more papers that draw on the same clinical or laboratory experience but shape their content for different audiences. An example might be a report in an internal medicine journal on the clinical consequences of an industrial toxin but with no detail—only a brief text mention—of an unusual radiographic appearance of the lungs, with illustrations of this lesion omitted to minimize the paper's length. A parallel report published in a radiology journal would give only brief descriptions of the clinical effects of the toxin but illustrate in detail the novel radiographic features. This type of repetitive publication could be considered ethical, notably if all authors and the editors of both journals have agreed on its validity because of the two papers' serving two different audiences and if each paper unequivocally cites the other. Nevertheless, this type of publication has been defined as topically divided publication and can be criticized as wasting limited resources.

A fourth type of repetitive publication is related review articles. When is the repetition of textual content in review articles by the same author undesirable repetition? A well-known expert is likely to be asked again and again to write reviews on topics within his or her expertise (Reaven 1992). If the successive reviews cover the same or a closely related topic and passages in them closely resemble each other, is this undesirable repetitive publication? Before damning the author, some thought should be given to the difficulties in trying to convey much the same message again and again in different texts. This is not repetition of original data but, rather, a kind of *self-plagiarism* (if a pejorative term seems needed). The consequences to an author of such repetition are likely to be no more than getting charged with wasting journal space and arousing envy for his or her growing bibliography. As with the other three types of acceptable repetitive publication, however, the author of a series of review articles may be able to deflect charges of deceptive republication by unequivocally citing his or her own preceding sources.

These analyses should help to emphasize that undesirable repetitive publication may represent either the mindless failure of an author to identify repetition of content and the identities of the repetitive papers or an intent to conceal the repetitive reporting. Such behavior can be tagged *mindless* or *deliberate deception*. It is not simply deception to which the scientific community can object, however, but the possible damage to the scientific enterprise that could ensue.

The Rate of Occurrence of Repetitive Publication

How frequently repetitive publication occurs is hard to identify. Repetitive publication can be identified to an editor but not called to the attention of the journal's audience because the editor prefers simply to reprimand the guilty author. The potentially most firm evidence of repetitive publication in medical journals is the listing in MEDLINE of notices of identified repetitive publication. In a search of the 1994–97 MEDLINE file for notices of "duplicate publication" (the NLM's preferred term), 41 notices turned up. These seem to be attached to pairs of repetitive papers, so the number of cases of paired repetitive papers must have been about 20. In the same period, the NLM indexed in MEDLINE almost 1,200,000 papers. A calculation based on these data yields a rough estimate of the occurrence of pairs of repetitive papers of 1.7 episodes of repetitive publication per 100,000 papers, or one episode per 59,000 papers.[3] Is this rate high enough to define repetitive publication as a problem that calls for action to reduce its occurrence? Or is this estimate too low?

Evidence for a higher rate comes from some editorials written by editors to call attention to the phenomenon (Berk 1992; Bevan 1991; Bier et al. 1990a, 1990b; Dobson 1990; Hanke et al. 1990, 1991; Smith et al. 1991; Smith 1992). A rate higher than that deduced from the MEDLINE data is suggested in part by their calling attention to instances of repetitive publication detected by them or some of their readers but not identified publicly by the victimized journals and hence not noted in MEDLINE. Some editors also pointed to experiences with authors' failed attempts at repetitive publication, the submission of manuscripts representing the same material already published in a full paper.

Additional evidence for more repetitive or attempted repetitive publication comes from the numbers of journals represented by these eight editorials. Three are signed by the editors of more than one journal: one editorial represents four different journals in anesthesia; one represents six different journals in dermatology; and one represents seven different journals in pediatrics. Hence, these eight editorials actually represent 19 different journals, and they are major journals in their fields. One gets the sense from these numbers that repetitive publication is more frequent and widespread than the evidence in MEDLINE seems to suggest.

Further evidence for a much higher rate than one can estimate from the MEDLINE notices comes from studies of the phenomenon in individual journals. Waldron (1992) examined papers published in the *British Journal of Industrial Medicine* for evidence that they had been also published elsewhere. Of 364 main articles published in 1988, 1989, and 1990, 31 had been published elsewhere, an occurrence of 8.5% and a rate of 85 pairs of repetitive papers per 1,000 papers published in this journal. This was not what could be strictly called duplicate publication; Waldron noted that "few of the papers were published in their entirety in another journal, the great majority (about 80%) reporting the findings in a slightly modified form, usually with the authors listed according to the specialty of the journal" (Waldron 1992, 1029).

A slightly higher rate was found in a study conducted by the *Nederlands Tijdschrift voor Geneeskunde* (Barnard and Overbeke 1993). The research considered articles appearing in this journal and already published elsewhere and articles originally published in the journal and then published elsewhere. They found an occurrence rate of 14%, or 140 pairs of repetitive papers per 1,000 papers in their journal.

Some additional data come from a study of nursing literature (Blancett, Flanagin, and Young 1995). Among 642 articles published in five years, 181 were duplicate, and of these, 59 did not give a reference to the duplicated article. These data indicate an occurrence of 9.19% of unacceptably repetitive pairs of papers, or 92 repetitive pairs per 1,000 papers.

There may be a higher rate of unacknowledged repetitive publication among authors publishing in two languages. Egger and colleagues (1997) carried out a study of possible English-language bias for publication of statistically significant positive findings. They incidentally identified among 62 English-language and German-language pairs of papers by the same authors reporting clinical trials 19 (30.6%) pairs of papers representing repetitive publication. This percentage equals 306 repetitive pairs per 1,000 papers.

These data suggest that the occurrence rate of repetitive papers in the clinical medical literature probably lies between 0.017 and 306 repetitive papers per 1,000 papers published. The lower figure must be too low an estimate because it depends on the NLM's indexers being able to identify published notices of repetitive publication. For better estimates we need additional specific investigations such as those of Waldron (1992), Barnard and Overbeke (1993), Blancett, Flanagin, and Young (1995), and Egger et al. (1997) but covering more journals in more fields. As Susser and Yankauer (1993, 792) pointed out, "Surprisingly little accurate information about the incidence and prevalence of duplicate publication has been published in the biomedical literature." Journal editors could contribute greatly to what we know about the frequency and extent of repetitive publication through systematic studies aimed at identifying the numbers of papers they have published that have already appeared or subsequently appear in another version in another journal. If, before accepting papers for publication, they also carried out MEDLINE searches for evidence of prior publication of essentially the same paper, they could also strengthen estimates of the phenomenon as represented by attempted repetitive publication.

The Causes of Repetitive Publication

Whatever the exact rate of repetitive publication, it has been occurring. Why? The causes can only be inferred from the culture of medical science in the years in which this phenomenon has come to wide attention.[4] What has been the culture that seems to have given rise to a perhaps still-growing rate of repetitive publication?

Before World War II the academic medical establishment in the United States was made up of a small fraction of full-time faculty and a large fraction of affiliated "volunteer" faculty; academic medical centers in some other countries had similar staffs. Thanks to the federal subsidy of research, U.S. medical centers were able to enlarge radically their full-time staffs. Similar trends developed in other countries investing heavily in medical education and research. Many persons who could not have remained in an academic center before the war sought academic posts. Competition for these posts began to rise, so criteria for selecting who would get tenure or promotion in the faculty were needed. One criterion for candidates has been the number and quality of publications (Angell 1986), and the advice "publish or perish" efficiently described the drives of candidates to get the numbers, if not the quality, of published papers. The competition for faculty appointments in the United States, Canada, the United Kingdom, and other countries with major academic medical centers heated up even more when government subsidies for medical research and education not only failed to keep up with the growth of medical centers, but even shrank. Consequently, in many clinical departments faculty turned to financial support through multicenter clinical trials paid for by pharmaceutical firms. Such arrangements increased the possibilities for multiplying reports as single-center reports of data also published in a multicenter single report.

This view of causes for repetitive publication is my conjecture.[5] No one seems to have queried authors responsible for repetitive publication and published broadly secured findings that might illuminate causes. Published comments from authors identified as responsible for undesirable repetitive publication usually rely on justifications such as their "naïveté," their "not understanding the rules," and similar immediate causes. Some authors have rationalized repetitive publication as justified in some circumstances (Barnard and Overbeke 1993), as when aiming to reach different target groups or adding data to already reported data. An explanation of and perhaps an excuse for such responses may lie in the fact that most definitions of acceptable and unacceptable conduct of authors have appeared only in information-for-authors pages of journals and in editors' editorials. Some professional societies and medical centers have published and disseminated rules for acceptable conduct in publication (Huth 1997); this point is discussed further below, under "The Prevention of Repetitive Publication."

Another cause of repetitive or divided publication could be advice from editors. If pressed for space in their journals and facing a decision on a paper that seems to them to be excessively long, they may advise an author to drop some content in the present version and, perhaps, even suggest that the dropped content could be published elsewhere. Such a step by the author might lead to divided publication (*salami science*), as defined above. But the editor who made the suggestion may not know whether some of the data in the first paper will reappear in the second as undesirable repetitive publication. Further, there may be editors of low-rank journals so hungry for papers to publish that they are willing to collaborate in repetitive publication.

The Consequences of Repetitive Publication

Given that undesirable repetitive publication occurs at a disturbing rate, why are editors concerned and why do they comment on the problem editorially? Why do readers of their journals write to them to object to it? Why have editors worked to define unacceptable and acceptable conduct in publishing previously published information? What do they see as consequences of undesirable repetitive publication?

Simply tagging repetitive publication as *unethical* is not an adequate explanation. Tagging motives and consequences with pejorative terms such as *greed* and *deception* fails to explain why such tags should be used. What are the actions and effects that may be thus tagged? Ethical issues seem invariably to represent situations in which the desires, needs, wants, and preferences of one party, if served, conflict with and deny the attainment of at least one other party's desires, needs, wants, and preferences. In the case of repetitive publication, authors' desires for the greatest possible yield—economic, political, social—from their work have led them to seek the highest possible visibility for their work. What are the desires, needs, wants, and preferences of editors and readers? How do they conflict with those of authors engaging in repetitive publication?

Editors work within financial constraints defined by their publishers, whether professional societies or commercial publishers. Hence, editors strive to make the best use of their journals for their readers and for their journal's reputation, which can determine not only the journal's financial footing but, more important for the editor, the journal's capacity to attract the best possible content for its audience. Giving space to information that has been or will be published elsewhere may be a waste of space in the journal. Additional wastes occur as the editor expends clerical effort, postage, and the services of reviewers in coming to decisions on repetitive papers.

The more important concern of the editor is that the journal supports the needs of readers for useful, reliable, and honest scientific information. Repetitive publication can seriously distort scientific information needed for critical judgments in many aspects of medicine. This is a concern the editor shares with readers and thus ultimately the entire scientific community.

Science cannot proceed productively if the information it works with is unreliable. In medicine we come to many important decisions on the basis of quantitative information relevant to sound judgments in answering the questions we face. Is drug A more effective in reducing or delaying mortality in AIDS than drug B? How different are they in effects? From how many subjects do the data come? What are the statistical characteristics of the data that define their certainty? The effect of repetitive publication of research findings when they are not identified as repeated is to multiply the apparent amount of scientific evidence bearing on the particular question. Three papers reporting data from the same clinical trial, none of which identifies the study and the data as reported or to be reported elsewhere, have provided three times the amount of apparent evidence bearing on the answer to the question the research investigated. That this is not just a potential problem is illustrated by comments in a quantitative systemic review of the treatment of postoperative nausea and vomiting with ondansetron: "Results from one multicentre trial with data from 500 patients treated with three different doses of ondansetron compared with placebo were assumed to have been published on two later occasions, in 1993 and in 1994 (first study). All contacted authors confirmed that one single dataset had been reported in three publications. Only data from the first publication [were] analysed for the purpose of this systematic review" (Tramer et al. 1997, 1089).[6] The authors go on to comment on the problem of multiple reportings from the same dataset.

> We are concerned that data from a large, sponsored, multicentre trial were published three times. Inclusion of the two duplicates in the analysis would have

increased the number of analysed reports by a quarter and doubled the number of analysed patients. Systematic reviewers are at risk of failing to recognise duplicates of an original report. The danger is that unrecognised duplicates will bias the estimates of an intervention's efficacy. Two duplicates were published in journal supplements, and the quality of supplement reports may be lower than reports in the parent journals. Both supplement articles declared that intravenous ondansetron 4 mg was the optimal dose to treat postoperative nausea and vomiting, although there was no good evidence to support this. Subsequent uncritical repetitions underline the potential influence of such unchallenged assertions. (Tramer et al. 1997, 1091–92)

The overreporting in this episode was readily detected. This may occur when the literature on the question is small and authorships are identical or overlapping so that the overreporting is easily detected. But with a large amount of literature and no, or little, overlap of authors on repetitively reporting papers, the overreporting could be undetected. There can be great difficulties in making clear assessments of which data can be properly used in a meta-analysis and which cannot. Another example of the problem was given to me by an analyst at Oxford.[7] In an ongoing analysis of drug trials relevant to the treatment of prostate cancer, two papers with apparently relevant data were found to, in fact, contain repetitive data from the same patients.

Such potential consequences of repetitive publication have been discussed in further detail elsewhere; for examples, see the letter by Leizorovicz, Haugh, and Boissel (1992) and the paper by Huston and Moher (1996), quoted above, who give an especially strong and clear summary of consequences:

> Everybody is affected by these practices. To abuse the honour system central to medical publications with the aim of overstating one's case undermines the integrity of science. It also calls into question author and investigator integrity. If authors are not explicit about multiple publications of the same results can they be trusted about other aspects of their trial conduct? . . .
>
> . . . the practices of redundancy and disaggregation have begun to subvert the role of medical publications from the unbiased reporting of data to the dissemination of information that carries with it a personal or corporate agenda. (Huston and Moher 1996, 1025, 1026)

Such reported instances of repetitive publication point only to identified instances; the repetitive data have been detected. The damage was not in any repeated use of the same data in a meta-analysis but was in the burden on the analysts of identifiying the repetitive reporting. Unfortunately, we know little or nothing of failures to identify repetitive reporting and hence biasing of an analysis by overuse of the same data. But the risk of failure is clear.

Undesirable consequences from repetitive publication do not stem only from reporting of clinical research. Repetitive reporting of laboratory experiments, especially when the repetition is disguised by extensive changes in text and illustrations, can multiply the apparent evidence in support of new developments in basic medical science and discourage replicative research. But the evidence thus far suggests that undesirable repetitive publication may be far more frequent in reports of clinical research.

Authors tempted to report data repetitively can readily discount some of the arguments of editors (CBE 1996) against repetitive publication (Susser and Yankauer 1993, 793): "Arguments such as adding needlessly to an overburdened scientific literature; wasting trees as well as the time and money of reviewers, editors, and publishers; and compounding communication problems fall on [authors'] deaf ears." But authors who believe they are responsible members of the scientific community cannot dismiss the damage that repetitive publication may inflict on scientific evidence if it is not detected.

Ultimately, it is not only the scientific community that suffers from misrepresentation of data resulting from repetitive publication. The public can also suffer when medical judgments are based on faulty data; that public includes you and me as patients or potential patients. Hence, authors' dismissing the consequences of repetitive publication affecting readers and the wider scientific community are pitting their self-centered needs against those of most of the rest of society. Authors can sometimes build a legitimate case for publishing the same data in more than one paper but only when they take precautions against possibly misleading readers; this point is discussed in more detail under "The Prevention of Repetitive Publication."

The Detection of Repetitive Publication

What is done and can be done to detect potential and actual repetitive publication? Peer review can detect attempted repetitive publication. A reviewer returns a comment such as, "This paper is little more than an expanded version of what the author published in the proceedings of the Ninth International Congress of Xxxxxology." Or a reviewer reports that

"This paper is essentially the same as what the authors published on new developments in xxxxxology in a supplement to the *Scandinavian Journal of Xxxxxology.*" Such comments may lead to prompt rejection of the paper under consideration. The first comment might lead the editor to look more closely at what was published in the proceedings; the expanded version may, in his judgment, merit publication. There is no question that the peer-review process has been and will continue to be a valuable resource for editors seeking to detect potential repetitive publication. A reviewer's ability to detect attempted repetitive publication depends on his or her wide scanning of literature relevant to personal scientific interests. Hence, editors could help in this kind of prevention by noting in the journal's consultant file any evidence of a reviewer's having an especially broad knowledge of the literature in his or her field.

Detecting repetitive publication that has actually occurred is more difficult. Readers who regularly scan several journals in their field may detect repetitive publication and report it to the editors of the involved journals. Perhaps little can be done to stimulate readers into such reporting, but if an editor responds promptly to the reporter, that action may help to support further awareness of that kind and hence future reporting by that reader or by his or her colleagues. Such detection and reporting seem not to be frequent, and better means of detection are needed.

Editors may be able to detect repetitive publication in which their journals were unwitting participants by searching a bibliographic database such as MEDLINE (Livesley 1992) for other papers by the same author(s) published either shortly before or after the editor's acceptance and the journal's publication of the author's paper. Such searches could be effective in preventing repetitive publication if the editor proceeds then to publish a notice of repetitive publication; this tool is discussed below. But thus detecting repetitive publication could be expensive and time consuming if published papers have to be visually examined for resemblances to a paper the journal published. Computer software called *autosummarizers* (in development) might be able to provide concise summaries (abstracts) of published papers for quick comparisons of contents. But to use such programs the searching editor would need digitized versions of both his journal and the paper or papers published by the author in another journal. At present, meeting this need would probably require scanning of other journals' papers suspected of being instances of repetitive publication. In the not too distant future, the suspected papers might be readily downloaded in digital form from electronic versions of journals. Whether the effort needed to detect repetitive publication occurring at a rate of roughly 100 pairs of papers per 1,000 papers or less would be worth a journal's investing in such searches is debatable. Detecting repetitive publication more frequently through such searches and publicizing it might be an effective means of discouraging future attempts, but perhaps other means of prevention might be less costly.

The Prevention of Repetitive Publication

What are the present and potential means of preventing undesirable repetitive publication? As noted above, detecting and publicizing repetitive publication might deter authors from trying to carry it out, but trying to detect it through literature searches could be too costly. Some of the effort needed for such searches would be reduced if possibly suspect papers could be identified more efficiently. Simply searching MEDLINE by author names or subjects could bring up papers in the same topical field but still too many for speedy analysis for possible repetitive publication.

What is needed is a simple tag that would efficiently identify papers probably generated from the same research study. A tag of this kind has for some time been required by various granting agencies, such as the National Institutes of Health and private disease-oriented organizations. Such requirements specify that the source and its specific grant-identifier be credited in papers resulting from the supported research. A similar tag would be the register number used in one or more of the existing or proposed clinical-trials registries (Making clinical trialists register 1991). Such tags may be buried within the texts of papers (in title-page footnotes or a closing acknowledgments section), and the entire text of a paper must be scanned to find them. A simple solution might be having MEDLINE citations include such tags, which could then serve as the sole search term. The present MEDLINE file carries for individual papers such bibliographic data as the keywords (MeSH terms), the type of paper, the authors' institution, and so on; it does carry grant identifiers for some papers. Such identifiers can be searched for in the MEDLINE command system in a search specifically looking for "Secondary Source" identifiers, but this approach could be difficult to use for unsophisticated searchers. The NLM might facilitate the more frequent representation of grant identifiers in MEDLINE files by asking journals to place such identifiers in a standard location, perhaps at the end of an article's abstract.

Whether adding such identifiers might greatly facilitate finding repetitive publications I cannot guess. Some of the egregious repetitive or divided publication seems to have involved industrial support not specifically identified by some tag, such as a trial number, and pharmaceutical firms could be reluctant to register trials they support (Making clinical trialists register 1991). Hence, repetitive publication emerging from their trials might not be identifiable through such tags as register numbers. But at least one British pharmaceutical firm, Schering Health Care UK, has registered its ongoing trials in the Cochrane Controlled Trials Register.[8]

Editors have led in taking preventive steps by trying to make authors aware of their journals' positions on repetitive and divided publication. Many journals have published commentaries on the problem or editorials discussing the issues and defining the journal's position; only a few have been cited here. Many journals have included statements in their information-for-authors pages requesting that authors, when submitting manuscripts, include in their submission letter any information bearing on possible prior publication of the paper's content. Such information is needed by an editor in coming to a decision on whether any possible repetitive publication of any content in the paper would be, in the journal's view, acceptable or unacceptable repetitive publication.

The statements in information-for-authors pages relevant to repetitive publication have generally been derived from or resemble the pioneering statement issued in 1978 by the International Committee of Medical Journal Editors (ICMJE). The most recent version reads as follows:

> Redundant or duplicate publication is publication of a paper that overlaps substantially with one already published.
>
> Readers of primary source periodicals deserve to be able to trust that what they are reading is original unless there is a clear statement that the article is being republished by the choice of the author and editor. The bases of this position are international copyright laws, ethical conduct, and cost-effective use of resources.
>
> Most journals do not wish to receive papers on work that has already been reported in large part in a published article or is contained in another paper that has been submitted or accepted for publication elsewhere, in print or in electronic media. This policy does not preclude the journal considering a paper that has been rejected by another journal, or a complete report that follows publication of a preliminary report, such as an abstract or poster displayed for colleagues at a professional meeting. Nor does it prevent journals considering a paper that has been presented at a scientific meeting but not published in full or that is being considered for publication in a proceedings or similar format. Press

reports of scheduled meetings will not usually be regarded as breaches of this rule, but such reports should not be amplified by additional data or copies of tables and illustrations.

When submitting a paper, the author should always make a full statement to the editor about all submissions and previous reports that might be regarded as redundant or duplicate publication of the same or very similar work. The author should alert the editor if the work includes subjects about which a previous report has been published. Any such work should be referred to and referenced in the new paper. Copies of such material should be included with the submitted paper to help the editor decide how to handle the matter.

If redundant or duplicate publication is attempted or occurs without such notification, authors should expect editorial action to be taken. At the least, prompt rejection of the submitted manuscript should be expected. If the editor was not aware of the violations and the article has already been published, then a notice of redundant or duplicate publication will probably be published with or without the author's explanation or approval. (ICMJE 1997, 36–37)

A following statement defines an acceptable form of repetitive publication, "secondary publication in the same or another language, especially in other countries" (ICMJE 1997, 37). The definition indicates that the prior publication must be stated and specified with a citation. The need for journals to develop clear policies on repetitive publication was emphasized by the CBE:

> Journals that publish original work should develop policies . . . regarding requirements of sole submission. . . . Once a journal has a policy about redundant publication, it should develop procedures to evaluate potential violations. . . . Once a journal has a policy . . . it should identify action(s) to be taken when a violation of the policy is determined to have taken place. . . . All of the above policies and procedures should be announced prominently in the journal and should be incorporated into the journal's instructions to authors. (CBE 1996, 77)

Table 5.1 outlines steps that can be taken by editors dealing with submitted papers that seem to represent attempted or actual repetitive publication.

Despite the ICMJE's successive statements in its "Uniform Requirements" documents, which have been published in hundreds of journals, and the related statements in journals' information-for-authors pages, efforts by authors to publish repetitively have continued. Some of these instances might represent misunderstandings of journals' positions or

Table 5.1. Steps Recommended to Editors for Dealing with Potential or Actual Repetitive Publication

Stage	Recommended Step
Presubmission and submission of a paper	Develop a policy on what kinds of submissions might represent attempted repetitive publication.
	Develop a policy defining requirements for "sole submission."
	State the journal's requirements for submissions in its information-for-authors page(s). This statement might include definitions of potential repetitive publication that the journal judges not to be attempted repetitive publication, such as prior publication of an abstract representing some or all of a submitted paper's content.
	Include information on what authors should supply with the submission of a paper if it might represent repetitive publication: statements about any prior publication of any of the paper's content, copies of any prior publications that might make the submission of the paper an attempt at repetitive publication (such as a proceedings report with similar content).
	Include statements on the journal's policy for actions on suspected attempted repetitive publication and identified repetitive publication (see steps below).
Suspected attempt at repetitive publication	Examine papers pointed to by reviewers as representing, in their opinion, prior publication of papers they have just reviewed for the journal. Have persons not already involved in the peer-review process carried out on the paper study the paper under review and any indicated prior publications. If a judgment of attempted repetitive publication is reached, communicate with the author to enable him or her to justify the submitted paper as not representing attempted repetitive publication ("due process" owed the author[s]).
Identified and confirmed repetitive publication	Publish a notice of repetitive (redundant, duplicate) publication in a prominent, page-numbered location in the journal (e.g., with editorials); list this notice in the table of contents of the issue; inform the National Library of Medicine of publication of the notice. The notice should identify with adequate bibliographic data (authors' names, article title, journal title, publication date, volume number, issue number, inclusive pages) all papers representing repetitive publication by the journal's definition.
Potential additional steps	Forbid submission of future papers by the responsible authors within a specified time.
	Share information on attempted repetitive publication with other journals at risk for the same offense, but note the legal risks in such a step.
	Inform appropriate academic superiors of the authors of identification of definite undesirable repetitive publication.

Source: This table is largely based on the statement "Redundant Publication" issued by the Council of Biology Editors (*CBE Views* 19[1996]:76–77). Reprinted with permission.

failure to consult journals' information pages, but others are probably willful disregard of what editors expect. If undesirable, abusive repetitive publication is to be sharply reduced or, even better, stamped out, steps are needed to make academic communities, the main habitats of authors, clearly aware of the problem. They should be made aware of the reasons for the undesirability of repetitive publication and of authors' responsibilities for avoiding it. Unfortunately, few professional societies in science have taken public positions on the problem. Recently, the ethics codes of 90 scientific societies were reviewed by two investigators for the National Science Foundation (NSF). Of these 90, only three seem to have substantive statements in their codes bearing on repetitive publication. A good example is that of the American Chemical Society (ACS):

> An author should recognize that journal space is a precious resource created at considerable cost. An author therefore has an obligation to use it wisely and economically. . . .
>
> In submitting a manuscript for publication, an author should inform the editor of related manuscripts that the author has under editorial consideration or in press. Copies of these manuscripts should be supplied to the editor, and the relationships of such manuscripts to the one submitted should be indicated.
>
> It is improper for an author to submit manuscripts describing essentially the same research to more than one journal of primary publication, unless it is a resubmission of a manuscript rejected for or withdrawn from publication. It is generally permissible to submit a manuscript for a full paper expanding on a previously published brief preliminary account (a "communication" or "letter") of the same work. However, at the time of the submission, the editor should be made aware of the earlier communication, and the preliminary communication should be cited in the manuscript. (ACS 1996, secs. B2, B7, and B8)

Especially relevant to divided publication is this statement: "Fragmentation of research reports should be avoided. A scientist who has done extensive work on a system or group of related systems should organize publication so that each report gives a well-rounded account of a particular aspect of the general study. Fragmentation consumes journal space excessively and unduly complicates literature searches. The convenience of readers is served if reports on related studies are published in the same journal, or in a small number of journals" (ACS 1996, sec. B6).

The "Ethical Principles of Psychologists and Code of Conduct" of the American Psychological Association (APA) has a shorter statement: "Psychologists do not publish, as original data, data that have been previously published. This does not preclude republishing data when they are accompanied by proper acknowledgment" (APA 1992, 1610, sec. 6.24). A detailed, extensive statement on standards for authorship and publication is that published by the Association of University Radiologists. Its section on "Credit, Citations, Re-publication, and Re-use of Data" merits quotation here: "The same or substantially the same paper should not be published twice. This may be a temptation if a paper has been published as part of a symposium or if an author wishes to use a submitted manuscript to satisfy the requirement of a symposium" (Friedman 1993, 34). Many journals published by scientific societies that have not made explicit statements on publication ethics do carry appropriate statements in their information-for-authors pages.

At least one additional association in the medical sciences not represented in the NSF survey has published explicit statements relevant to repetitive or divided publication. These are the statements in the detailed, explicit document published by the American Diabetes Association (ADA). It first briefly defines authors' responsibilities for maintaining "the traditional standards of intellectual integrity called for in any scholarly publication." Two of these responsibilities are especially relevant to questions of repetitive publication: (1) "Citing accurately and completely. The author must acknowledge all debts to other investigators and accurately represent their earlier work." (2) "Disclosing to editors the existence of similar publications previously submitted or under consideration by another publisher" (ADA 1992, 1059). The document goes on to define the guidelines that should be followed by authors submitting articles to the journals of the ADA.

> —Authors of reviews or articles submitted as part of symposia proceedings must directly notify the editors of American Diabetes Association journals when they have previously published or submitted the same article, in whole or in part, in another journal. Disclosure must be made directly to the publisher; authors are not relieved of the obligation to disclose similar publications by informing the sponsoring company or a medical communications firm associated with it. The editor of the American Diabetes Association journal should be provided with a copy of the primary version of the paper.
> —Authors must cite any similar previous publications when submitting articles to American Diabetes Association journals. This includes citing illustrations or tables reprinted or adapted from other journals. Again, this responsibility remains with the authors and cannot be assigned to a sponsor or communications firm. . . .

> ... Unacceptable publishing practices [include]:
>
> —Submitting a previously published original research paper or review as part of the proceedings of a sponsored symposium. (Such a submission would only be acceptable if both the editor of the journal in which the article first appeared and the editor of the American Diabetes Association journal were fully informed and agreed to the duplicate publication.)
>
> —Failing to cite the original source for the data contained in a review or symposium proceeding. . . .
>
> —Representing to an editor that a submission is original when in fact it has been previously published or submitted elsewhere in whole or in part. (ADA 1992, 1060)

But even if many more scientific societies were to publish such standards, what would be their effect? Would they change the ethos, the spirit, the consensual standards of authors' communities so as to sharply reduce the incidence of undesirable practices in publishing and, in particular, repetitive publication? Such standards can be seen in print once and promptly forgotten just as information-for-authors pages can be scanned and the fine print relevant to repetitive publication ignored. I have commented elsewhere on the need for a spirit in a scientific community supporting desirable practices: "Editors cannot build an ethos alone. Not until deans, departmental chairmen, section heads, and all other mentors in research and medical education see their responsibilities for efficient and honest science and set standards in their own places will we have the ethos we need. . . . The day might even come when we leave behind the 'shalt not' of editors' rules and enter the ethos of 'thou shalt' support responsible science" (Huth 1992, 1063). Everyone in the scientific community must agree that we all need efficient science, science we all can trust. Such science can exist only if some individual desires are kept in check, if we have a "fair balance between individual needs and those of science as a reliable system" (Huth 1992, 1062).

Medical schools could lead in developing the needed ethos. Only a few seem to have developed their own standards for publishing practices. Harvard Medical School first issued its "Guidelines for Investigators in Scientific Research" in 1988. Under the heading "Publication Practices" is noted the undesirability of repetitive or divided publication: "Certain practices . . . make it difficult for reviewer and reader to follow a complete experimental sequence: . . . the publication of fragments of a study, and the submission of multiple similar abstracts or manuscripts differing only slightly in content" (Faculty of Medicine, Harvard University 1988, p. 5, sec. IV). Similar statements have been issued by a few other medical schools.

Some research institutions active in aspects of medical science have stated policy positions on repetitive publication. A document issued by the National Institutes of Health (1997) takes this position: "Timely publication of new and significant results is important for the progress of science, but fragmentary publication of the results of a scientific investigation or multiple publications of the same or similar data are inappropriate. Each publication should make a substantial contribution to its field." Some medical school documents were probably prepared and issued as a consequence of widespread attention to particular episodes involving members of their faculties. How many other medical institutions with responsibilities for responsible science have developed, issued, and disseminated their own policy statements on publication practices I do not know.

What else might medical schools and other organizations do to heighten awareness among potential authors of ethical standards for publication? They can develop policies akin to those quoted above. They can adopt already published policies. But are policies likely to make their staffs more aware of standards? I am skeptical. Some more constant stimulus to authors' attention to standards may be needed. One device would be having institutional review boards or other similar intramural groups track papers emerging from research they have approved. The board could review them for evidence of unjustified repetitive or divided publication. For papers clearly repetitive or divided into fractional reports of single studies, authors could be expected to provide documents justifying such publication (e.g., letters from editors of participating journals indicating their agreement that such publication is justified). Such a device could keep authors constantly aware that their publication practices are being monitored.

Conclusions

Undesirable repetitive publication occurs in medical journals published in Europe and the United States and probably in journals published in other parts of the world. The rate of its occurrence is not clear; the estimates here are based on data at least two years old and represent a very wide range of rates. A new survey of editors on the question might yield mainly perceptions of occurrence or attempts, not firmly identified actual repetitive publication. If editorials such as those cited here, society policies such as that issued by the American Diabetes Association, and policy documents issued by medical institutions are reducing the problem, new preventive action may not be needed. Critical to a judgment on whether new action may be needed is more information, not only on the current occurrence rates, but also on the current ethos in medical schools and research institutions. Are the dangers for the scientific community in repetitive publication widely known and appreciated? If the only bases for objecting to repetitive publication were wastes of publication space and the envy of authors with shorter personal bibliographies, repetitive publication might not seem to be such an offense against science. But the potential dangers from improperly multiplied, inadequately identified evidence bearing on medical and research decisions should be reason enough for medical institutions to work on developing the ethos needed among their faculties and staffs to prevent distortions of scientific evidence.

Acknowledgments

I thank Iain Chalmers, Michael Clarke, Matthias Egger, David Moher, and John Overbeke for supplying me with information highly relevant for this paper. They are not responsible, however, for any statements or interpretations in it; the responsibility for the paper is entirely mine.

Notes

1. The "Ingelfinger rule" represented Ingelfinger's unwillingness to consider for publication in his journal a paper whose main data or other evidence had already been published in a news medium. This policy as originally stated seemed to be limited in its referents, but it had ambiguities that were not entirely dispelled by a subsequent restatement (Relman 1981). Relman did make clear, however, that the prior publication of an abstract did not disqualify a paper based on the work reported in the abstract from being considered for publication. Relman conceded that the policy was based in part on the journal's desire to maintain its newsworthiness.

2. The acceptability of such dual-language publication is defined in the policy statement of an international body of medical editors (ICMJE 1997, 37).

3. In this calculation, the apparent number of repetitive papers, 41, is rounded down to 40. The assumption is made that 40 represents 20 pairs of repetitive papers; some ambiguities about the listing suggest that the actual number of undesirably repetitive papers may be fewer than 40, but 40 can be taken as a maximal estimate from the MEDLINE data.

4. We know little or nothing of the rate of repetitive publication in the years before 1980.

5. This view has also been expressed by too many other persons for citation and reference here. I have set forth a similar view (Huth 1996) in a recently published book on conflicts of interest.

6. This paper was called to my attention by Iain Chalmers, Cochrane Collaboration, Oxford, United Kingdom.

7. Michael Clarke, Imperial Cancer Research Fund Research Scientist, Clinical Trials Service Unit, University of Oxford, Oxford, United Kingdom. Personal communication, ca. April 1997.

8. Iain Chalmers, personal communication, 24 March 1997.

References

American Chemical Society (ACS), Publications Division. 1996. Ethical guidelines. http://pubs.acs.org/instruct/ethic.html. Site accessed 6 November 1998.

American Diabetes Association (ADA), Publications Policy Committee. 1992. Duplicate publication in American Diabetes Association journals: Challenges and recommendations. *Diabetes Care* 15:1059–61.

American Psychological Association (APA). 1992. Ethical principles of psychologists and code of conduct. *American Psychologist* 47:1597–1628. See also http://www.apa.org/ethics/code.html. Site accessed 4 January 1999.

Angell, M. 1986. Publish or perish: A proposal. *Annals of Internal Medicine* 104:261–62.

Barnard, H., and J. A. Overbeke. 1993. [Duplicate publication of original articles in and from the *Nederlands Tijdschrift voor Geneeskunde*]. *Nederlands Tijdschrift voor Geneeskunde* 137:593–97. I am reporting these data from an English translation of this article kindly supplied to me by the second author.

Berk, P. D. 1992. Redundant publication: Deja vu all over again. *Hepatology* 16:840–42.

Bevan, D. R. 1991. Duplicate and divided publication. *Canadian Journal of Anaesthesia* 38:267–69.

Bier, D. M., V. A. Fulginiti, J. M. Garfunkel, J. F. Lucey, J. Spranger, H. B. Valman, M. L. Chiswick, and R. Zetterstrom. 1990a. Duplicate publication and related problems. *American Journal of Diseases of Children* 144:1293–94.

———. 1990b. Duplicate publication and related problems. *Archives of Diseases in Childhood* 65:1289–90.

Blancett, S. S., A. Flanagin, and R. K. Young. 1995. Duplicate publication in the nursing literature. *Image—The Journal of Nursing Scholarship* 27:51–56.

Broad, W. J. 1981. The publishing game: Getting more for less. *Science* 211:1137–39.

Council of Biology Editors (CBE), Editorial Policy Committee. 1996. Redundant publication. *CBE Views* 19:76–77.

Dobson, R. L. 1990. Dual publication and manipulation of the editorial process. *Journal of the American Academy of Dermatology* 23:1181–82.

Egger, M., T. Zellweger-Zähner, M. Schneider, C. Junker, C. Lengeler, and G. Antes. 1997. Language bias in randomised controlled trials published in English and German. *Lancet* 350:326–69.

Faculty of Medicine, Harvard University. 1988. Guidelines for investigators in scientific research. In *Faculty policies on integrity in science,* 4–5. Boston: Harvard Medical School, 1996. See also http://www.hms.harvard.edu/integrity/index.html. Site accessed 17 March 1999.

Flanagin, A., R. M. Glass, and G. D. Lundberg. 1992. Electronic journals and duplicate publication: Is a byte a word? *JAMA* 267:2374.

Friedman, P. J. 1993. Standards for authorship and publication in academic radiology. Association of University Radiologists' Ad Hoc Committee on Standards for the Responsible Conduct of Research. *Radiology* 189:33–34; *Investigative Radiology* 28:879–81; *AJR American Journal of Roentgenology* 161:899–900.

Hammerschmidt, D. E. 1992. Echoes in the halls: Thoughts on double publication. *Journal of Laboratory and Clinical Medicine* 119:109–10.

Hanke, C. W., K. A. Arndt, R. L. Dobson, L. M. Dzubow, L. C. Parish, and J. S. Taylor. 1990. Dual publication and manipulation of the editorial process. *Archives of Dermatology* 126:1625–26.

——. 1991. Dual publication and manipulation of the editorial process. *Journal of Cutaneous Pathology* 18:145–46.

Huston, P., and D. Moher. 1996. Redundancy, disaggregation, and the integrity of medical research. *Lancet* 347:1024–26.

Huth, E. J. 1986. Irresponsible authorship and wasteful publication. *Annals of Internal Medicine* 104:257–59.

——. 1992. Journals and authors: Rules, principles, and ethos. *Diabetes Care* 15:1062–64.

——. 1996. Conflicts of interest in industry-funded clinical research. In *Conflicts of interest in clinical practice and research,* ed. R. G. Spece, D. A. Shimm, and A. E. Buchanan, 389–406. New York: Oxford University Press.

——. 1997. Authorship standards: Progress in slow motion. *CBE Views* 20:127–32.

International Committee of Medical Journal Editors (ICMJE). 1997. Uniform requirements for manuscripts submitted to biomedical journals. *Annals of Internal Medicine* 126:36–47. See also http://www.acponline.org/journals/resource/unifreqr.htm. Site accessed 5 February 1999.

Leizorovicz, A., M. C. Haugh, and J.-P. Boissel. 1992. Meta-analysis and multiple publication of clinical trial reports. *Lancet* 340:1102–3.

Livesley, B. 1992. Duplicate publication. *BMJ* 304:1314.

Making clinical trialists register. 1991. *Lancet* 338:244–45.

National Institutes of Health (NIH). 1997. Guidelines for the conduct of research in the intramural research programs of NIH. 3d ed. http://www.nih.gov/news/irnews/guidelines.htm. Site accessed 12 January 1999.

National Library of Medicine (NLM). 1998. Fact sheet: Errata, retraction, duplicate publication, and comment policy. http://www.nlm.nih.gov/pubs/factsheets/ errata.html. Site accessed 12 January 1999.

The new shorter Oxford English dictionary on historical principles. 2 vols. 1993. s.v. "redundant."

Reaven, G. M. 1992. An open letter to the editor. *Diabetes Care* 15:1057–58.

Relman, A. S. 1981. The Ingelfinger rule. *New England Journal of Medicine* 305:824–26.

Smith, G. 1992. Dual publication of abstracts. *British Journal of Anaesthesia* 68:5.

Smith, G., R. Miller, L. J. Saidman, and M. Morgan. 1991. Ethics in publishing. *British Journal of Anaesthesia* 66:421–22.

Susser, M., and A. Yankauer. 1993. Prior, duplicate, repetitive, fragmented, and redundant publication and editorial decisions. *American Journal of Public Health* 83:792–93.

Tramer, M. R., R. A. Moore, J. M. Reynolds, and H. J. McQuay. 1997. A quantitative systematic review of ondansetron in treatment of established postoperative nausea and vomiting. *BMJ* 314:1088–92.

Waldron, T. 1992. Is duplicate publishing on the increase? *BMJ* 304:1029.

Conflict of Interest 6

Annette Flanagin

Concern about financial conflict of interest has increased considerably during the last two decades. Allegations of public officials' failure to uphold their sworn duties to society because of financial ties and greed are now common forage for investigative news reports, criminal investigations, political strategies, cocktail party gossip, and Internet chats. Simultaneously, biomedical science has moved away from its altruistic truth-seeking roots toward commercial enterprise with economic motives and incentives. Why, then, were we surprised when what was first recognized as a problem for politicians, bankers, and investors also became a problem for biomedical researchers, whose scientific pursuits could be tainted by financial interests in their own work? Certainly, we need not have been so amazed, for conflicts of interest are to be expected among all people. However, problems arise when competing interests result in conflict that causes bias or inappropriate decisions.

In biomedical publication, academic, professional, institutional, and financial interests may bias judgments and interfere with the dissemination of scientific information. Although these multiple interests affect all stages of biomedical research and publication, financial conflicts of interest will serve as the primary focus of this chapter. Financial conflicts have been the focus of much discourse involving biomedical publication, perhaps because financial associations and equity are easily defined and measured when compared with nonfinancial interests. Although quantifiable, financial interests are not as readily identifiable as specific academic and professional interests. For example, an author's academic degrees and professional affiliations often make discernible a number of personal and institutional interests. The desire for recognition and advancement encourages authors to identify themselves, their professional expertise and education, and their institutional affiliations. Government granting agencies and educational institutions require identification of their support in published articles. Yet authors do not volunteer many types of financial interest, primarily because of concerns about invasion of privacy, unwanted competition, the desire to stake a scientific claim, personal and institutional interests, agreements with sponsors and funding sources, employment contracts, and the effect of perceived or actual conflicts and biases on their ability to publish.

What Is a Conflict of Interest?

Friedman (1992) described a *conflict of interest* as that which occurs when a decision maker allows a selfish interest to influence judgment by favoring self-interested goals over altruistic, professional, and societal trusts. *Merriam-Webster's Collegiate Dictionary* (1994) defines *conflict of interest* as "a conflict between the private interests and the official responsibilities of a person in a position of trust." Stephen J. Welch (1997, 865) extrapolated from *Merriam-Webster's* definition to the broader and more practical context of biomedical publication:

> In the peer review publishing arena . . . the "position of trust" is that of author, reviewer, . . . or editor. The "private interests" can be financial, professional, academic, ethical, and even political. The "official responsibilities" comprise the authors reporting results of scientific research and/or medical practices, reviewers assessing the quality and relevance of that report, . . . and the editor-in-chief making decisions on journal policy and acceptance and rejection of reports, editorials, letters, and reviews.

A conflict may be real or perceived, potential or actual, inconsequential or harmful. Each of these states depends on the interests involved, their relative importance and value, and the potential for harm or bias that may result if one interest outweighs another.

Conflict of interest is related to but different from a *conflict of commitment*, a phrase often used in academic settings to describe competing demands on a person's time. For example, a conflict of commitment may arise when a faculty member's ability to meet the obligations of academic appointment (e.g., teaching, research, patient care) becomes impaired because of his or her commitment to outside activities (e.g., professional consulting, authorship, involvement with professional societies, participation on review panels) (Association of American Medical Colleges [AAMC] 1990).

The Origins of the Phrase *Conflict of Interest*

The origin of the phrase *conflict of interest* is not known. However, contrary to claims that it entered the English-language lexicon relatively recently (*Merriam-Webster's Collegiate Dictionary* puts the date of 1951 on its definition), the phrase has ancient roots, probably dating to the beginning of civilized politics (or at least to Caesar's wife). The *Oxford English Dictionary (OED)* (1989) cites its definition—"to come into collision, to clash; to be at variance, be incompatible"—as the chief sense of the term today. The *OED* (1989) traces the first use of the phrase to Joshua Sprigge (1618–84) in a 1647 publication of *Anglia Rediviva*, in "England's Recovery Being the History of the Motions, Actions and Success of the Army under the Immediate Conduct of His Excellency SR Thomas Fairfax." Thomas Hill Green (1836–82) is noted to have referred to a more philosophical conflict in the following phrase from his 1883 *Prolegomena to Ethics:* "the perplexities of conscience . . . in which duties appear to conflict with each other." Contemporary usage of the phrase *conflict of interest* has emerged from its beginnings in military and civil politics to apply to anyone who holds a public trust. Biomedical researchers and health professionals enjoy a significant public trust, although such confidence is in jeopardy.

Conflict of Interest in Biomedical Research

Huth (1996) identified six parties with interests in the results of biomedical research: (1) the investigator, whose successful research leads to career advancement, academic promotion, future research funding, and personal financial gains; (2) the investigator's institution or employer, whose reputation and financial standing or profitability can be enhanced by the success of the investigator's research; (3) the commercial sponsor of the research, who relies on positive research results to enhance return on investment and corporate profits; (4) the patient, who desires personal benefit; (5) the scientific community, which needs reliable information and public respectability; and (6) the public, who pays for biomedical research through taxes and charitable donations. The interests of each of these parties may conflict with the interests of any of the other parties.

The AAMC (1990, 491) offered the following useful description of conflict of interest in the biomedical arena:

The term *conflict of interest* in science refers to situations in which financial or other personal considerations may compromise, or have the appearance of compromising, an investigator's professional judgment in conducting or reporting research. The bias such conflicts may conceivably impart affects not only collection, analysis and interpretation of data, but also the hiring of staff, procurement of materials, sharing of results, choice of protocol, and use of statistical methods. Conflicts of interest can affect other scholarly duties as well, but are particularly important to consider in biomedical and behavioral research because of the impact such conflicts can have on human health.

The AAMC (1990) provided a list of situations that may lead to bias, inappropriate interests, and unacceptable conflicts of interest in the academic biomedical community (table 6.1). Horton (1997) published another useful list of interests commonly facing biomedical investigators (table 6.2).

Financial interests, the primary focus of this chapter, may be the easiest to quantify and may be difficult to identify if not disclosed or if purposefully concealed. Financial interests in biomedical research include the following:

- salary and benefits of employment
- consultancies
- payment for service on boards of directors, advisory boards, review panels, and consensus groups
- sponsored research agreements
- donations of research-related funds, materials, or equipment
- payment for recruitment or referral of study subjects
- stock ownership and other forms of commercial equity
- current and pending research grants
- current and pending patents
- licensing agreements
- paid royalties
- paid expert testimony
- honoraria
- financial support for education and meeting attendance
- paid travel and accommodations

Academic-Industry Relationships

A commonly cited reason for concern about financial conflicts of interest in biomedical research is the growth in academic-industry relationships, which developed after World War II, as large amounts of government fund-

Table 6.1. Situations Possibly Leading to Bias, Inappropriate Interests, and Unacceptable Conflicts of Interest in the Academic Biomedical Community

Situations that may . . .	Examples
Impart bias in research	Undertaking basic or clinical research when the investigator or the investigator's immediate family has a financial, managerial, or ownership interest in the sponsoring company or in the company producing the drug or device under evaluation.
	Accepting gratuities or special favors from research sponsors.
	Entering into a consultantship arrangement with an organization or individual having an economic interest in related research.
Involve inappropriate use of institutional assets and resources in research	Using students or employees of the institution to perform services for a company in which a faculty member has an ownership interest or from which he or she receives any type of remuneration.
	Using institutional resources (such as equipment, supplies, and facilities), without reimbursement or authorization, for personal purposes or to support the activities of an independent entity in which an investigator holds a financial or other interest.
	Associating one's name or one's work with the institution in such a way as to profit monetarily by trading on the reputation or goodwill of the institution, rather than on one's professional competence.
Involve inappropriate use of information	Using, without authorization, privileged information acquired in connection with one's professional responsibilities.
	Accepting support for basic or clinical research under terms and conditions that results be held confidential, unpublished, or significantly delayed in publication.
	Providing privileged access to information, developed with university resources or supported by independent sponsors, to an entity in which the faculty member has a financial interest.
Involve self-dealing	Purchasing equipment, instruments, or supplies for research or teaching from a firm in which the investigator or faculty member has a financial or other interest.
	Influencing the negotiation of contracts between the academic institution and outside organizations with which the investigator or faculty member has a financial interest or other relationship.
	Requiring or recommending one's own textbook or other teaching aids.
Involve special considerations in consulting to federal agencies	Consulting to a federal agency when one is also conducting federally sponsored research.

Source: Association of American Medical Colleges, "Guidelines for Dealing with Faculty Conflicts of Commitment and Conflicts of Interest in Research," *Academic Medicine* 65(1990):492. Reprinted with permission.

Table 6.2. Interests (Commitments) Facing an Investigator

Professional (e.g., personal, specialty, departmental, or institutional status)

Financial (e.g., personal reward; research funding)

Patient-related (e.g., as a personal physician; payment for study recruitment)

Institutional (e.g., ethics committee)

Grant-related

Regulatory (e.g., FDA)

Scientific publication

Mass media

Legal (e.g., patent protection)

Sociopolitical

Public interest (e.g., research support through taxes, charitable donations)

Source: Richard Horton, "Conflicts of Interest in Clinical Research: Opprobrium or Obsession," *Lancet* 349(1997):1112, © by The Lancet Ltd. Reprinted with permission.

ing for clinical and basic science began to be replaced with support from industry (pharmaceutical, biotechnology, and equipment firms) (Huth 1996; Steiner 1996). In the United States, growth in the relationship between industry and academia followed federal legislative initiatives in the early 1980s—the Stevenson-Wydler Technology Act (1982, U.S. Code, vol. 15, sec. 3702, 3) and the Bayh-Dole Amendments to the U.S. patent laws (1980, U.S. Code, vol. 35, sec. 201a–i). The Bayh-Dole Amendments gave small businesses, nonprofit organizations, and academic institutions the right to own, license, and profit from scientific advances funded by the federal government (AAMC 1990; Steiner 1996). Such legislation led to the removal of previous barriers to partnerships between academic institutions and industry, allowing both partners to benefit financially if the research leads to commercially viable products (AAMC 1990; Frankel 1996). Academic-industrial relationships continue to grow in the wake of reductions in annual increases of government funding of research, increased competition for such support, increased interdisciplinary collaboration, competitive economic incentives for more rapid advances, and approval of joint ventures between private institutions and federal government laboratories (National Academy of Sciences [NAS] 1992; Shimm and Spece 1996; Huth 1996).

Innovative approaches to technology transfer result in many types of partnerships among faculty, students, and industry. These partnerships include corporate researchers working with faculty and graduate students in university laboratories, corporations establishing offices and laboratories in university-owned research parks, universities owning new technologies and licensing these technologies to corporations, and universities licensing new technologies to spin-off corporations created, owned, and operated by university faculty and employees (Gunsalus 1989). In these situations, both conflicts of interest and conflicts of commitment are common, and the potential risks to all parties are substantial. Thus, detailed conflict-of-interest policies, requiring disclosure of conflicts by all persons involved and monitoring by the university, are typically recommended.

Scientific Investigators and Financial Interests

During the 1980s, a number of public scandals and investigations into the financial interests of biomedical researchers emerged. The cases involving clinical research were damaging to the public image of biomedical researchers. In many of these cases, it became apparent that some researchers' financial interests in the drugs they were investigating and the accompanying denial or biased enthusiasm (at best) or self-serving greed (at worst) resulted in the minimization, delay in dissemination, and suppression of negative research results. In a few cases, the researchers may have sacrificed the health of the public for their own financial gains.

An early, well-publicized case of biomedical financial conflict (and one that clearly involved publication) was aptly described by a news reporter as "a story about a drug study at Harvard Medical School that went awry. . . . a morality play about what happens to researchers with stock options or a cautionary tale about the dangers of careless enthusiasm" (Booth 1988, 1497). In this case, a Harvard-affiliated ophthalmologist, Scheffer C. G. Tseng, had been investigating an experimental ophthalmic ointment containing vitamin A (tretinoin) as a possible treatment for keratoconjunctivitis sicca, a dry-eye disorder that then affected approximately ten million people in the United States (Booth 1988; Shulman 1988; Lichter 1989). Tseng's research began with animal models in the early 1980s, and he published the preliminary results of the first human trial in the journal *Ophthalmology* in June 1985 (Tseng et al. 1985). Two months earlier, in April 1985, Tseng had received approval from the U.S. Food and Drug Administration (FDA) to use the ophthalmic ointment as an orphan drug, which gave Tseng exclusive rights to market the drug for seven years. This financial interest was not disclosed in the article Tseng published in *Ophthalmology* in 1985.

During the same period, a group of ophthalmologists formed a company, Spectra Pharmaceutical Services, to market ophthalmic drugs. Spectra purchased the rights to Tseng's tretinoin ointment, paying him $310,000 in July 1985, one month after the publication of his preliminary results in *Ophthalmology* (Booth 1988). Five months later, in December 1985, Spectra conducted a public stock offering. According to Paul R. Lichter (1989, 576), then editor-in-chief of *Ophthalmology*, "Considerable publicity, based largely on the results of the study published in *Ophthalmology* in June 1985, surrounded the stock sale." Holding 530,000 shares of stock in Spectra, Tseng had a major stake in the company's financial success, as did one of his co-investigators and his supervisor at Harvard Medical School (Booth 1988; Lichter 1989).

Subsequent studies conducted by Tseng and others were not as promising as the initial report. In early 1986, because of concerns over the effectiveness of the drug and knowledge that Tseng and his co-investigator were major stockholders in the company that owned the ointment (Tseng had informed his department chair of his equity in Spectra after he had purchased the stock), both the Massachusetts Eye and Ear Infirmary and Harvard began investigations into Tseng's research and the possibility that results of negative trials had been suppressed. These independent investigations revealed that Tseng had treated at least four times the number of patients the FDA had approved for treatment and that study patients had not experienced a clinical benefit from the tretinoin ointment (Booth 1988; Lichter 1989). The publicity following the sale of the stock had created unexpected public demand for treatment, and Tseng did not limit the number of patients he treated with the tretinoin ointment. Because of the increase in patients, Tseng had changed the trial's design several times, making it difficult to assess accurately the effectiveness of the ointment. He also minimized negative findings. It was during this time that Tseng's financial interest in the drug grew, and he sold his stock at a significant profit (Booth 1988).

Although Harvard's investigation into Tseng's research determined that scientific misconduct was not a factor and that no patient was harmed by the study, Harvard concluded that "a significant conflict of interest developed . . . and proper safeguards were not in place to protect the study from potential bias" (Lichter 1989, 576). Harvard also determined that Tseng had failed to make timely and complete disclosures about changes in his study design and his financial interest in the subject of his investigations (Booth 1988; Shulman 1988; Lichter 1989). During the 1986 investigations of Tseng's research, Spectra launched a national clinical trial to test the ointment's effectiveness. In 1988, the results of this trial were published in *Ophthalmology* (Soong et al. 1988). This report concluded that the ointment was no better than placebo and did not reduce clinical signs and symptoms of keratoconjunctivitis sicca, except in those patients with severe dry-eye disorders (Soong et al. 1988; Lichter 1989). In October 1988, the *Boston Globe* ran a news story describing many of the details of Tseng's financial interest and biased investigations (Booth 1988). This news story was followed by investigative reports published in major newspapers and scientific journals.

Similarly prominent cases of alleged abuse involving investigators' financial conflicts of interest and their failure to disclose such interest when reporting the results of their research have occurred among researchers investigating thrombolytics, antibiotics, and biogenetic material (Shimm and Spece 1996; Altman 1991; Curran 1991). Although perhaps less common among students, junior investigators, and junior faculty, financial interests are not uncommon among biomedical investigators and senior faculty. In many respects, biomedical research has become an economic enterprise. As summarized by Dorothy Nelkin (1998, 893), "Science is a big business, a costly enterprise commonly financed by corporations and driven by the logic of the market. Entrepreneurial values, economic interests, and the promise of profits are shaping the scientific ethos."

In this regard, a study by Krimsky and colleagues (1996) of the financial interests of authors publishing in scientific and medical journals is worth reviewing. Krimsky et al. (1996) examined 789 articles published by 1,105 university-affiliated authors in 14 leading scientific and medical journals in 1992. Thirty-four percent of the articles (267/789) in this study had a lead author (indicated as first or last author in the byline) who possessed a significant financial interest. *Significant financial interest* was defined as being listed on a patent or patent application closely related to the work described in the article; serving on the scientific advisory board of a biotechnology company; or being an officer, director, or major shareholder in a company that had a commercial interest in the author's research. None of the 267 articles included a statement of the author's financial interest. This study was conducted in 1992, when only one of the 14 journals had instituted a policy on disclosure of conflicts of interest. By 1996, only four of the 14 journals had done so. Krimsky et al. (1996) concluded that further research was needed to determine the effectiveness of mandatory disclosure requirements established by academic institutions, governmental agencies, and journals.

Additional concern arose after publication of several studies demonstrated associations between the financial interests of authors and what they publish as reports of research, reviews, and editorial comment. For example, a study by Stelfox and colleagues (1998) found an association between authors' published positions about a controversial drug therapy and their financial relationships with pharmaceutical companies. In this study, authors who published articles that supported the use of calcium-channel antagonists were more likely to have financial relationships with the companies that manufacture these drugs than were authors who published articles that were neutral or critical toward use of calcium-channel antagonists. (The safety of calcium-channel antagonists, used in the treatment of heart disease, has been the subject of much research, conflicting results, and controversy.) The study did not determine that the financial relationships resulted in bias among the authors who support the use of these drugs. Stelfox et al. (1998, 105) concluded that "authors are naive about public perceptions concerning such relationships" and wondered "how the public would interpret the debate over calcium-channel antagonists if it knew that most of the authors participating in the debate had undisclosed financial ties with pharmaceutical manufacturers."

The Development of Policies and Guidelines by Academic Institutions, Professional Societies, and Government Agencies

After the publicity over Tseng's financial conflicts, Harvard Medical School appointed a committee to set up new rules governing financial conflicts of interest for Harvard faculty (Booth 1988; Shulman 1988). Today, Harvard Medical School has a detailed policy on conflict of interest for faculty and employees (Faculty of Medicine, Harvard University 1996). Most U.S. academic institutions have rules governing financial support for faculty activities, when faculty must disclose particular interests, and when they must divest themselves of particular financial interests. Some institutions have specific rules on management of conflict that may result from financial relationships.

In 1990, the U.S. Congress held public hearings on conflicts of interest in biomedicine (U.S. House 1990). During the hearings, guidelines for regulation of financial conflict of interest in biomedicine were discussed, including the AAMC's 1990 advice to faculty to disclose all relevant conflicts of interest (AAMC 1990). The American Federation for Clinical Research (AFCR) (1990) recommended that researchers publicly disclose all research funding and not hold equity in any commercial entity that makes a product the researcher is investigating. Such public disclosure pertains to all presentation of research results, including both oral presentation (e.g., in educational or professional meetings, testimony, and press briefings) and written presentation (e.g., submission of abstract or manuscript).

Other organizations that, in the early 1990s, developed guidelines on conflicts of interest in recommendations for biomedical research include the American College of Cardiology, the American College of Physicians, the American Medical Association, the American Psychological Association, the Royal College of Physicians, the U.S. National Academy of Sciences, the U.S. Institute of Medicine, and Canada's National Council on Bioethics in Human Research (established by the Medical Research Council of Canada and the Royal College of Physicians and Surgeons of Canada). Huth (1996) published a critical analysis of each of these guidelines as well as a proposal for ideal guidelines to help prevent scientific or ethical lapses due to conflicts of interest in industry-funded clinical research.

In 1995, after many years of debate and acrimony, the U.S. Public Health Service (PHS) and the National Science Foundation (NSF) adopted guidelines to regulate government-funded researchers' financial interests in their work (PHS 1995; NSF 1995). The PHS guideline requires investigators to disclose significant financial interests that are or would be affected by their government-funded research. The guideline defines *significant* as "anything of monetary value, including, but not limited to, salary or other payments for services (e.g., consulting fees or honoraria); equity interests (e.g., stocks, stock options or other ownership interests); and intellectual property rights (e.g., patents, copyrights and royalties from such rights)" that exceeds $10,000 in monetary value or 5% equity interest of a single entity (NSF 1995, 35822). All U.S. academic institutions that receive federal funding for research are required to include this disclosure policy in their institutional guidelines for faculty. In addition, the PHS guideline requires investigators to disclose conflicts of interest "in each public presentation of results" (PHS 1995, 35817). In 1999, the FDA began requiring pharmaceutical companies, when submitting applications for new drug licenses, to disclose whether clinical investigators involved in drug trials have received financial compensation from the company. Such compensation includes stock and patents or options for stocks and patents, research grants, equipment or other material gifts, consultant fees, and honoraria (FDA 1998; Josefson 1998).

The policies of government agencies and those of specific academic institutions may differ in terms of the lowest monetary value defined as a significant financial interest that requires disclosure (e.g., $10,000 versus $250). These policies may cause confusion for faculty and students. In addition, academic institutions may prohibit certain financial relationships, or they may have more restrictive rules regarding the management of conflict once a significant financial interest is disclosed.

A new risk for biomedical researchers surfaced in the United States in the 1990s, after the U.S. Security and Exchange Commission's prosecution of several researchers who used their knowledge of the results of research to benefit personally in the stock market. These researchers conducted illegal insider trading before the results of the research were made public (e.g., via publication, presentation at a scientific or regulatory meeting, or press release). In these cases, the researchers' financial interests caused them to commit criminal acts for which they were sent to prison (Skolnick 1998).

Financial Interests and Restrictions on Biomedical Publication

A conflict of interest may arise when a researcher agrees to receive funding from a commercial entity under conditions that may restrict the dissemination of the results of that research. Although unethical, the suppression of undesired negative results by the biotechnology industry is not uncommon and is often "justified" in terms of commercial propriety and profitability. A researcher who is not employed by a for-profit company but who receives research funding from the company (or whose institutional employer receives the research funding) can be caught in a difficult conflict if the researcher agrees to restrictions on the dissemination of findings.

In a highly publicized case, a pharmaceutical company attempted to suppress the results of a study conducted by university-affiliated researcher Betty Dong and colleagues (King 1996; Rennie 1997). Dong, an employee of the University of California, San Francisco, agreed to receive research funds from a pharmaceutical company to conduct a bioequivalence trial of several drugs intended for the treatment of thyroid disease, provided that the company controlled the publication of any findings, an ominous provision. From the beginning of their collaboration, both Dong and the company expected that the research would prove that the company's bestselling drug, Synthroid, would be shown to be superior to the other drugs in the study. However, Dong's research determined that a less expensive generic drug was as effective as the company's proprietary drug. As described by Drummond Rennie, from the time of Dong's first communication of preliminary results to the sponsoring pharmaceutical company in 1990 through 1994, the company "waged an energetic campaign to discredit the study and prevent publication of the drafts Dong and colleagues sent to them for comment, claiming that the study was seriously flawed." Company representatives also claimed that Dong's research had "deficiencies with patient selection criteria and compliance, with assay reliability, with study administration, with measuring bioequivalence, and with statistical analysis," as well as "unspecified ethical problems" (Rennie 1997, 1238).

The University of California, San Francisco, conducted two investigations after these allegations surfaced and found only "minor and easily correctible problems" (Rennie 1997, 1238). The university concluded that the study had been conducted appropriately, that the actions of the sponsoring pharmaceutical company constituted "harassment" (Rennie 1997, 1238), and that the actions of the company's representatives were "deceptive and self-serving" (Rennie 1997, 1239). At that time, the university saw no reason to suppress the results of Dong's research.

In April 1994, Dong and colleagues prepared a manuscript based on the research and submitted it to the *Journal of the American Medical Association (JAMA)* for publication. The editors of *JAMA* were unaware of Dong's previous conflict with the sponsoring pharmaceutical company. After review and revision, *JAMA* accepted the manuscript for publication. In January 1995, *JAMA* received a letter from Dong withdrawing the manuscript from publication because of pending legal action by the pharmaceutical company against Dong, her research colleagues, and the University of California, San Francisco, and because university officials refused to support Dong against this legal action (Rennie 1997). At the time, *JAMA* was preparing to publish Dong's study; the article was already in proof stage. The editors of *JAMA* complied with Dong's request and did not publish the article. Subsequently, a group of investigators employed by the pharmaceutical company (Mayor, Orlando, and Kurtz 1995) reanalyzed the data from Dong's study and reached a conclusion that opposed that of Dong and colleagues (i.e., that the generic preparation was therapeutically nonequivalent to the company's top-selling drug). Mayor, Orlando, and Kurtz (1995) published this reanalysis, without acknowledging the work of Dong and colleagues (who conducted the study and collected the data), in the *American Journal of Therapeutics,* a new journal of which Mayor was an associate editor (Rennie 1997).

After news of this leaked to the newspapers (King 1996), resulting in negative publicity for the pharmaceutical company, the company agreed to allow Dong to publish her article, but this was seven years after Dong had conducted the research. *JAMA* published the article in April 1997 (Dong et al. 1997) with an accompanying editorial by Drummond Rennie summarizing the entire affair.

In the editorial, Rennie (1997, 1241) offered the following advice for researchers and faculty: "Even if researchers have been approached by sponsors, investigators should not assume that the sponsors will encourage publication of unfavorable results and should never allow sponsors veto power." Researchers should carefully evaluate any sponsorship or funding agreements before signing them, and they should not sign agreements that allow sponsors to suppress publication of the results of the sponsored research.

In an attempt to quantify the extent of this particular aspect of conflict of interest, Blumenthal et al. (1997) surveyed 2,100 life-science faculty and found that 20% (410) of these faculty reported delaying the publication of their research results for more than six months. Of these 410 respondents, 28% (114) reported that the delay was intended to slow the dissemination of undesired research results. Thus, 5% of these life-science researchers admitted to intentionally withholding results because the data did not produce desired results.

In this study, Blumenthal and colleagues (1997) identified specific conflicts of interest that caused faculty to delay publication. These included allowing time for patent application (46%), protecting the proprietary or financial value of the results by means other than patent application (33%), protecting the investigator's scientific lead (31%), allowing time for license agreement (26%), and resolving disputes over ownership of intellectual property (17%). Of the faculty who reported delaying publication, 27% reported that they were involved in an academic-industry research relationship and 31% reported that they were involved in some form of commercialization of the results of their research (e.g., patents, trade secrets, regulatory review of product, marketing of product, or starting of a new company).

Recognizing the profit-motivated interests of commercial sponsors of research and the interests of investigators who desire to publish the results of their research (although, for some, not until after securing their scientific lead and potential for financial reward for themselves or their institutions), the AFCR included recommendations in its 1990 guideline on conflict of interest to address the restrictive and suppressive influences on scientific publication: "If an investigator makes an observation about a product or a potential product, these observations, whether positive or negative, should be published in a timely manner. This guideline should not preclude the normal and customary delay in reporting required to allow the sponsoring company to file for patent rights" (AFCR 1990, 240). Other guidelines on conflicts of interest in biomedical research that specifically address restrictions on publication or delays in the dissemination of research include those proposed by the American College of Cardiology, the Royal College of Physicians, the American Psychological Association, the U.S. Public Health Service, and the International Committee of Medical Journal Editors (ICMJE) (Huth 1996; ICMJE 1998).

Biomedical Journal Policies

Biomedical journals have developed specific policies to guide investigators, when they become authors, about financial interests and research funding. In 1984, the *New England Journal of Medicine* announced to authors that the journal would "routinely acknowledge in a footnote *all* funding sources supporting their submitted work," including "relevant direct business associations . . . by a corporation that has a financial interest in the work being reported." Arnold S. Relman, then editor of the *New England Journal of Medicine,* considered other types of financial interests, "such as part-time service as a consultant, ownership of stock or other equity interest, or patent-licensing arrangements," to be more complicated and, thus, required consideration of the need for disclosure to the readers on an individual basis (Relman 1984, 1183). To allow for individual consideration of financial conflicts of interest by the editors, the journal asked authors to volunteer such information in a cover letter submitted with the manuscript. The manuscript would be sent for peer review without including such information, so as not to bias the review process, and if the manuscript was accepted, the editors would decide how much, if any, of the disclosed information needed to be published in the article. The editors emphasized the importance of such disclosure being voluntary, with final responsibility resting with the author.

In 1985, *JAMA* instituted a similar policy for its authors (Knoll and Lundberg 1985; Southgate 1987). In 1988, the ICMJE, with members representing both the *New England Journal of Medicine* and *JAMA,* as well as editors of other major general medical journals published in North America, Europe, Australia, and New Zealand, adopted a statement encouraging, but not requiring, authors to acknowledge financial interests that "may pose a conflict of interest" (ICMJE 1988, 260).

In 1989, recognizing that inadequate education of investigators and authors and lack of formal policies at many journals resulted in confusion for authors and allowed some intentionally to deceive, *JAMA* began requesting authors to sign a statement of financial disclosure (along with a statement of authorship responsibility and transfer of copyright) when submitting manuscripts for publication and requiring them to do so before publication (Lundberg and Flanagin 1989). Since the late 1980s, *Annals of Internal Medicine* also has included a statement requiring disclosure of financial conflicts of interest in its Authors' Form (1998) that all authors must sign. These policies continue to leave the responsibility of disclosure with the author, but they also assist the author by providing a simple mechanism for self-monitoring and disclosure. These journals publish authors' relevant financial interests in articles (in the information about author affiliation, which usually appears at the bottom of the first page; in the acknowledgment, which usually appears at the end of the article; or in the methods section of research articles).

After a survey of members of the Council of Biology Editors (CBE) on ethics and policy in scientific publication, the Editorial Policy Committee of CBE organized a conference, with support from NSF, in 1988 (CBE 1990). Conflicts of interest was one of the topics of the conference. The committee determined that conflicts of interest were causing problems for authors, editors, and journals, and it recommended the following:

> The best tool to be used to prevent questions of bias due to authors' financial affiliations is disclosure by authors to editors and, when appropriate, disclosure by editors to reviewers and readers. At the time of initial submission of a manuscript, authors should provide editors with adequate information regarding their commercial or financial ties to products and regarding financial support of the work presented.
>
> Journals should include in their information for authors a requirement for statements from authors citing all sources of support for the research reported and possible conflicts of interest. Publishing such a statement moves responsibility from a journal to the authors. (CBE 1990, 35)

A subsequent survey of 735 medical journals conducted during 1994 and 1995, with a 57% response rate, demonstrated that 34% of responding journals had written policies regarding conflicts of interest (Glass and Schneiderman 1997). Most of these policies involved a requirement of authors to disclose financial interests. In this study, higher-circulation journals based in the United States were more likely to have such policies than were lower-circulation journals and journals based outside the United States. In the early 1990s, after reports of increasing numbers of scientific investigators holding financial interests in companies with stakes in cutting-edge science (e.g., molecular biology, genetics, neuroscience), the leading basic-science journals (e.g., *Science*) began to consider adopting similar policies (Koshland 1992). But at that time, the majority of science journals did not have formal policies on conflict of interest to guide authors and editors (Barinaga 1992).

A journal's policy of disclosure does not allege wrongdoing or conclude that a conflict of interest necessarily results in the loss of objectivity. Rather, it encourages honesty and truthfulness, both of which are essential for the progress of science and public trust in the scientific enterprise. According to Friedman (1992, 246), "Disclosure is the key method of managing conflicts of interest, by inhibiting deliberate improprieties and alerting others to the risk of bias, but it does not and cannot remove a conflict." Shortly after the initial editorial policies on conflict of interest for authors were announced, the major general medical journals instituted similar policies for peer reviewers, editorial board members, and editors.

Kenneth J. Rothman (1991, 1993), editor of the journal *Epidemiology*, has expressed opposition to editorial policies requiring authors to disclose conflicts of interest. According to Rothman, such policies presume wrongdoing on the part of the author. Rothman (1993, 2782) argued that rules requiring authors to disclose conflicts of interest "thwart the principle that a work should be judged solely on its merits. By emphasizing credentials, these policies foster an ad hominem approach to evaluating science." Rothman has equated policies on conflict of interest of biomedical journals with editorial McCarthyism and censorship.

The editors of *Nature* have labeled such policies "financial 'correctness.'" In an editorial defending its policy of not requiring authors to disclose financial affiliations, *Nature* declared, "It would be reasonable to assume, nowadays, that virtually every good paper with a conceivable biotechnological relevance emerging from the west and east coasts of the United States, as well as many European laboratories, has at least one author with a financial interest—but what of it? The measurements and conclusions are in principle unaffected, as is the requirement that uncertainties be made clear." Perhaps naïvely or perhaps reflecting the lack of governmental and academic regulations concerning conflicts of interest among basic scientists in the United Kingdom at the time, the editors of *Nature* proclaimed in the same editorial, "This journal will persist in its stubborn belief that research as we publish it is indeed research, not business" (Avoid financial "correctness" 1997, 469).

Most journals do not ban publication of articles because of the financial interests of authors. However, in 1990 the *New England Journal of Medicine* changed its initial policy to one that prohibits editorialists and authors of review articles (including book reviews) who have financial interests in a product discussed in the editorial or review from publishing in the journal (Relman 1990). This policy does not apply to authors of scientific reports that present original data; in these cases, the editors reason that disclosure is sufficient. However, the editors of the *New England Journal of Medicine* believe that authors of editorials and reviews, which are not based on self-contained data, cannot provide an objective and disinterested evaluation or opinion. In 1994, the editors extended the policy further to authors of cost-effectiveness analyses, declining to consider such reports if any of the authors has a personal financial interest in the subject of the analysis (Kassirer and Angell 1994).

Rothman (1993) argued that such policies result in scientific censorship. For example, in 1995, the American Lung Association and American Thoracic Society announced that their journals, the *American Journal of Respiratory and Critical Care Medicine* and the *American Journal of Respiratory Cell and Molecular Biology,* would no longer publish articles funded by the tobacco industry. The ethicist Arthur L. Caplan (1995, 273) praised the journals' ban, stating that "any organization committed to the goal of preventing respiratory illness and disability and to working with government agencies who seek to do everything in their power to reduce the use of tobacco products among children and adults cannot remain credible if it permits research sponsored by the tobacco industry in its publications." Another ethicist, H. Tristram Engelhardt Jr. (1995), countered that a ban against research funded by the tobacco industry could harm the basic foundation of scientific freedom. Citing the "slippery slope" argument, Engelhardt (1995, 271) questioned why, if receiving tobacco money is unacceptable, it would be "acceptable to take governmental money if acquired through unjust taxation policies or to publish articles that contradict specific health-related policies" of the journals' owners. In an editorial urging a reversal of this policy, John Roberts and Richard Smith (1996, 134) of the *British Medical Journal (BMJ)* wrote: "The ban of tobacco funded research by the two American journals turns two respected scientific journals into publications with political agendas. In the end, this will make them little more than house organs for one group. And no matter how praiseworthy the goals of that group, it and its publications will be diminished."

A concern regarding policies prohibiting publication because of financial interest is that authors may feel justified in purposefully hiding financial interests and denying or minimizing potential conflicts (Flanagin and Rennie 1995). Another more common concern is that authors may misinterpret the meaning of disclosure and disqualifying policies. For example, if an author had a relevant financial interest last year or ten years ago, should that information be disclosed or should that disqualify the author from writing an editorial for a journal that bans editorialists with financial interests?

In 1997, the editors of the *New England Journal of Medicine* and two authors of an editorial found themselves in public arguments over the authors' apparent financial interests and the journal's decision to publish their editorial without disclosing these interests (Pham 1996; Angell and Kassirer 1996; Manson and Faich 1996a). The authors, JoAnn Manson and Gerald Faich (1996b), experts in endocrinology, pharmacology, and epidemiology, were invited by the editors of the *New England Journal of Medicine* to write an editorial to accompany an article that described a case-control study showing that appetite-suppressant drugs, such as dexfenfluramine, were associated with a risk of pulmonary hypertension (Abenhaim et al. 1996). The editorialists concluded that the risks of dexfenfluramine seemed to be outweighed by its benefits (Manson and Faich 1996b).

In the letter inviting the authors to write the editorial, the editors of the *New England Journal of Medicine* included a statement of their standard policy: "Because editorials involve interpretation and opinion, we ask that authors not have ongoing financial associations (including equity interest, regular consultancies, or major research support) with a company that produces a product (or its competitor) discussed in the editorial" (Angell and Kassirer 1996, 1056). Apparently, the authors and editors had different interpretations of the words *ongoing* and *regular* (Pham 1996; Angell and Kassirer 1996, 1056). Both authors had served as consultants to pharmaceutical companies that manufactured or marketed dexfenfluramine. The authors interpreted their consultancies as neither "ongoing" nor "regular" and believed that the opinions expressed in their editorial were "entirely independent" and not influenced by industry or the financial compensation they had received (Manson and Faich 1996a, 1064–65).

After news reports and allegations that Manson and Faich had failed to disclose their financial interests and that either the authors had violated the journal's conflict-of-interest policy or the journal had failed to enforce its policy properly, the editors of the journal published an editorial "to set the record straight" (Angell and Kassirer 1996, 1055; Pham 1996). The editors wrote that they "did not appreciate until it was too late . . . that Dr. Manson and Dr. Faich had both been paid consultants for companies that stood to gain from the sale of one of the antiobesity agents studied" (Angell and Kassirer 1996, 1055). The editors explained that Manson's consultancy "was in a gray area not explicitly covered by the language of our policy and therefore required further discussion. Dr. Faich's connection, however, was in no such gray area, and if we had known the facts of his consultancy we would not have permitted him to coauthor an editorial on the subject" (Angell and Kassirer 1996, 1056). The editors defended the *New England Journal of Medicine*'s policy and revised it slightly to make it more explicit: "Because editorials involve interpretation and opinion, we require that authors be free of financial associations (including equity interest, consultancies, or major research support) with a company that stands to gain from the use of a product (or its competitor) discussed in the editorial" (Angell and Kassirer 1996, 1056). The journal has always included the following: "If there are any questions about this policy, please phone us" (Angell and Kassirer 1996, 1056). In its revised policy, the journal added a requirement for authors of editorials to attest, in writing, that they have no financial associations (Angell and Kassirer 1996). Other medical journals (e.g., *Annals of Internal Medicine* and *JAMA*) have required authors to identify, in writing, their financial interests or indicate that they have had no relevant financial interests since the mid-1980s.

In an editorial criticizing the *New England Journal of Medicine*'s policy, Stephen J. Welch, the managing editor of *Chest,* concluded that such policies "set very dangerous precedents and are outright censorship. They assume that potential conflict equates to actual conflict. . . . Journals and organizations that refuse to consider papers because of *potential* conflicts of interest are sending a message that they do not trust certain authors, they do not trust their peer review system to make sound judgments about those papers, and they do not trust the readers to make judgments for themselves" (Welch 1997, 867).

The *New England Journal of Medicine* has received criticism for failing to enforce its policy effectively and failing to publish relevant financial interests of authors of editorials, drug reviews, and a book review (Politics of disclosure 1996; Horton 1997; Monmaney 1999; Tye 1998). In light of such criticism and studies demonstrating that financial interests can influence publication (Rochon et al. 1994; Barnes and Bero 1998), the *BMJ* modified its policy in 1998 (Smith 1998). In 1994, the *BMJ* had begun requesting authors to sign forms declaring conflicts of interest, but authors did not always volunteer their relevant conflicts. Explaining that the *BMJ* focuses on disclosure of conflict of interest rather than prohibition, editor Richard Smith (1998, 292) described the *BMJ*'s policy:

> We simply don't think prohibition is feasible, although we try to avoid having an editorial written by somebody with a major conflict of interest. We send authors of all original papers, editorials, and review articles and of selected letters a form in which we define what we mean by conflict of interest and ask them to sign to say whether they have one. . . . Competing interests will be disclosed [to the readers], and if authors tell us they have none (the usual case) we will write "none declared."

With this modification, the *BMJ* replaced the term *conflict of interest* with the term *competing interests,* hoping to dissociate disclosure from the sense of wrongdoing and to encourage authors freely to disclose these interests. The *BMJ* also changed its policy to focus on financial interests. Smith explained this decision: "Narrowing the range may make it more likely that authors will declare competing interests. If authors want to disclose other competing interests then we will disclose them to readers" (Smith 1998, 292).

Guidelines for Authors

Whether a journal's policy on conflicts of interest requests or requires disclosure or is restrictive and prohibits authors with financial interests from publication and whether the policy focuses on financial interests or addresses nonfinancial interests as well, the policy should be clearly communicated to all prospective authors. Authors should be able easily to locate a copy of such polices in journals' instructions for authors, which should be indexed, published in print at least once a year, and included on the journal's Web site (if available). Authors should read such policies carefully and contact a journal's editorial office if they have any questions about the policy, specific terms within the policy, or the policy's applicability to any financial interests. Journals should remind authors of their policies by describing them in manuscript solicitation and acceptance letters.

The *Lancet* provides authors the following advice: "The right to comment freely must be qualified by a duty to declare your interests" (Anything to declare 1993, 728). In an editorial continuing support for disclosure in light of author-editor misunderstandings of the meaning of disclosure, the *Lancet* concluded: "We rely on the conscience and judgment of the author to draw our attention to such a personal conflict. In the end, this must be the person with whom the responsibility lies." The *Lancet* also follows a simple test, which could be used by both editors and authors: "Would a non-disclosed commercial interest, should it be revealed later, prove embarrassing to an author?" (Politics of disclosure 1996, 627).

The ICMJE offers the following guidance for authors, which includes specific advice about commercially sponsored research agreements:

> Scientists have an ethical obligation to submit creditable research results for publication. Moreover, as the persons directly responsible for their work, scientists should not enter into agreements that interfere with their control over the decision to publish the papers they write.
>
> When they submit a manuscript, whether an article or a letter, authors are responsible for recognizing and disclosing financial and other conflicts of interest that might bias their work. They should acknowledge in the manuscript all financial support for their work and other financial or personal connections to the work. (ICMJE 1998, 615)

Guidelines for Peer Reviewers

Many journals request peer reviewers to identify the existence of a conflict of interest (financial or otherwise) when asked to review a manuscript submitted for publication. Some journals request reviewers who believe they have a conflict of interest with the subject of the manuscript to decline to review the paper. Other journals recognize that in some instances a reviewer with a conflict of interest is best suited to review the paper, if the reviewer believes that an objective review can be offered and always provided that the reviewer discloses the conflict to the editor (Rennie, Flanagin, and Glass 1991). Reviewers with a potential conflict of interest who are uncertain of a journal's policy should contact the editorial office before conducting the review. As part of the privileged nature of the current peer-review process, a reviewer's disclosure of a conflict of interest to the editorial office should remain confidential (Iverson, Flanagin, and Fontanarosa 1998).

In 1993, the ICMJE revised its conflict-of-interest statement to include conflicts of peer reviewers:

External peer reviewers should disclose to editors any conflicts of interest that could bias their opinions of the manuscript and they should disqualify themselves from reviewing specific manuscripts if they believe it appropriate. The editors must be made aware of reviewers' conflicts of interest to interpret the reviews and judge for themselves whether the reviewer should be disqualified. Reviewers should not use knowledge of the work, before its publication, to further their own interests. (ICMJE 1993, 743)

Guidelines for Editors

With regard to editors and editorial staff, the following recommendations from the ICMJE (1998, 615–16) are useful:

Editors who make final decisions about manuscripts should have no personal financial involvement in any of the issues they might judge. Other members of the editorial staff, if they participate in editorial decisions, should provide editors with a current description of their financial interests, as they might relate to editorial judgements, and disqualify themselves from any decisions where they have a conflict of interest. Published articles and letters should include a description of all financial support and any conflict of interest that, in the editors' judgement, readers should know about. Editorial staff should not use for private gain the information gained through working with manuscripts.

Editors should require authors to describe the role of outside sources of project support, if any, in study design; in the collection, analysis and interpretation of data; and in the writing of the report. If the supporting source had no such involvement, the authors should so state. Because the biases potentially introduced by the direct involvement of supporting agencies in research are analogous to methodological biases of other sorts (e.g., study design, statistical and psychological factors), the type and degree of involvement of the supporting agency should be described in the Methods section. Editors should also require disclosure of whether or not the supporting agency controlled or influenced the decision to submit the final manuscript for publication.

Journals with disclosure policies should also have a policy defining action in the event that an individual fails to declare a relevant financial interest (Iverson, Flanagin, and Fontanarosa 1998; Smith 1998). Failure to declare financial interests has caused problems for authors and editors (Angell and Kassirer 1996; Manson and Faich 1996a; Correction 1990). When such failure is discovered after the publication of an article, a journal may publish an editorial or notice of the author's failure to disclose. In such cases, an author's failure to communicate a financial interest in the subject of the article is often brought to the editor's attention by readers or news reporters. The *American Medical Association Manual of Style* (Iverson, Flanagin, and Fontanarosa 1998) recommends that editors ask such authors for a written explanation of their failure to disclose financial conflicts of interest and, if appropriate, publish the explanation in the correspondence column. In the event that an author's financial disclosure is not published because of editorial or production error, the journal should publish a formal correction and explanation.

Conclusions: What Do We Really Know?

Biomedical science has become a commercial enterprise fueled by economic interests, yet financial conflicts of interest in scientific publication continue to be the subject of debate (Bero 1998). Studies have demonstrated the effects of authors' financial interests on publication quality and outcome (Rochon et al. 1994; Krimsky et al. 1996; Blumenthal et al. 1997; Barnes and Bero 1998; Stelfox et al. 1998). Other studies have documented that reports of commercially funded clinical trials with negative results are less likely to be published than are reports with positive results (Davidson 1986; Dickersin, Min, and Meinert 1992). Reports of sponsoring companies suppressing publication of negative trials are disturbing reminders of the power of commercial financial interests (Rennie 1997; King 1996; O'Hara 1998). In addition, some authors continue to fail to disclose financial interests even to journals with policies requiring such disclosure. Finally, disagreement and complacency among editors of biomedical journals; a lack of universally accepted uniform policies governing disclosure, disqualification, and divestment in biomedical publication; and confusion over the definitions of *interest* and *conflict* continue to plague the scientific community.

After nearly two decades of confusion, however, the discourse of conflict of interest is showing signs of enlightenment. Unlike their predecessors, today's faculty, students, researchers, authors, and journal editors can rely on government-, institution-, professional society-, and journal-based policies that define conflicts of interests (financial and otherwise) and provide guidance on divestiture, disclosure, and disqualification. These policies acknowledge that all individuals have multiple, secondary, self-directed interests that may conflict with a primary altruistic interest and that such a conflict can lead to improper judgments or bias. Many of these policies provide ways to monitor and manage conflicts and identify disclosure as the mechanism for balancing integrity and motivation.

References

Abenhaim, L., Y. Moride, F. Brenot, S. Rich, J. Benichou, X. Kurz, T. Higgenbottam, C. Oakley, E. Wouters, M. Aubier, G. Simmoneau, and B. Begaud. 1996. Appetite-suppressant drugs and the risk of primary pulmonary hypertension. International Primary Pulmonary Hypertension Study Group. *New England Journal of Medicine* 335:609–16.

Altman, L. K. 1991. Hidden discord over right therapy. *New York Times,* 24 December, B6.

American Federation for Clinical Research (AFCR). 1990. Guidelines for avoiding conflict of interest. *Clinical Research* 38:239–40.

Angell, M., and J. P. Kassirer. 1996. Editorials and conflicts of interest. *New England Journal of Medicine* 335:1055–56.

Anything to declare? 1993. *Lancet* 341:728.

Association of American Medical Colleges (AAMC). 1990. Guidelines for dealing with faculty conflicts of commitment and conflicts of interest in research. *Academic Medicine* 65:488–96. See also http://www.aamc.org/research/dbr/coi.htm. Site accessed 8 November 1998.

Authors' form. 1998. *Annals of Internal Medicine* 128:I-23.

Avoid financial "correctness." 1997. *Nature* 385:469.

Barinaga, M. 1992. Confusion on the cutting edge. *Science* 257:616–19.

Barnes, D. E., and L. A. Bero. 1998. Why review articles on the health effects of passive smoking reach different conclusions. *JAMA* 279:1566–70.

Bero, L. 1998. Disclosure policies for gifts from industry to academic faculty. *JAMA* 279:1031–32.

Blumenthal, D., E. G. Campbell, M. S. Anderson, N. Causino, and K. S. Louis. 1997. Withholding research results in academic life science: Evidence from a national survey of faculty. *JAMA* 277:1224–28.

Booth, W. 1988. Conflict of interest eyed at Harvard. *Science* 242:1497–99.

Caplan, A. L. 1995. Con: The smoking lamp should not be lit in ATS/ALA publications. *American Journal of Respiratory and Critical Care Medicine* 151:273–74.

Correction. 1990. *JAMA* 263:2182.

Council of Biology Editors (CBE), Editorial Policy Committee. 1990. *Ethics and policy in scientific publication.* Bethesda, Md.: Council of Biology Editors.

Curran, W. J. 1991. Scientific and commercial development of human cell lines: Issues of property, ethics, and conflict of interest. *New England Journal of Medicine* 324:998–99.

Davidson, R. A. 1986. Source of funding and outcome of clinical trials. *Journal of General Internal Medicine* 1:155–58.

Dickersin, K., Y.-I. Min, and C. L. Meinert. 1992. Factors influencing publication of research results: Follow-up of applications submitted to two institutional review boards. *JAMA* 267:374–78.

Dong, B. J., W. W. Hauck, J. G. Gambertoglio, L. Gee, J. R. White, J. L. Bubp, and F. S. Greenspan. 1997. Bioequivalence of generic and brand-name levothyroxine products in the treatment of hypothyroidism. *JAMA* 277:1205–13.

Engelhardt, H. T., Jr. 1995. Pro: The search for untainted money. *American Journal of Respiratory and Critical Care Medicine* 151:271–72.

Faculty of Medicine, Harvard University. 1996. Policy on conflicts of interest and commitment. In *Faculty policies on integrity in science*. Boston: Harvard Medical School. See also http://www.hms.harvard.edu/integrity. Site accessed 17 March 1999.

Flanagin, A., and D. Rennie. 1995. Cost-effectiveness analyses. *New England Journal of Medicine* 332:124.

Food and Drug Administration (FDA), Department of Health and Human Services. 1998. Financial disclosure by clinical investigators [Docket No. 93N-0445], 21 CFR part 54. See also http://www.fda.gov. Site accessed 5 March 1999.

Frankel, M. S. 1996. Perception, reality, and the political context of conflict of interest in university-industry relationships. *Academic Medicine* 71:1297–1304.

Friedman, P. J. 1992. The troublesome semantics of conflict of interest. *Ethics & Behavior* 2:245–51.

Glass, R. M., and M. Schneiderman. 1997. A survey of journal conflict of interest policies. Paper presented at the 3d International Congress on Biomedical Peer Review and Global Communications, 18 September, Prague. http://www.ama-assn.org/public/peer/apo.htm. Site accessed 8 November 1998.

Gunsalus, C. K. 1989. Considerations in licensing spin-off technology. *Society of Research Administrators Journal* (summer):13–25.

Horton, R. 1997. Conflicts of interest in clinical research: Opprobrium or obsession? *Lancet* 349:1112–13.

Huth, E. J. 1996. Conflicts of interest in industry-funded clinical research. In *Conflict of interest in clinical practice and research,* ed. R. G. Spece Jr., D. S. Shimm, and A. E. Buchanan, 389–406. New York: Oxford University Press.

International Committee of Medical Journal Editors (ICMJE). 1988. Uniform requirements for manuscripts submitted to biomedical journals. *Annals of Internal Medicine* 108:258–65.

———. 1993. Conflict of interest. *Lancet* 341:742–43.

———. 1998. Statement on project-specific industry support for research. *Canadian Medical Association Journal* 158:615–16. See also http://www.cma.ca/cmaj/vol-158/issue-5/0615e.htm. Site accessed 25 September 1999.

Iverson, C., A. Flanagin, and P. Fontanarosa. 1998. *American Medical Association Manual of Style: A Guide for Authors and Editors.* 9th ed. Baltimore: Williams & Wilkins.

Josefson, D. 1998. FDA rules that researchers will have to disclose financial interest. *BMJ* 316:493.

Kassirer, J. P., and M. Angell. 1994. The journal's policy on cost-effectiveness analyses. *New England Journal of Medicine* 331:669–70.

King, R. T. 1996. Bitter pill: How a drug company paid for university study, then undermined it. *Wall Street Journal*, 25 April, 1, 33.

Knoll, E., and G. D. Lundberg. 1985. New instructions for *JAMA* authors. *JAMA* 254:97–98.

Koshland, D. E., Jr. 1992. Conflict of interest policy. *Science* 257:595.

Krimsky, S., L. S. Rothenberg, P. Stott, and C. Kyle. 1996. Financial interests of authors in scientific journals: A pilot study of 14 publications. *Science and Engineering Ethics* 2:395–410.

Lichter, P. R. 1989. Biomedical research, conflict of interest, and the public trust. *Ophthalmology* 96:575–78.

Lundberg, G. D., and A. Flanagin. 1989. New requirements for authors: Signed statements of authorship responsibility and financial disclosure. *JAMA* 262:2003–4.

Manson, J. E., and G. A. Faich. 1996a. Conflicts of interest: Editorialists respond. *New England Journal of Medicine* 335:1064–65.

——. 1996b. Pharmacotherapy for obesity: Do the benefits outweigh the risks? *New England Journal of Medicine* 335:659–60.

Mayor, G. H., T. Orlando, and N. M. Kurtz. 1995. Limitations of levothyroxine bioequivalence evaluation: Analysis of an attempted study. *American Journal of Therapeutics* 2:417–32.

Merriam-Webster's Collegiate Dictionary. 10th ed. 1994. s.v. "conflict of interest."

Monmaney, T. 1999. Medical journal may have flouted own ethics 8 times. *Los Angeles Times*, 21 October. See also http://latimes.com/news/state/updates/lat_journal991021.htm. Site accessed 21 October 1999.

National Academy of Sciences (NAS), Panel on Scientific Responsibility and the Conduct of Research. 1992. In *Responsible science: Ensuring the integrity of the research process,* 1:72–77. Washington, D.C.: National Academy Press.

National Science Foundation (NSF). 1995. Investigator financial disclosure policy. *Federal Register* 60:35820–23. See also http://frwebgate1.access.gpo.gov/cgi-bin/waisgate.cgi?WAISdocID=7165820026+0+0+0&WAISaction=retrieve. Site accessed 26 March 1999.

Nelkin, D. 1998. Publication and promotion: The performance of science. *Lancet* 352:893.

O'Hara, J. 1998. Whistle-blower: A top researcher says a drug under trial poses a risk to patients. *Maclean's*, 16 November, 64–69.

Oxford English Dictionary (OED). 2d ed. 1989. s.v. "conflict of interest."

Pham, A. 1996. Journal admits conflict: Authors of editorial had links with drug firms. *Boston Globe*, 29 August, C11.

The politics of disclosure. 1996. *Lancet* 348:627.

Public Health Service (PHS), Department of Health and Human Services. 1995. Objectivity in research. *Federal Register* 60:35810–19 (42 CFR part 50 and 45 CFR part 94). See also http://frwebgate3.access.gpo.gov/cgi-bin/waisgate .cgi?WAISdocID=694491288+0+0+0WAISaction=retrieve. Site accessed 26 March 1999.

Relman, A. S. 1984. Dealing with conflicts of interest. *New England Journal of Medicine* 310:1182–83.

———. 1990. New "Information for Authors" and readers. *New England Journal of Medicine* 323:56.

Rennie, D. 1997. Thyroid storm. *JAMA* 277:1238–43.

Rennie, D., A. Flanagin, and R. M. Glass. 1991. Conflicts of interest in the publication of science. *JAMA* 266:266–67.

Roberts, J., and R. Smith. 1996. Publishing research supported by the tobacco industry. *BMJ* 312:133–34.

Rochon, P. A., J. H. Gurwitz, M. Cheung, J. A. Hayes, and T. C. Chalmers. 1994. Evaluating the quality of articles published in journal supplements compared with the quality of those published in the parent journal. *JAMA* 272:108–13.

Rothman, K. J. 1991. The ethics of research sponsorship. *Journal of Clinical Epidemiology* 44(suppl 1):25S–28S.

———. 1993. Conflict of interest: The new McCarthyism in science. *JAMA* 269:2782–84.

Shimm, D. S., and R. G. Spece Jr. 1996. An introduction to conflicts of interest in clinical research. In *Conflicts of interest in clinical practice and research,* ed. R. G. Spece Jr., D. S. Shimm, and A. E. Buchanan, 361–76. New York: Oxford University Press.

Shulman, S. 1988. Conflict of interest over Harvard drug. *Nature* 335:754.

Skolnick, A. A. 1998. SEC going after insider trading based on medical research results. *JAMA* 280:10–11.

Smith, R. 1998. Beyond conflict of interest. *BMJ* 317:291–92.

Soong, H. K., N. F. Martin, M. D. Wagoner, E. Alfonso, S. H. Mandelbaum, P. R. Laibson, R. E. Smith, and I. Udell. 1988. Topical retinoid therapy for squamous metaplasia of various ocular surface disorders: A multicenter, placebo-controlled double-masked study. *Ophthalmology* 95:1442–46.

Southgate, M. T. 1987. Conflict of interest and the peer review process. *JAMA* 258:1375.

Steiner, D. 1996. Competing interests: The need to control conflict of interests in biomedical research. *Science and Engineering Ethics* 2:457–68.

Stelfox, H. T., G. Chua, K. O'Rourke, and A. S. Detsky. 1998. Conflict of interest in the debate over calcium-channel antagonists. *New England Journal of Medicine* 338:101–6.

Tseng, S. C. G., A. E. Maumenee, W. J. Stark, I. H. Maumenee, A. D. Jensen, W. R.

Green, and K. R. Kenyon. 1985. Topical retinoid treatment for various dry-eye disorders. *Ophthalmology* 92:717–27.

Tye, L. 1998. Journal fuels conflict-of-interest debate. *Boston Globe,* 6 January, B1.

U.S. Code. http://www4.law.cornell.edu/uscode. Site accessed 26 March 1999.

U.S. House. 1990. Subcommittee on Human Resources and Intergovernmental Relations of the Committee on Government Operations. *Are scientific misconduct and conflicts of interest hazardous to our health?* 101st Cong., 2d sess., H.R. 101–688. Washington, D.C.: Government Printing Office.

Welch, S. J. 1997. Conflict of interest and financial disclosure: Judge the science, not the author. *Chest* 112:865–67.

Ethics in Cyberspace
The Challenges of Electronic
Scientific Publishing

Faith McLellan

Perhaps the most serious challenge to prevailing notions about the ethics of biomedical publication is the Internet—not just because the scientific community must modify some of its procedures to accommodate to it, but also because it forces us to reformulate our conception of publication. The electronic medium invites examination of conventional standards for publication ethics to determine those that can merely be transferred to this new medium, those that require modification, and those that must be newly created (LaFollette 1997; Lock 1986). The strongest ethical framework must encompass the whole scope of electronic communication in science and medicine, for this is where health and public policy, research ethics, medical ethics, communication ethics, and publication ethics intersect.

Forms of Electronic Communication
Journals

An array of types of biomedical communication exists on the Internet. Peer-reviewed journals come in several varieties: the electronic adjunct to a print journal, whether indexed or nonindexed, which may not include the full text of all articles; hybrid, parallel, or mixed forms (electronic versions of print journals that also contain some electronic-only features and journals that are mainly electronic but also publish, for archival purposes only, a paper version); and journals that exist only online (Taubes 1996b). Other combinations of print and electronic versions, some involving dual modes of publication but separated in time, also exist (Harter and Kim 1996). The *British Medical Journal (BMJ)* has recently begun publishing shorter versions of some papers in the paper journal and a longer version in the electronic journal, a process they call ELPS (electronic long, paper short) (Delamothe, Müllner, and Smith 1999).

The electronic version of a peer-reviewed, indexed journal poses the fewest new problems for publication ethics. Because the articles merely appear in an additional medium, they have been subjected to the traditional reviewing and editing processes. Some journals that have electronic-only sections may modify their peer-review procedures for these articles, but they usually follow an established convention of rapid communication or priority publication based on the novelty or urgency of the findings. Analogous to meeting abstracts or proceedings, these reports must be construed in some sense as preliminary.

Nonjournal Sites

The death of the traditional journal has been proclaimed in several quarters (LaPorte and Hibbitts 1996; Odlyzko 1994), a pronouncement that has led to new forms of research communication. Non-peer-reviewed communication includes original research reports that authors post on their own home pages or others' Web sites, submit to a preprint archive, or contribute to a nonreviewed journal. Databases, informational Web sites, e-mail lists, and discussion groups are examples of other forms. These forms may figure prominently in contemporary biomedical research, clinical practice, and the patient-physician relationship, and they often have ethical ramifications as important as those affecting more familiar types of publication.

Some forms of research communication are ultimately intended for print or electronic journals. The electronic preprint, one such example, was pioneered in the physics community in an archive at Los Alamos National Laboratories as "a means of 'author empowerment'" (Taubes 1996a, 767). Electronic communication has been enthusiastically embraced in physics, in part because high-energy physics already had a "preprint culture" in which researchers mailed copies of papers to large numbers of colleagues simultaneously with submission of the paper to a journal (Taubes 1996a, 767; Ginsparg 1994).

The only form of review envisioned in the Los Alamos e-print archives was one of open commentary. "Any commentary that any legitimate physicist chose to make" (Taubes 1996a, 768) could be attached to the e-print. This very qualification, however, immediately raises questions: What is a "legitimate physicist"? How do we know people online are who they claim to be? Peer review traditionally depends upon those considered experts on the subject written about; thus, just being a physicist, even if identities and affiliations could be verified, might not be sufficient for effective commentary. Further, such a system does not allow the author to revise the article to improve it in light of the review, the hoped-for result of effective reviewing in the traditional system.

Some have argued that stringent peer review is simply not necessary in some disciplines. In medicine, however, there has been great reluctance to give up this entrenched tradition. One of the dividing lines of attitudes toward the electronic medium is clearly whether the data reported are clinical or nonclinical. This concern has been one of the strongest objections made to *E-biomed*, an initiative for electronic publications proposed by Harold Varmus, director of the National Institutes of Health, which is being actively debated as this volume goes to press (Varmus 1999). The proposal currently includes two levels for submission of scientific reports, one of which bypasses conventional peer review. This "general repository" is one aspect of E-biomed that has caused concern in clinical medicine. Research with potentially critical effects on clinical practice and public health may require a different electronic model and a different ethical framework than other kinds of scientific information (Horton 1996; Lundberg 1996).

Paul Ginsparg, the founder of the Los Alamos archive, dismissed the contention frequently made in medicine that peer review is the best method for keeping preliminary or incorrect information out of the literature. He pointed out the consequences of discovering one's preprint work to be flawed: "Posting a preprint to an electronic archive instantly publicizes it to thousands of people, and so the embarrassment over incorrect results and the consequent barrier to distributing material prematurely are, if anything, increased. Such submissions cannot be removed but can only be replaced by a note that the work has been withdrawn as incorrect, leaving a more permanent blemish than a hard copy of limited distribution, which is soon forgotten" (Ginsparg 1994, 394). A plan to experiment with peer review of submissions to the Los Alamos archive included a ban on anonymous reviewing and the institution of a postsubmission scoring system. Allowing one's paper to be scored would, however, be voluntary, and comments would first be screened by the authors to avoid "flame wars" (Taubes 1994a, 967), those heated, sometimes uncontrolled online arguments.

Given the review and comment practices of some electronic journals, it is difficult to know how an author could ever achieve a final version of an article. The review process for an article submitted to *Behavioral and Brain Sciences,* for example, begins with about five referees from at least three different disciplines. If the article passes their review, it is then sent to up to

100 other people for further critique before being posted with up to 30 commentaries, to which the author responds (Stix 1994; Harnad 1995). Although readers of the journal are apparently used to this system, the model may not be applicable to other fields. Some authors and readers might feel overwhelmed by opinions.

Postpublication scoring systems, also proposed for biomedical articles, have been criticized as mere popularity contests (Pitkin 1995), with the frequency of online "hits" no more than an "appeal to the lowest common denominator" (Gellert 1995, 507) that is unlikely to provide reliable information about real use of the site (Cowie 1995). One suggestion has been a "'social recommender' system," in which readers' ratings of papers would be weighed based upon whether the searcher considers the reader a peer whose judgment is close to the searcher's own (Varian 1997). More substantive ways to assess electronic documents have been developed and are discussed below.

Depositing preprint data into an archive is not the only way researchers are exchanging information on the Internet. Two innovative forms that come from clinical medicine also undergo peer review or other forms of filtering and take advantage of the same interactive functions often touted for less formal sites. These Web sites involve large clinical trials, both peer-reviewed reports of finished trials and data collection for ongoing trials. The Cochrane Collaboration, for example, has proposed electronic publication of lengthy adjuncts to print reports of clinical trials (Chalmers and Haynes 1994). Print reports necessarily include extensive evaluation of previously published data. The electronic adjuncts, which lend themselves to frequent updating, are systematic reviews of all trials related to the one being reported in a print journal. As new trials are reported, the electronic document can be revised and updated to incorporate the additional data. Readers who consult the online database can also append comments to the systematic reviews. As evidence-based medicine increases in importance, electronic databases of synthesized knowledge will become even more critical to clinical practice (Anderson et al. 1996).

The ability to post articles of substantial length online is not limited to systematic reviews. Because space is not a primary consideration, as it is in print publications, much more data can be included in articles, a development that may reduce error and fraud (Heller 1995). Other items impossibly large for print journals, such as complete genome maps, can be posted electronically (Bloom 1995). Electronic forms may also permit the publication of more innovative studies than might appear in traditional journals and of more negative studies, thus reducing a bias against the writing up and submission (bias created by researchers) or publication (bias created by reviewers and editors) of negative results (Dickersin et al. 1987; Easterbrook et al. 1991; Chalmers, Frank, and Reitman 1990; Dickersin, Min, and Meinert 1992).

The Internet is also being explored as a vehicle for multisite data collection (Subramanian, McAfee, and Getzinger 1997) and for conducting randomized controlled trials. One experiment is the prototype Internet Trials Service, based at the University of Leeds, in conjunction with the Growth Restriction Intervention Trial, in which early delivery of growth-restricted babies to prevent damage from intrauterine hypoxia is being compared with delayed delivery (Lilford 1994). A Web site describes the trial and provides a mechanism for research groups to become trial centers. The trial coordinator, after verifying the identify and qualifications of the group, registers the center and issues identity codes and passwords, which the centers then use to enter patient data into the database (Kelly and Oldham 1996). Confidentiality, authentication, and security of the data are only some of the ethical and technical issues that must be worked out. However, the Internet can greatly enhance access, which will increase the sample sizes of randomized controlled trials to achieve statistically significant results more quickly and efficiently than is possible through conventional methods.

Case reports are ubiquitous on e-mail lists and discussion groups. Cases that would not appear in formal publications, combined with other anecdotal reports, are producing a unique contribution to the literature of some specialties. In the anesthesia community, a form of cross-pollination is occurring, in which two peer-reviewed journals plan to publish "selected case reports and topic threads" from electronic e-mail lists (A. J. Wright, personal communication, 1996). Some academic medical departments also compile cases from their practice for posting on their Web sites, in readily searchable formats, as a resource for clinicians (Susan Eastwood, personal communication, 1998).

Issues
Anonymity, Confidentiality, Privacy, and Patient Concerns

The Internet partakes of well-documented assumptions about anonymity, identity, and self-representation (Turkle 1995). Electronic interaction *feels* anonymous, your presence is not obvious, and usually no one can hear what you sound like or see what you look like. Pseudonyms and electronic addresses can also obscure identity. People often feel that they are talking to a small group of their peers online when, in fact, a whole host of other participants may be lurking. This is obviously less true of moderated lists or those that require subscribers to meet certain criteria, but even within a closed group, members may copy and disseminate portions of discussions to others not on the list, and subscribers may write about or use the exchanges in ways that are unknown to other participants. Conventions for the use of online postings are not yet firmly established; therefore, ethical use of such materials is largely in the hands of individual consciences.

The confidentiality of sensitive information is at particular risk online. Information that could easily compromise confidentiality can be contained in multimedia, some features of which are only beginning to be exploited in electronic journals. Before these additions become ubiquitous, especially in the clinical literature, we need to consider what kinds of ethical standards must be in place to deal with them. Video of interventional procedures or video or audio of interviews with patients, for example, may require modification of existing standards of consent to publication. Further, the process of a patient's consent to publication in an electronic forum may involve different assumptions and psychological factors than consent to traditional publication. Patients who would consent to having their photographs or other identifying information published in a print journal may feel differently about publication in an electronic journal. Computer-literate patients may be especially enthusiastic or especially reluctant to permit such reports. Conversely, patients who are not familiar with the Internet may not be able to give real consent to electronic publication, and thus the possibilities for exploitation increase.

Some of the ethical issues that arise in other, nonjournal discussions of clinical cases involve potential breaches of confidentiality and privacy, as well as the critical question of how to evaluate the interchanges. One widely known case in which the Internet was used to solve a clinical dilemma gave many identifying details about the patient, including her name, blood type, occupation, and hobbies (Sharma 1995). Students at Peking University who were friends of Zhu Ling, a 21-year-old university student, posted an urgent e-mail message that was widely disseminated to medicine and science newsgroups on the Internet (Li, Aldis, and Valentino 1996). Zhu was acutely ill with an undiagnosed condition, and her friends asked anyone who knew of similar cases or what the diagnosis might be to contact them. The description of her illness elicited a diagnosis, e-mailed on the same day the message was posted, of thallium poisoning. The diagnosis was confirmed in China approximately two weeks after the posting, a period in which some 84 e-mail correspondents from around the world suggested the same diagnosis. Interestingly, the chair of the Neurology Department at Peking had made the correct diagnosis two days after Zhu was hospitalized but had been rebuffed by local toxicologists.

Exactly what those who posted the case did with the diagnostic and therapeutic information they received is not entirely clear. There is evidence from the recounting of the story that telemedicine practiced in this way (filtered through nonprofessionals) was confusing and time-consuming. The liability to which the patients' physicians might have exposed themselves by acting on advice from these sources is also an open question. After the diagnosis was made, Zhu's mother posted a message in which she thanked the many people who had helped her daughter, and neither she nor anyone else mentioned any misgivings about the identifying details given over the Internet. Nor was there discussion about how to assess the advice given by strangers whose qualifications were apparently accepted at face value (though there were requests for "informed suggestions" and a warning that photographs of Zhu were meant "only for doctors"). Those concerned with her case were so desperate that these considerations may have been clearly secondary to the clinical issues. Still, alongside the responsibility for accurate diagnosis lies the burden of an ethical patient-physician relationship, a balancing of interests that led one writer to declare, "Hippocrates should also be in cyberspace" (Sharma 1995, 250).

Breaches of confidentiality and invasions of patients' privacy that occur on the Internet are even more serious than those in nonelectronic environments because of the vastly larger audience and the speed at which such information can be disseminated. The best course of action is for participants to adhere to the same—or stricter—standards as those that prevail in print. Patients must not be able to be identified from the information given. Some journals now require the consent of patients for the publication of any report arising out of the patient-physician relationship (Smith 1998). Thus, even if patients described in case reports are thoroughly anonymous, obtaining consent may be the most ethical course of action. Expending the effort necessary to obtain consent may be unrealistic in urgent situations, however, since part of the Internet's appeal is its speed of interaction. Further, it is unclear whether truly informed consent is possible in this medium, given its evolving nature and incompletely known consequences.

Patients are getting medical information directly from databases and other online sources, instead of having it filtered through their physicians; physicians are using the technology to communicate with their patients; and patients are certainly using it to talk to each other, with mixed results (McLellan 1998). Information obtained in these ways may "empower a public with increasing medical savvy to make more of its own medical choices" (Kassirer 1995b, 1100). One example of such a choice came to light in a discussion group for people with amyotrophic lateral sclerosis. Anecdotal experience reported there resulted in the U.S. Food and Drug Administration being pressured to authorize an experimental treatment that had not been shown to be efficacious (Bulkeley 1995).

Administrators of a molecular genetics network have developed a system for dealing with patients' requests for information. The messages are reviewed for relevance to the network's topic and then transmitted without the patient's address to the network members for responses, which are screened for accuracy before being sent back to the requestor. When the responses contain potentially devastating information, the network administrators attempt to contact the patient and "try to deliver the information through his or her physician" (Gambacorti-Passerini, Ott, and Bergen 1995, 1573). Exactly how this is accomplished is not specified, and the potential risk incurred by the administrators is unknown.

Some medical centers and managed care organizations are using the medium to provide information to patients and link them with health-care providers (Kassirer 1995a; Stevens 1998). The positive consequences of these developments are obvious, but the negatives are sometimes overlooked. Information is useless without the ability to evaluate and apply it, and one can only imagine the potential disparities in the information and quality of care that could be provided to patients in managed-care networks who are and are not electronically connected.

Certain Internet developments may be plagued by concerns about liability, malpractice, and the legal status of the documents. Suppose the video of a novel surgical procedure also gives evidence of surgical error or some other irregularity in the operating suite: What parties are then open to litigation? Suppose a case report would be greatly enhanced by a link to laboratory values in an electronic medical record: What are the boundaries of the consent the patient has given? The electronic medical record itself raises serious ethical concerns, especially about confidentiality, which is often breached by people with a legitimate "need to know" the information accessed (Lundberg 1996). How the information is used and disclosed is critical in determining the legitimacy of access.

Some concerns about the use of electronic information are shaped by specific disciplines and specialties. Psychiatrists have called attention to the special needs for protecting the confidentiality of information about their patients in an increasingly electronic environment (Huang and Alessi 1996). These concerns are heightened by pressures from managed care organizations to change psychiatric practice in a number of ways: (1) the construction of clinical practice guidelines to establish standards of practice that eventually may be distributed through the Internet, with potential legal risks and clinical consequences for the unconnected; (2) the electronic medical record and the use of computer networks for transmission of this information; and (3) computerized screening tools for patients to do preliminary self-evaluation and referral (Huang and Alessi 1996). These developments have the laudable goals of reducing costs and administrative burdens while efficiently providing information to patients and practitioners, yet they must all be designed with a wary eye toward violations of privacy and untoward effects on the patient-physician relationship.

Plagiarism, Attribution, and Citation

The use and respectful appropriation of the work of others is an integral part of the culture of biomedical publication, whether paper-based or electronic. Quotation, citation, and attribution have practical and ethical dimensions. Ethical use of others' work fulfills the traditional principle of respect for persons.

Certain aspects of plagiarism—especially defining it and understanding cultural forces that shape it—are widely understood as problematic. Established definitions of plagiarism usually include several elements: "(1) use of *another's* words, text, ideas, or illustrations; (2) failure to credit the original ('real') author; (3) the implication (or statement), uncontradicted elsewhere in the work, that the plagiarist first wrote these words or had these ideas; and (4) the failure to seek the original author's consent for use, including obscured use" (LaFollette 1994, 27). Different academic communities, however, may interpret these elements differently. Julliard (1994) showed that physicians, including medical editors, had very different notions of what constituted plagiarism than did university English teachers, editors in the humanities, and medical students. A majority of the physicians surveyed believed that no plagiarism had occurred in three variations of a sample, one of which was a 48-word verbatim copy of text that was not enclosed in quotation marks but did include a citation to the source. Apparently, they considered the attribution to be enough acknowledgment of another's work.

The problem of plagiarism becomes even more complex when language skills and other cultural conventions are thrown into the mix. Some Chinese authors, for example, have maintained that poor English skills were the root cause of allegations of plagiarism against them and that copying of verbatim text did not constitute plagiarism because they had not falsified original data, which they produced in their laboratory (Li and Xiong 1996). These instances suggest that the global biomedical community must make better known its own standards for ethical conduct in publication. One practical effort is the translation into Chinese of a pamphlet on conduct in research (Li and Xiong 1996); the Internet is an obvious vehicle for disseminating such standards even more widely.

Electronic communication makes widespread replication and dissemination of others' words and ideas practically effortless, but search and archive functions also make it easier to detect instances of potential plagiarism and repetitive publication. Hypertext makes linking of information possible, but long chains of electronic links also make it easy to get "lost" online, to lose track of one's originating point and thus, perhaps, original sources in a document. As a practical matter, still-developing standards for citing electronic documents may hamper accurate citation. The existence of multiple electronic versions of documents and documents that once had a URL but subsequently disappeared from the Web makes it important for the citation to include a date on which the document was accessed.

A citation analysis of references in articles appearing in electronic, peer-reviewed journals showed that only 1.9% of the citations were to online sources, including Web pages, e-mail messages, electronic journal articles, and newsgroup and mailing-list postings (Harter and Kim 1996), a curiously low percentage, given that the articles containing them were themselves electronic. The format of these citations was frequently inconsistent, incomplete, or erroneous, with the result that more than half of the online sources could not be found. Inaccurate bibliographic citation is not a new problem in scientific publication, but a lack of widely known standards for citation of electronic documents, combined with the constant flux of online sources, exponentially increases the difficulty of accurate electronic citation.

What is the ethical dimension of citation in an electronic environment? If we accept that authors have a moral duty to place their work in the context of related studies, then clearly there are ethical responsibilities of citation. But how are authors to deal with a seemingly endless supply of online documents that may or may not need to be evaluated in light of their own work? Particularly Internet-savvy reviewers may point to electronic documents they believe authors should have consulted, thus placing additional burdens upon researchers simply to locate these sources and upon the designers of search engines, whose job it will be to make such searching more targeted and useful in the first place. Then the question of how to evaluate the documents found becomes critical, especially if the sites are not reviewed.

Peer Review

The development of peer review in biomedicine and a trial adaptation of its procedures for online use have been described in earlier chapters. Problems specific to certain types of electronic documents have been discussed. Whatever models are ultimately implemented for peer review of electronic documents, it would be useful for journals and other sites to have explicit statements of the review procedures they use for their electronic publications. These statements may be necessary even for established journals whose procedures are well known, as some conventions of publication that are evident in traditional forms may not be so obvious in electronic versions. If print journals have physical divisions of peer-reviewed and non-peer-reviewed information, for example, these distinctions may not be so clear online. If reviewers' comments are appended to the articles, reviewers may need to sign their reviews. The anonymity of traditional peer review may have to disappear once persons besides authors and editors become privy to the reviews and these materials are posted in a medium in which anonymity itself is an intrinsic feature. Anonymous review may provide the most insightful and critical feedback for authors, but it may decrease credibility among readers of online articles. Likewise, where the commented-upon article stands relative to the review—whether it is an original or revised version—should be specified through date stamping. This convention already exists in journals that print receipt dates for the original and revised versions of papers they publish.

In short, readers' ability to evaluate electronic publications may require the use of more cues, more specification of the process by which they have been created and modified. And the most effective cues may require that we move beyond print models, where a statement of the journal's procedures is buried in an appendix or a banner at the top of the page categorizes the article, or even beyond a model where the journal provides a hyperlink to this information on its home or table of contents page, to a system of icons attached to each article. These icons could specify the type of document (peer-reviewed report of original research, invited review, news, letter, commentary, etc.) to reinforce the reader's ability to evaluate the content.

Quality

Biomedical Internet sites raise troubling questions about the accuracy and quality of the information posted: How can it be verified? How can readers be assured of the legitimacy of the claims made? Concerns about the quality of electronic information have led to the development of several evaluative tools, some as aids to researchers and some specifically to assist patients seeking medical advice.

One checklist for evaluating Web pages divides them by function and sponsorship and then describes five criteria—authority, accuracy, objectivity, currency, and coverage—for judging their quality and usefulness (table 7.1) (Alexander and Tate 1999). The document containing the checklists could serve as a model for Web publication. The first page contains a short abstract and description of the contents of the document, a citation to the print version, the names and postal and e-mail addresses of the authors, the date on which the document was mounted on the server and the date of its latest revision, and the complete URL of the page being viewed.

Other projects assessing the quality of online resources include the University of Southern California's Infofilter Project, which uses peer-review procedures to evaluate, besides content and authority criteria, the search capabilities of resources (Engstrom 1996). A National Library of Medicine project is developing similar criteria for nonjournal resources, including bibliographies and image and factual databases (Engstrom 1996). Medical Matrix is a project of the American Medical Informatics Association (AMIA) Internet Working Group. Its specific task is to evaluate online resources for clinicians. An editorial board of AMIA members and a large number of other contributors grade Web sites according to the categories listed in table 7.2. What all of these efforts suggest is that a first level of immersion in the biomedical literature of the Internet is access to information. The next level of concern involves, appropriately, shifting the focus to the quality of that information (Frisse 1997).

Table 7.1. Checklist for an Informational Web Page

Criterion 1: AUTHORITY

1. Is it clear who is responsible for the contents of the page?
2. Is there a link to a page describing the purpose of the sponsoring organization?
3. Is there a way of verifying the legitimacy of the page's sponsor? That is, is there a phone number or postal address to contact for more information? (Simply an e-mail address is not enough.)
4. Is it clear who wrote the material, and are the author's qualifications for writing on this topic clearly stated?
5. If the material is protected by copyright, is the name of the copyright holder given?

Criterion 2: ACCURACY

1. Are the sources for any factual information clearly listed so they can be verified in another source?
2. Is the information free of grammatical, spelling, and other typographical errors? (These kinds of errors not only indicate a lack of quality control, but also can actually produce inaccuracies in information.)
3. Is it clear who has the ultimate responsibility for the accuracy of the content of the material?
4. If there are charts or graphs containing statistical data, are they clearly labeled and easy to read?

Criterion 3: OBJECTIVITY

1. Is the information provided as a public service?

2. Is the information free of advertising?
3. If there is any advertising on the page, is it clearly differentiated from the informational content?

Criterion 4: CURRENCY

1. Are there dates on the page to indicate:
   a. When the page was written?
   b. When the page was first placed on the Web?
   c. When the page was last revised?
2. Are there any other indications that the material is kept current?
3. If material is presented in graphs or charts, is it clearly stated when the data were gathered?
4. If the information is published in different editions, is it clearly labeled from which edition the page is derived?

Criterion 5: COVERAGE

1. Is there an indication that the page has been completed and is not still under construction?
2. If there is a print equivalent to the Web page, is there a clear indication of whether the entire work or only parts of it are available on the Web?
3. If the material is from a work that is out of copyright (as is often the case with a dictionary or thesaurus), has there been an effort to update the material to make it more current?

Source: Adapted from the Web site "Evaluating Web Resources" (http://www.widener.edu/ libraries.html, select "Evaluating Web Resources"), which complements the book *Web Wisdom: How to Evaluate and Create Information Quality on the Web,* by Janet E. Alexander and Marsha Ann Tate of Widener University, Chester, Pennsylvania. Published in Mahwah, N.J.: Lawrence Erlbaum Associates, 1999. Reprinted with permission.

Standards have been suggested as guides to assessing Internet medical information (table 7.3); further, the instruments used to assess quality have themselves been scrutinized recently (Jadad and Gagliardi 1998). Several organizations, joining forces as the Health on the Net Foundation, have developed a preliminary set of criteria for medical and health Web sites to serve as an imprimatur of quality (Selby et al. 1996; Boyer et al.

Table 7.2. Medical Matrix Evaluation Categories

Category	Scoring	Assessment
Application	1–20 points	How well does the resource enhance the knowledge of primary care clinicians and specialists at the point of care?
Peer review	1–10 points	How current is the information? Does it appear to be verifiable and authentic? Does it include references? Do endorsements accompany the information, and do visitors know how old it is?
Media	1–5 points	Does the site offer text, hypertext, or multimedia, including images, video, and sound?
Feel	1–5 points	How do the search features, navigation tools, tools for hypertext markup language, composition, and integration within a larger database rate?
Ease of access	1–5 points	Is clinical content highlighted? What are the reliability and speed of the links there? How many bytes are on the page?
Dimension	1–5 points	How large is the site? How much effort does it require? How important is it to the discipline?

Source: From P. Engstrom, "How Quality-Minded Groups Sift through the Rubble for Online Gems," *Medicine on the Net* 2(1996):1–5 (COR Healthcare Resources 805-564-2177). Reprinted with permission.

1998). The impetus for the initiative was "evidence that recently diagnosed patients were seeking medical information and details of potential treatments [from the Internet], recognition that some patients were seeking information while in a state of stress/anxiety, examples of questionable claims for unproven treatments, [and] examples of medical advice being offered by individuals lacking formal medical training and qualifications" (Selby et al. 1996; Boyer et al. 1998, 605).

The result of this multiorganization collaboration was a draft version of the Health on the Net Code of Conduct (HONcode), which embodies eight principles designed to ensure quality information on cooperating Web sites. The principles involve authors' credentials; protection of the patient-physician relationship; confidentiality; references to data sources; claims about treatments, products, and services; contact information; and disclosure of funding and advertising policies. These sites may display an HONcode logo that must be linked to the HONcode home page. The foundation's quality assurance process includes regular searches for sites that bear the HONcode logo but have not registered with the site, review of registered sites, procedures for dealing with sites that violate the principles, and procedures for legal action against trademark and copyright infringement for sites that continue to violate the principles.

Table 7.3. Assessing the Quality of Medical Information on the Internet

Authorship	Authors and contributors named
	Clearly labeled as medical professionals or not
	Affiliations and credentials specified
	Contact information, including Webmaster's e-mail address, given
Attribution	References and sources given
	Any relevant copyright notices specified
Confidentiality	No disclosure of confidential information about individual patients or Web site visitors
	Legal requirements for medical and health information privacy in location of Web site and mirror sites met or exceeded
Currency	Dates of creation of content and of last modification posted
	Links to mirror sites provided
Disclosure	Web site ownership stated, all commercial interests specified, including sponsorship, advertising, underwriting, funding agreements
	Potential conflicts of interest noted
	Advertising differentiated from original site content
Legitimacy	Claims about treatments, products, or services supported by balanced evidence
Purpose	Information provided supports but does not replace patient-physician relationship

Source: Adapted from Silberg, Lundberg, and Musacchio in *JAMA* 277:1244–45, copyrighted 1997, American Medical Association (1997, 1245); Health on the Net Foundation (1997); HONcode 1996–99.

There have been a few studies about patients' use of sites designed for professionals (Widman and Tong 1997) and about the quality of medical advice given in online discussion groups and on Web sites (Culver, Gerr, and Frumkin 1997; Impicciatore et al. 1997). Biomedical journals may have significant roles in the dissemination of information specifically for the public. The American Medical Association (AMA) estimates that more than half the users of its Web site are not medical professionals (Chi-Lum, Lundberg, and Silberg 1996); thus, their site provides "carefully structured access" to other medical information sites that have been subjected to editorial and peer review by professionals and members of the community (Aversa, Silberg, and Wilkes 1996, 121). This procedure is designed to protect readers as well as the reputation of the AMA. The journal also initiated the "*JAMA* Patient Page," a page of noncopyrighted information about various diseases written in lay language and intended for widespread copying and distribution (Glass, Molter, and Hwang 1998). The page appears both in the print journal and on the *JAMA* Web site.

Repetitive Publication

Some journals, such as the *New England Journal of Medicine,* have explicit policies that the posting of a manuscript on the Internet constitutes publication and thus precludes the manuscript's submission to the journal (Kassirer and Angell 1995). Sending the paper "by e-mail to a limited number of colleagues" does not constitute prior publication (Kassirer and Angell 1995, 1709); however, care must be taken in determining the number of recipients and the instructions given to them about what they may do with the material. The policy of the *New England Journal of Medicine* also exends to the posting of abstracts and posters, despite arguments that these constitute "a virtual meeting," presentations from which would normally be exempt from the prior-publication rule (Gardner and Barbarash 1995, 1078). The International Committee of Medical Journal Editors (ICMJE) also considers its statements on prior publication to extend to electronic media (ICMJE 1992).

Other forms of research communication may also be subject to similar policies. Some organizations mandate the release of non-peer-reviewed findings, such as DNA sequence data, directly to Internet databases (Adams and Venter 1996). This practice creates problems when the data are later incorporated into a paper for publication, since the policies of some journals consider the availability of the data to constitute prior publication.

Economics

Economic issues loom large for publishers and editors of electronic journals. The costs of producing and distributing an electronic journal have been shown to be lower than those of print versions; however, this reduction can be offset by a decline in subscriptions (Jog 1995). Marketing an electronic journal may incur greater than normal costs to convince current and potential subscribers that the quality controls of counterpart print journals carry over to electronic versions.

The economics of electronic publication are also affected by advertising, the nature of which may change dramatically online because of the possibilities of hypertext. Should advertisements be linked to the journal's home page? Should those ads be linked to specific content? "Inline" advertising also enables authors' citation of scientific companies' equipment, reagents, and supplies to be linked from the methods section of a paper to the home page of the manufacturer. Is this process potentially unsavory or merely a help to busy researchers trying to replicate the methods? What is the journal's responsibility, if any, for the quality of the sites to which its articles are linked? Does a reader's perception of this practice change if the author is also the principal of the company, as when a development has led to the creation of a commercial spin-off? One way of looking at these issues demonstrates that their substance is not new to biomedical publication; the relationship of science to industry has always been uneasy, as has the separation of editorial from advertising content. But the particular practices in which they are embedded are novel, created in part by the non-linear, nonhierarchical construction of hypertext.

Academic-Industry Relationships

If the future of biomedical research is one of greater competition for fewer sources of public funds, then academic-industry relationships are likely to increase. Such relationships often carry restrictions on scientific communication (Anderson 1994b), which would presumably extend to electronic sources of communication. Restrictions on communication are antithetical to the "traditional openness and sharing among scientists" (Frankel 1996, 1297) but are a particular affront to the open exchange of the Internet. The interchange between academic-industry relationships, intellectual property challenges, and the traditional procedures of scientific publication is complex and sometimes contentious. Adding electronic publication to the mix will doubtless increase the number of problems requiring legal remedies.

Intellectual Property

The status of intellectual property—copyright, patent, and trademark—on the Internet can be summed up by a short quotation in a report on the physics e-print archive: "The situation is very confusing" (Bederson 1994). Case law on the relationship of electronic publication to intellectual property concerns is not yet well developed, and the issues involved are further obscured by the multiplicity of overlapping "cultures" in electronic publication: those of cyberspace, academic disciplines, publishers, and countries.

How much current copyright law, which evolved to meet the needs of print, will have to change to accommodate cyberspace is in debate. Most problematic is the mode by which the Internet distributes information, "copying packets from node to node" (Godwin 1987, 102). Some common features of Internet distribution may be interpreted as violations of existing copyright law, including downloading a copy to a computer's random access memory, creating a link from one Web site to another, and sending a text file by e-mail (Koren-Elkin 1995). Where an "original" document even exists in a networked environment is often unclear. However, the inability of creators to control distribution of their electronic works, a control authorized by copyright, does not seem to have stemmed the flood of Internet communication.

Copyright is governed by federal law in the United States, but the United States is also a party to an international copyright treaty (the Berne Convention, discussed in chap. 8), as are most European countries, Japan, and Canada (Stern and Westenberg 1995), with China a notable exception. The World Intellectual Property Organization (WIPO) created a copyright treaty that is a special agreement to the Berne Convention. This treaty specifies that databases, but not the actual data, constitute an intellectual creation protected by copyright (WIPO 1996), a conclusion that has generated substantial controversy.

Because the Internet is a form of global communication, law in many countries greatly complicates consensus about intellectual property in a digital environment. China, for example, does not have an indigenous intellectual property law, especially with regard to copyright, although it has been under great pressure, from the United States in particular, to formulate such protections (Alford 1995, vii–8).

Rights to Data

For the scientific community, the ability to link articles with raw data and data analysis engines is one of the most exciting and problematic aspects of electronic publication. The development of "collaboratories" (Makulowich 1995, 148), which use MOO (Multiple-user dimension, Object Oriented) technology, allows scientists to work in each other's labs through electronic connection. These innovations raise questions about the use of data in general, as well as about intellectual property and foreign copyright (Stix 1994; Anderson 1994a; Makulowich 1995). Researchers' capacity to have access to the data of other laboratories may lead to quicker confirmation of controversial findings, suggest other interpretations resulting from different types of analysis, and point toward further areas of investigation. These interactions can serve as a kind of postpublication peer review and as a double-check on the validity of the authors' conclusions. All of these potentially positive results emerge from the heightened collaborative, interactive nature of science on the Internet.

Yet there are serious issues to be resolved, including securing the raw data so it cannot be changed. Further, questions about rights to data in an electronic environment quickly become complex. What if researchers re-analyze interpreted data, reach a conclusion different from that of the originators of the data, and then wish to publish it? What if they add to the data set, using work from their own laboratory? What is the meaning of authorship of papers that use primary data generated by others (Adams and Venter 1996; Kassirer 1992)? This type of interaction with data is not entirely unique to the Internet—indeed, in an ideal world it is the way science is done, with an ethos that combines sharing and collaboration with spontaneity and independent discovery—but the ease of access and linkages it provides greatly expand gray areas in ownership of and rights to data. The scientific community and its journals need specific policies that address these questions (Adams and Venter 1996; Kassirer 1992), as do institutions that are reconsidering systems of academic reward and credit.

Digital Images

Digital images have ethical implications, particularly since figures created entirely by computer have no negatives with which to compare subsequent copies, thus tempting unscrupulous researchers to manipulate the images. The easy availability of images in large databases is another potential source of modification and fraud. Images created from conventional negatives may also be digitally enhanced, and some journals have explicit policies about what kinds of manipulation are allowable. Enhancement is usually allowed only for purposes of clarification or correction of incorrect exposures (Richardson, Frank, and Stern 1995) and may not alter the "scientific content" of the image, a change that "constitutes scientific fraud" (Berk 1995, 230). Proposed standards for digital illustration include a stipulation that researchers must create a graphic "audit trail" by maintaining "some archival record of how the graphic was obtained and what has been done to it" (Anderson 1994b, 317). Such a record may eventually be created through technological advancements that store original archived image data or by a "digital 'signature'" or authenticated timestamp (Taubes 1994b, 318). None of these developments is as critical, however, as the integrity of the individual researcher.

The ethical use of digital images extends beyond conventional and electronic journal publishing, encompassing other sites that may contain confidential information. The University of Iowa's Virtual Hospital site (http://vh.radiology.uiowa.edu/), a medical education resource, contains a thoracic imaging teaching file that enables readers to access a variety of radiologic and pathologic images (Gavin et al. 1995). The images have been cropped to remove patient identification data, a key consideration in protecting patients' privacy. The site also contains an extensive disclaimer about accountability for and the accuracy of the information posted.

Information Management

The management of electronic information involves a host of complex tasks, some technical and others with profound implications for the conceptual and theoretical bases of research and publication. Archiving electronic biomedical publications is complicated by the endless revisions made possible by the medium. "One true copy" of an article may be necessary for "patent examination, for judicial decision-making, [and] for scientific debate" (LaFollette 1997). Specific international standards for authenticating and archiving scientific and medical information have been called for (Electronic publishing in science 1996). Effective search tools for all documents on the Web must overcome formidable technical problems in indexing, tagging, and the development of tools for concept searching across databases; current projects are hampered by the necessity for intensive human intervention (Schatz 1997).

Those who extol the virtues of the research paper as an "ever changing story" (LaPorte et al. 1995, 1389) dismiss the virtues of a permanent original record, whatever its eventual flaws. These virtues include "the original vision, quality, integrity, and moment of time captured" in the original document (Gellert 1995, 507). Serious attention to archiving is critical for the construction and maintenance of a record of progress, error, and discovery.

Cultural Considerations

The Internet, despite its open, chaotic, and democratic nature, still divides the haves from the have-nots. Graphical and other tools that depend on increasingly sophisticated technology will continue to separate researchers with fewer resources from those with more assets. Further, as the cost of equipment decreases, the cost of information itself is becoming a greater barrier than the cost of the technology (Zielinski 1995). One position that balances a number of interests is for electronic journals to remain available in plain text or ASCII format, which does not require cutting-edge technology for viewing. Such a format would potentially remove one obstacle to access for some readers, particularly those from developing countries (Hitchcock, Carr, and Hall 1996) and others whose technology may be dated. Ironically, the format would not remove some language barriers if plain-text English articles were also translated into other languages, for "the ASCII character set does not permit the use of accents or other diacritical marks" (Readings 1996).

Governmental, political, and social pressures on the control of information should not be underestimated. Governments and state-owned telecommunications companies may be quite wary of giving citizens access to the open information exchange of the Internet. Some countries, currently including China, Sri Lanka, Malaysia, and Singapore, restrict what may be transmitted electronically, and the question of censorship of the Internet is being energetically debated in the United States, the United Kingdom, and New Zealand (Gimon 1998). Scientific information in an electronic world can be a two-way street. As more researchers are connected around the globe, it is critical to formulate goals beyond getting Western science to the developing world to enable the open exchange of information from all sources (Zielinski 1995).

Changing Roles

In addition to changing our ideas about publication, the Internet changes traditional notions about reading and writing and thus challenges the roles and skills of authors, readers, and editors. The ability to evaluate resources critically takes on greater importance as the explosive growth of the Internet continues. Efforts toward improved search engines and selective filtering of relevant sites based on personal interests and the movement of many scientists away from open online discussion into private groups suggest that ways to organize and evaluate Internet information are critical next steps in the use of this technology. But some scientists worry that attempts to narrow their focus into ever more specific topics will be at the expense of general knowledge and that connections with colleagues around the world, many of whom will never be met face to face, will come at the price of decreased interactions with those down the hall. Thus, the Internet may create "both the global village and the virtual Balkans of scientific collaboration" (Van Alstyne and Brynjolfsson 1996, 1480).

Some aspects of authorship of electronic papers must be solved at an institutional level. Committees that review candidates for promotions and tenure often measure academic success by quantity of publications in quality journals, with quality sometimes measured by the journal's impact factor, a measure of the frequency with which articles from that journal are cited throughout the biomedical literature. Electronic-only journals currently have no such methods of assessment. What will the status of electronic publications be for career development, and how will it be determined? In highly interactive communications, how will credit be assigned (Odlyzko 1994; Winograd and Zare 1995)?

Further, what will count as a real scholarly article in a world of increasingly electronic scholarship? Will value be placed on work that increasingly crosses disciplinary lines, in part simply because more diverse audiences have access to electronic publications than the narrower readerships of specialized print journals? The medium itself, not just the audience, contributes to the expansion, interrelatedness, and open-endedness of electronic publications (Unsworth 1996). Paradoxically, given the range of electronic information, the Internet may also lead to the decline of the general reader (Readings 1996) and place a greater burden of evaluation on readers. Far from becoming obsolete, as everyone with computer access becomes a potential publisher, editors will remain "the primary source for ethical responsibility among professional publications" (Lundberg 1992, 111). Their roles will become even more critical, not only in the evaluation of quality for professional audiences, but also in the education of new readers about the interpretation and application of the information they publish.

Conclusions

Electronic communication, given its mutability of content and form, profoundly calls into question the nature of the scientific knowledge it describes—whether definitive conclusions based on unchanging data are possible. The capacity of electronic biomedical publications to "be updated, revised, expanded, altered, [and] corrected indefinitely" (Shoaf 1993) is both boon and bane. Research findings and clinical reports can become living communication, products of interactive exchange by thinkers around the globe who have been brought together in ways that no other medium has ever before made possible. Developments that have so much power—over lives, careers, policy, and knowledge—deserve our best and deepest ethical reflection to ensure that this technology remains a tool in the service of the scientific community and the public. At the end of the day, the sound and fury of still-emerging forms of biomedical communication in cyberspace ought to signify something quite meaningful indeed.

References

Adams, M. D., and J. C. Venter. 1996. Should non-peer-reviewed raw DNA sequence data release be forced on the scientific community? *Science* 274:534–36.

Alexander, J., and M. Tate. 1999. Evaluating web resources. http://www.science .widener.edu/~withers/inform.htm. Site accessed 23 March 1999.

Alford, W. P. 1995. *To steal a book is an elegant offense: Intellectual property law in Chinese civilization.* Stanford: Stanford University Press.

Anderson, C. 1994a. Cyberspace offers chance to do "virtually" real science. *Science* 264:900–901.

———. 1994b. Easy-to-alter digital images raise fears of tampering. *Science* 263:317–18.

Anderson, M. F., H. Moazamipour, D. L. Hudson, and M. E. Cohen. 1996. The role of the Internet in medical decision making. Presented at the European Congress of the Internet in Medicine, 15 October 1996. http://www.mednet.org.uk/mednet/dl5.htm. Site accessed 23 March 1999.

Aversa, E. S., B. Silberg, and R. Wilkes. 1996. Maintaining editorial quality and integrity online. *CBE Views* 19:121.

Bederson, B. 1994. Report to council on e-print archive workshop. Meeting of the American Physical Society, Los Alamos, 14–15 October 1994. http://www .publish.aps.org/EPRINT/losa.html. Site accessed 7 July 1999.

Berk, R. N. 1995. Policy regarding electronic manipulation of radiologic images. *AJR American Journal of Roentgenology* 164:230.

Bloom, F. E. 1995. Wired or wary? *Science* 269:1323.

Boyer, C., M. Selby, J.-R. Scherrer, and R. D. Appel. 1998. The Health on the Net Code of Conduct for medical and health Websites. *Computers in Biology and Medicine* 28:603–10.

Bulkeley, W. M. 1995. E-mail medicine: Untested treatments, cures find stronghold on on-line services. Doctors fret the gravely ill may share information and skew drug testing. No miracles from Neurontin. *Wall Street Journal,* 27 February, A1, 7.

Chalmers, I., and B. Haynes. 1994. Reporting, updating, and correcting systematic reviews of the effects of health care. *BMJ* 309:862–65.

Chalmers, T. C., C. S. Frank, and D. Reitman. 1990. Minimizing the three stages of publication bias. *JAMA* 263:1392–95.

Chi-Lum, B. I., G. D. Lundberg, and W. M. Silberg. 1996. Physicians accessing the Internet, the PAI project: An educational initiative. *JAMA* 275:1361–62.

Cowie, J. 1995. The death of biomedical journals: Journals are not yet obsolete. *BMJ* 311:507–8.

Culver, J. D., F. Gerr, and H. Frumkin. 1997. Medical information on the Internet: A study of an electronic bulletin board. *Journal of General Internal Medicine* 12:466–70.

Delamothe, T., M. Müllner, and R. Smith. 1999. Pleasing both authors and readers. *BMJ* 318:888–89. See also http://www.bmj.com/cgi/content/full/318/ 7188.888. Site accessed 9 December 1999.

Dickersin, K., S. Chan, T. C. Chalmers, H. S. Sacks, and J. Smith Jr. 1987. Publication bias and clinical trials. *Controlled Clinical Trials* 8:343–53.

Dickersin, K., Y.-I. Min, and C. L. Meinert. 1992. Factors influencing publication of research results: Follow-up of applications submitted to two institutional review boards. *JAMA* 267:374–78.

Easterbrook, P. J., J. A. Berlin, R. Gopalan, and D. R. Matthews. 1991. Publication bias in clinical research. *Lancet* 337:867–72.

Electronic publishing in science. 1996. *European Science Editing* 59:10–11.

Engstrom, P. 1996. How quality-minded groups sift through the rubble for online gems. *Medicine on the Net* 2:1–5.

Frankel, M. S. 1996. Perception, reality, and the political context of conflict of interest in university-industry relationships. *Academic Medicine* 71:1297–1304.

Frisse, M. E. 1997. Re-imagining the medical informatics curriculum. *Academic Medicine* 72:36–41.

Gambacorti-Passerini, C., J. Ott, and A. Bergen. 1995. The human molecular genetics network. *New England Journal of Medicine* 333:1573.

Gardner, J. D., and R. A. Barbarash. 1995. The Internet and the *Journal*. *New England Journal of Medicine* 333:1078.

Gavin, J. R., M. P. D'Alessandro, Y. Kurihara, W. E. Erkonen, T. A. Knutson, and D. L. Lacey. 1995. Distributing an electronic thoracic imaging teaching file using the Internet, Mosaic, and personal computers. *AJR American Journal of Roentgenology* 164:475–78.

Gellert, G. A. 1995. The death of biomedical journals: Electronic journals supplement their paper cousins. *BMJ* 311:507.

Gimon, C. A. 1998. Internet censorship around the world.http://www.skypoint .com/members/gimonca/foreign.html. Site accessed 23 March 1999.

Ginsparg, P. 1994. First steps towards electronic research communication. *Computers in Physics* 8:390–96.

Glass, R. M., J. Molter, and M. Y. Hwang. 1998. Providing a tool for physicians to educate patients: The *JAMA* patient page. *JAMA* 279:1309.

Godwin, M. 1987. Copyright crisis: Copyright holders, with some reason, fear the Net's threat to intellectual property, but the laws being proposed go too far in restricting rights. *Internet World*, March, 100–102.

Harnad, S. 1995. Implementing peer review on the Net: Scientific quality control in scholarly electronic journals. In *Electronic publishing confronts academia: The agenda for the year 2000*, ed. R. Peek and G. Newby, 103–18. Cambridge: MIT Press. See also ftp://cogsci.ecs.soton.ac.uk/pub/harnad/harnad95.peer.review. Site accessed 5 April 1999.

Harter, S. P., and H. J. Kim. 1996. Electronic journals and scholarly communication: A citation and reference study. http://www.press.umich.edu/jep/archive/harter.html. Site accessed 25 March 1999.

Health on the Net Foundation. 1997. Health on the Net (HON) code of conduct (HONcode) for medical and health Web sites: Version 1.6. http://www.hon.ch/HONcode/Conduct.html. Site accessed 23 March 1999.

Heller, S. R. 1995. Chemistry on the Internet—the road to everywhere and nowhere. http://www.ch.ic.ac.uk/internet/heller.html. Site accessed 23 March 1999.

Hitchcock, S., L. Carr, and W. Hall. 1996. A survey of STM online journals, 1990–95: The calm before the storm. In *Directory of electronic journals, newsletters and academic discussion lists,* 6th ed., ed. D. Moggee, 7–32. Washington, D.C.: Association of Research Libraries. See also http://journals.ecs.soton.ac.uk/survey/survey.html. Site accessed 5 April 1999.

Horton, R. 1996. Rights, wrongs, and journals in the age of cyberspace: A colourless conveyor belt? *BMJ* 316:1609–12. See also http://www.bmj.com/archive/7072fd2.htm. Site accessed 25 March 1999.

Huang, M. P., and N. E. Alessi. 1996. The Internet and the future of psychiatry. *American Journal of Psychiatry* 153:861–69.

Impicciatore, P., C. Pandolfini, N. Casella, and M. Bonati. 1997. Reliability of health information for the public on the World Wide Web: Systematic survey of advice on managing fever in children at home. *BMJ* 314:1875–79.

International Committee of Medical Journal Editors (ICMJE). 1992. Statements on electronic publication and on peer-reviewed journals. *Annals of Internal Medicine* 116:1030.

Jadad, A. R., and A. Gagliardi. 1998. Rating health information on the Internet: Navigating to knowledge or to Babel? *JAMA* 279:611–14.

Jog, V. 1995. Cost and revenue structure of academic journals: Paper-based versus e-journals. http://www.schoolnet.ca/vp-pv/phoenix/e/vijayjog.html. Site accessed 23 March 1999.

Julliard, K. 1994. Perceptions of plagiarism in the use of other authors' language. *Family Medicine* 26:356–60.

Kassirer, J. P. 1992. Journals in bits and bytes: Electronic medical journals. *New England Journal of Medicine* 326:195–97.

———. 1995a. The next transformation in the delivery of health care. *New England Journal of Medicine* 332:52–54.

———. 1995b. The next transformation in the delivery of health care. *New England Journal of Medicine* 332:1100.

Kassirer, J. P., and M. Angell. 1995. The Internet and the *Journal. New England Journal of Medicine* 332:1709–10.

Kelly, M. A., and J. Oldham. 1996. The Internet and randomised controlled trials. Presented at the European Congress of the Internet in Medicine, 10 October

1996, Brighton, U.K. http://www.mednet.org.uk/mednet/ca16.htm. Site accessed 23 March 1999.

Koren-Elkin, N. 1995. The challenges of technological change to copyright law: Copyright reform and social change in cyberspace. *Science Communication* 17:186–200.

LaFollette, M. C. 1994. Avoiding plagiarism: Some thoughts on use, attribution, and acknowledgment. *Journal of Information Ethics* 3(fall):25–33.

———. 1997. An accelerated rate of change—journal publishing. *Science Communication* 18:182–93.

LaPorte, R. E., and B. Hibbitts. 1996. Rights, wrongs, and journals in the age of cyberspace: "We all want to change the world." *BMJ* 313:1609–10. See also http://www.bmj.com/archive/7072fd2.htm. Site accessed 25 March 1999.

LaPorte, R. E., E. Marler, S. Akazawa, F. Sauer, C. Gamboa, C. Shenton, C. Glosser, A. Villasenor, and M. Maclure. 1995. The death of biomedical journals. *BMJ* 310:1387–90.

Li, X., J. W. Aldis, and D. Valentino. 1996. The first international telemedicine trial to China: ZHU Lingling's case. http://www.radsci.ucla.edu/telemed/zhuling/preface.html. Site accessed 23 March 1999.

Li, X., and L. Xiong. 1996. Chinese researchers debate rash of plagiarism cases. *Science* 274:337–38.

Lilford, R. 1994. Formal measurement of clinical uncertainty: Prelude to a trial in perinatal medicine. The Fetal Compromise Group. *BMJ* 308:111–12.

Lock, S. 1986. *A difficult balance: Editorial peer review in medicine.* Philadelphia: ISI Press.

Lundberg, G. D. 1992. Perspective from the editor of *JAMA, The Journal of the American Medical Association.* The future of biomedical communication: A symposium. *Bulletin of the Medical Library Association* 80:110–14.

———. 1996. Rights, wrongs, and journals in the age of cyberspace: A Christmas fairy tale. *BMJ* 313:1609–12. See also http://www.bmj.com/archive/7072fd2.htm. Site accessed 25 March 1999.

Makulowich, J. S. 1995. Labs online: Research on the Internet. *Environmental Health Perspectives* 103:148–50.

McLellan, F. 1998. Like hunger, like thirst: Patients, journals and the Internet. *Lancet* 352(suppl 2):39–43.

Odlyzko, A. M. 1994. Tragic loss or good riddance? The impending demise of traditional scholarly journals. http://www-mathdoc.ujf-grenoble.fr/textes/Odlyzko/amo94/amo94.html. Site accessed 25 March 1999.

Pitkin, R. M. 1995. The death of biomedical journals: Popularity does not equal peer review. *BMJ* 311:507.

Readings, B. 1996. Caught in the net: Notes from the electronic underground. http://tornade.ere.umontreal.ca/~guedon/Surfaces/vo14/readings.html. Site accessed 25 March 1999.

Richardson, M. L., M. S. Frank, and E. J. Stern. 1995. Digital image manipulation: What constitutes acceptable alteration of a radiologic image? *AJR American Journal of Roentgenology* 164:228–29.

Schatz, B. R. 1997. Information retrieval in digital libraries: Bringing search to the net. *Science* 275:327–34.

Selby, M., C. Boyer, D. Jenefsky, and R. D. Appel. 1996. Health on the Net Foundation code of conduct for medical and health web sites. Presented at the European Congress of the Internet in Medicine, 16 October, Brighton, U.K. http://www.mednet.org.uk/mednet/ip6.htm. Site accessed 25 March 1999.

Sharma, P. 1995. Popular medical information on Internet. *Lancet* 346:250.

Shoaf, R. A. 1993. Gonzo scholarship: Policing electronic journals. http://tornade.ere.umontreal.ca/~guedon/Surfaces/vol4/shoaf.html. Site accessed 25 March 1999.

Silberg, W. M., G. D. Lundberg, and R. A. Musacchio. 1997. Assessing, controlling, and assuring the quality of medical information on the Internet: *Caveant lector et viewor:* Let the reader and viewer beware. *JAMA* 277:1244–45.

Smith, R. 1998. Informed consent: Edging forwards (and backwards). *BMJ* 316:949–51.

Stern, E. J., and L. Westenberg. 1995. Copyright law and academic radiology: Rights of authors and copyright owners and reproduction of information. *AJR American Journal of Roentgenology* 164:1083–88.

Stevens, L. 1998. Involving the patient in medical decisions. *Medicine on the Net* 4:8–14.

Stix, G. 1994. The speed of write. *Scientific American* 271:106–11.

Subramanian, A. K., A. T. McAfee, and J. P. Getzinger. 1997. Use of the World Wide Web for multisite data collection. *Academic Emergency Medicine* 4:811–17.

Taubes, G. 1994a. Peer review in cyberspace. *Science* 266:967.

———. 1994b. Technology for turning seeing into believing. *Science* 263:318.

———. 1996a. Electronic preprints point the way to "author empowerment." *Science* 271:767–68.

———. 1996b. Science journals go wired. *Science* 271:764–66.

Turkle, S. 1995. *Life on the screen: Identity in the age of the Internet.* New York: Simon & Schuster.

Unsworth, J. 1996. Electronic scholarship; or, scholarly publishing and the public. *Journal of Scholarly Publishing* 28:3–12.

Van Alstyne, M., and E. Brynjolfsson. 1996. Could the Internet balkanize science? *Science* 274:1479–80.

Varian, H. R. 1997. The future of electronic journals. http://www.arl.org/scomm/scat/varian.html. Site accessed 22 March 1999.

Varmus, H. 1999. E-BIOMED: A proposal for electronic publications in the biomedical sciences. http://www.nih.gov/welcome/director/ebiomed/ebi.htm. Site accessed 8 July 1999.

Widman, L. E., and D. A. Tong. 1997. Requests for medical advice from patients and families to health care providers who publish on the World Wide Web. *Archives of Internal Medicine* 157:209–12.

Winograd, S., and R. N. Zare. 1995. "Wired" science or whither the printed page? *Science* 269:615.

World Intellectual Property Organization (WIPO). 1996. Diplomatic conference on certain copyright and neighboring rights questions. WIPO copyright treaty. http://www.wipo.org/eng/diplconf/index.htm. Site accessed 23 March 1999.

Zielinski, C. 1995. New equities of information in an electronic age. *BMJ* 310:1480–81.

II

Responses and Remedies:

Law, Policy, Education

When Ethics Fails

8

Legal and Administrative Causes of Action and Remedies

Debra M. Parrish

If ethics fails, one must look to laws, regulations, and institutional guidelines to establish and enforce appropriate conduct. When a researcher appropriates someone else's work and fails to provide appropriate attribution, fabricates or falsifies research, abuses the peer-review process, or violates human subjects regulations, he or she may be pursued through institutional processes, a relevant federal agency, the judicial court system, or a combination of these. This chapter focuses on the administrative and legal liabilities and remedies available when a researcher violates the ethical norms of the biomedical community. Specifically, the chapter examines forms of misconduct and, for each of the major forms of misconduct, offers a three-level analysis of federal agencies and their processes for responding to such misconduct, legal actions stemming from these violations, and publishers' issues associated with such violations.

The Failure to Provide Appropriate Attribution to a Contributor

It is important to distinguish failure to give credit for ideas from failure to give credit for words or failure to give credit for work the ideas or words generate or represent. All science is built on the sharing of ideas. It would be impossible for a scientist to acknowledge in every publication all the individuals who contributed to his or her scientific development. Such a list could include everyone from a grade school science teacher to those with whom the scientist had thoughtful hallway conversations. Nonetheless, if an idea, expression, or work is a significant contribution to a research project, the contributor is entitled to credit for that contribution. After all, credit for one's ideas, words, and work is the currency of professional scientific advancement. Such contributions should be acknowledged in publications, grant applications, presentations, research progress reports, and patent applications.

Copyright and Patents

Formal legal mechanisms exist to secure protection for words and ideas, the most important of which are copyrights and patents. If a researcher wants to protect the particular expression of an idea (e.g., the words used to describe the idea), he or she may seek copyright protection for that expression. Copyright protection protects only the particular expression of an idea from use by others; it does not protect the idea itself. *Work* here refers to a product to which copyright protection may be extended, not the sense of labor determined by contract and other norms.

Copyright

Since 1978, all copyrightable works created in the United States have federal statutory copyright protection from the moment of creation. Registering the work with the U.S. Copyright Office and attaching a notice of copyright protection are not required for copyright protection of a work.[1] However, such registration and notice provide significant advantages if an author must bring an action to enforce a copyright,[2] and registration is still required to bring a copyright infringement suit for works created in the United States.

In March 1989, the United States entered the Berne Convention, an international treaty that establishes minimum copyright standards for member countries and requires each member country to extend to works created in other member countries the same copyright protection accorded to domestic works.[3] Thus, the Berne Convention does not create an international copyright law; it simply provides that each country must accord the protection of its national copyright laws to both foreign and domestic works. Most publishers of scientific journals and textbooks require authors to assign the copyright of their works to the publisher. Publishers believe requiring such assignment is a service to researchers because it provides the researcher with the resources of a journal in responding to requests for use of the published material and enforcing the copyright against infringement. Unfortunately, it also means that researchers must request permission to reproduce or adapt their own work. Further, some publishers require authors to give the publisher the right to use the text in any way the publisher deems appropriate without providing the authors credit for their work.

Patents

To protect a unique idea, a researcher may file a patent application or may decide to keep the idea a trade secret and simply not share the idea with others. To secure a patent in the United States, the researcher must file with the U.S. Patent and Trademark Office a patent application that explains the idea and establishes that it is novel and unobvious. During the patent process, the researcher must aver that all the inventors (i.e., those who conceived the invention described in the patent application) are identified in the patent application. Most large companies and some universities require that inventors working for them assign the inventorship rights to the employing institution.

Despite the availability of these formal ways to protect words and ideas, they are not used by most researchers because they are expensive and impractical. For example, most researchers do not secure federal copyright protection for their laboratory notes, lecture notes, and interdepartmental memos on research progress. It would be too expensive and time consuming, and researchers would find themselves spending too much time each day sending off every scrap of paper to the U.S. Copyright Office. Accordingly, most scientists must address breaches in the ethical norms of the scientific community without their ideas and words having formal legal protection.

Administrative Remedies

Although mechanisms have been established by various scientific enterprises and national professional associations (Lock and Wells 1996),[4] only a small number of countries that conduct biomedical research have developed federal mechanisms for responding to allegations of breaches of the ethical norms of the scientific community, the most formal of which are the systems created by the United States and Denmark (Danish Committee on Scientific Dishonesty [DCSD] 1996).[5] Further, many of these models address only certain ethical breaches; that is, they have different and often limited definitions of *scientific misconduct*. For example, the Association of the British Pharmaceutical Industry defines *research fraud* as the generation of false data with an intent to deceive, while the Royal College of Physicians (RCP) (1991) defines *scientific misconduct* as piracy, plagiarism, and fraud. These terms are further defined as follows: "Piracy is the deliberate exploitation of ideas from others without acknowledgment. Plagiarism is the copying of ideas, data or text (or various combinations of the three) without permission or acknowledgment. Fraud involves deliberate deception, usually the invention of data" (RCP 1991, 3).

The Danish model (DCSD 1996) states:

Scientific dishonesty includes all deliberate fraudulent work at any time during the application-research-publication process as well as such extreme cases of negligence that the question of professional credibility becomes an issue. This corresponds to the legal concepts of intent and gross negligence.

The area of scientific dishonesty that is covered by the [DCSD] is characterized by falsification or distortion of the scientific message or a false credit or emphasis given to a scientist. This includes but is not limited to:

—construction of data
—selective and hidden rejection of undesirable results
—substitution with fictive data
—deliberate manipulation of statistics with the intention of drawing
 conclusions beyond what the data warrant
—distorted interpretations of results and distortion of conclusions
—plagiarism of other people's results or entire articles
—distorted representations of other scientists' results
—inappropriate credit as author
—misleading applications

The Australian model, developed jointly by the National Health and Medical Research Council (NHMRC) and the Australian Vice-Chancellors' Committee (AVCC), defines *misconduct* or *scientific misconduct* as

fabrication, falsification, plagiarism, or other practices that seriously deviate from those that are commonly accepted within the scientific community for proposing, conducting, or reporting research. It includes the misleading ascription of authorship including the listing of authors without their permission, attributing work to others who have not in fact contributed to the research, and the lack of appropriate acknowledgment of work primarily produced by a research student/trainee or associate. It does not include honest errors or honest differences in interpretation or judgements of data. (NHMRC 1997)

The U.S. Public Health Service (PHS) defines *scientific misconduct* as "fabrication, falsification, plagiarism, or other practices that seriously deviate from those that are commonly accepted within the scientific community for proposing, conducting, or reporting research. It does not include honest error or honest differences in interpretations or judgments of data" (Parrish 1994, 519). The U.S. National Science Foundation (NSF) defines *scientific misconduct* as "(1) fabrication, falsification, plagiarism, or other serious deviation from accepted practices in proposing, carrying out, or reporting results from activities funded by NSF; or (2) retaliation of any kind against a person who reported or provided information about suspected or alleged misconduct and who has not acted in bad faith" (Parrish 1994, 519).[6]

Because the United States has the most developed response to and experience with allegations of research misconduct, the following discussion focuses on American responses. Which U.S. federal agency has jurisdiction to address the misappropriation of ideas or words depends on which agency sponsored the relevant research. If a federal agency did not sponsor the research, no federal agency will have jurisdiction to address the misappropriation. However, if a researcher engages in theft of another's research, either ideas or words, in privately sponsored research, it is possible that the researcher will be deemed unfit to receive federal funds and may be declared ineligible to receive such funds for a period of time. If the research was funded by PHS, the Office of Research Integrity (ORI)[7] has jurisdiction over the case, and the case generally will proceed under ORI guidelines for investigating allegations of scientific misconduct. If the research was funded by NSF, NSF has jurisdiction. ORI and NSF may exercise prosecutorial discretion and decide not to pursue a case, although they have jurisdiction over it. Other federal agencies have slightly different responses to allegations of misappropriation of ideas and words, but ORI and NSF are the agencies most active in setting federal policy and responding to allegations of misappropriation of words or ideas. ORI and NSF deem some cases of the misappropriation of words and ideas to constitute plagiarism, a form of scientific misconduct (Parrish 1994). Because PHS is more involved in funding biomedical research than is NSF, the following discussion focuses on the ORI process.

The Institutional Phase

Under both ORI and NSF processes for responding to allegations of misconduct and in misconduct models used in countries other than the United States (e.g., Canada and Australia), the research institution employing the involved researcher(s) has primary responsibility for investigating an allegation of scientific misconduct. ORI or NSF may assume responsibility for the investigation [see editors' note, p. 218], however, if an institution is unable or unwilling to conduct it. Under PHS guidelines, the institutional process must include inquiry, investigational, and reporting phases.

During the inquiry phase, the institution must determine whether there is sufficient substance to the allegation to warrant an investigation. If there is no substance to the allegation, then the case is closed and the institution simply reports to ORI that it conducted an inquiry without finding sufficient substance to warrant an investigation and without identifying the accused party. Two important issues should be resolved during this phase: whether any federal funds are involved, to resolve the issue of whether the investigation must comply with federal regulations governing scientific misconduct and, if so, which federal regulatory body must be satisfied with the possibly ensuing investigation; and whether, if true, the alleged action would constitute scientific misconduct as defined by the institution and/or the relevant federal regulatory body. If the answer to either of those questions is negative, the institution may have flexibility regarding the nature of any subsequent investigation.

With respect to the second prong of the analysis, neither ORI nor NSF has deemed *authorship disputes* (as used herein *authorship dispute* does not include gift or ghost authorship) to constitute scientific misconduct (Office of Inspector General [OIG] 1994, 27–30; OIG 1996, 43–44; ORI 1994). (Under the Danish and Australian systems, however, authorship disputes are investigated.) An authorship dispute occurs when there has been a collaborative relationship between the alleged plagiarizer and the person whose work was copied (OIG 1994, 27–30; OIG 1996, 43–44; ORI 1994). Although some researchers believe that ORI should be involved in such authorship disputes and that an artificial line has been drawn between authorship disputes and plagiarism, ORI made a policy decision not to get involved in these cases (ORI 1994). Part of ORI's rationale was that involvement in such cases would require the expenditure of large amounts of resources to investigate unresolvable allegations, and because the institution is awarded the grant that supported the research, the institution may determine authorship rights among its researchers. For example, it is difficult to segregate the contributions of long-term collaborators. Further, during an ongoing collaboration, there usually is an implicit or explicit agreement that the collaborators will use and build upon each other's work. ORI has extended this understanding such that, even when it is possible to segregate the data or words contributed by one collaborator who has withdrawn from the collaboration, the remaining collaborators may continue to use the withdrawn collaborator's data and words.

If a federal agency such as ORI or NSF has jurisdiction and if the institution determines that there is substance to the allegation of scientific misconduct, the institution must conduct an investigation of the allegation. Two questions that often arise during an investigation are, What due process is the accused scientist entitled to receive during the investigation?

and, What level of proof is required to establish scientific misconduct? *Due process* generally means that the accused person will be told what the nature of the dispute is and will have the right to be heard by and defend himself in front of the tribunal deciding the issue. Further, the matter will be heard by the tribunal during an orderly proceeding adapted to the nature of the case, and it will be decided only after the decision-making tribunal has conducted a proceeding with the elements stated above. Simply put, due process means that a matter was decided in a manner that was fair to the accused. Different levels of due process can and do exist among institutions and federal agencies. Significant debate exists about how much due process scientists accused of scientific misconduct are entitled to receive, and scientists who believe they have not received sufficient due process have brought lawsuits against the relevant institutions and agencies (Hallum and Hadley 1991; Olswang and Lee 1984; Bersoff 1996; Association of American Medical Colleges [AAMC] 1992).

With respect to the level of proof required during the investigations, the federal agencies have required that scientific misconduct be established by a preponderance of evidence—that is, it is more likely than not that scientific misconduct occurred. This level of proof is substantially lower than levels of proof requiring "clear and convincing evidence" and evidence that establishes the conduct "beyond a reasonable doubt." At the conclusion of an investigation, the institution must send the report of its investigation to ORI for ORI's analysis and review.

Agency Oversight/Investigation

ORI reviews the institutional report to determine that the investigation was thorough, had appropriate expertise (was competent), and lacked bias. Whether or not the investigation found misconduct, ORI typically asks for the supporting documentation for the investigation, including transcripts and documents reviewed.

After reviewing the institutional investigation report, ORI may accept, reject, or modify the institutional findings as support for PHS findings of scientific misconduct. If ORI accepts an institutional report finding no misconduct, it notifies the institution and the case is closed by ORI, although it may continue in institutional and judicial forums. If ORI accepts an institutional report finding misconduct, ORI will determine which of those findings support a finding of scientific misconduct as defined by PHS, and those findings alone will underpin a federal finding of scientific misconduct. The distinction is important because some institutions have adopted a definition of scientific misconduct that includes conduct not included in the PHS definition, for example, violations of radiation safety, animal care, and human subjects regulations. ORI will issue an oversight report stating that, based on the institution's report, ORI concurs with the institution's findings that support a finding of misconduct as defined by PHS. Findings about conduct outside the PHS definition are left to the institution to handle.

Alternatively, ORI may reject the institutional findings. If so, ORI may require the institution to conduct an additional investigation or, if ORI believes that the institution is unable or unwilling to conduct an appropriate investigation, it may decide to conduct its own investigation [see editors' note, p. 218]. NSF follows a similar process.

Sanctions/Resolution

Institutions have applied a variety of sanctions for ethical breaches, ranging from a letter of reprimand to the sanctioned researcher to termination from the institution. ORI and NSF consider the institutional sanctions when determining whether federal sanctions should be applied.

If ORI finds that a researcher has committed scientific misconduct, it typically proposes federal sanctions. These range from prohibition from serving in an advisory capacity for PHS to debarment from receiving federal funds for a period of years, usually three.[8] ORI offers the accused scientist the option of entering into a Voluntary Exclusion Agreement (VEA), in which the accused scientist agrees to the federal findings and sanctions, or the opportunity to request a hearing before a hearing panel on the findings, sanctions, or both.[9]

A VEA states the federal sanctions, refers to the findings of misconduct, and may state that the accused either admits or denies the findings of misconduct. ORI has offered the accused scientist a VEA even after ORI's preliminary review of an institutional finding of misconduct and before a federal finding of misconduct has been made.[10] Most scientists who have been found by ORI to have committed scientific misconduct choose this option because it brings faster resolution of the case and avoids the expense of a protracted hearing.

The hearing offered to a scientist found by ORI to have committed scientific misconduct is a de novo hearing—that is, a hearing in which all the evidence must be presented to an impartial panel without any presumption in favor of ORI or institutional findings, investigation, or inquiry. ORI presents the case to the panel even when the case is based on an institutional investigation and report. The accused scientist is allowed to present witnesses and to cross-examine witnesses presented by ORI to support the findings of misconduct. The panel that hears the case is a panel of the Departmental Appeals Board (DAB) of the Department of Health and Human Services (DHHS) (Parrish 1997).[11] After both parties have presented their case, a decision is made by the hearing panel. The decision is PHS's final decision on the case. Only the accused scientist, not ORI, can appeal the ruling to the courts.

A very small fraction of the cases involving an allegation of scientific misconduct actually go through the hearing phase. For example, in 1994, although 185 allegations of scientific misconduct were made to ORI, only one went to a hearing (ten resulted in VEAs). The other cases did not result in findings of scientific misconduct by PHS. Between 1993 and 1997, ORI received approximately one thousand allegations of misconduct, made 76 findings of misconduct, and completed four hearings.

If scientific misconduct is established or conceded, either after a hearing on the issue or through a VEA, ORI publicizes the finding through notices in the *Federal Register,* the *NIH Guide to Grants and Contracts,* and the *ORI Newsletter.* Unless the scientist is debarred by NSF, NSF does not publicize its findings except through anonymous descriptions in its Office of Inspector General's *Semiannual Report to the Congress.* If the scientist is debarred, NSF provides the name of the scientist to the Government Accounting Office and Government Procurement Office. Similarly, the DCSD does not publish the names of scientists found to have committed scientific dishonesty.

Legal Remedies
Copyright Infringement

A copyright infringement action is available when a person can show ownership of a valid copyright and that another person copied those elements of the work that are original and protectable. As used in this section, in copyright law, *copying* is when the words between two works are exactly the same, while *substantial similarity* does not require identity of words. However, neither copying nor substantial similarity alone constitutes copyright infringement. Further analysis must be conducted. To prove infringement, a plaintiff must show a valid copyright, prove the infringer's access to the copied work, and demonstrate that the relevant works are substantially similar.

The ultimate question in all infringement cases is whether the portion of work that was copied was significant enough that the works are substantially similar. A common defense in copyright infringement actions is that the copying simply constitutes fair use. *Fair use* is a concept in intellectual property law that essentially holds all copying will not give rise to a copyright violation. The fair-use doctrine was established to permit the use of copyrighted works "for purposes such as criticism, comment, news reporting, teaching . . . , scholarship, or research" (Copyright Act, U.S. Code, vol. 17, sec. 107). The fair-use doctrine essentially creates a privilege to use copyrighted material in a reasonable manner despite the lack of the copyright owner's consent. To determine whether the copying constitutes fair use, the following factors are evaluated: "(1) the purpose and character of the use, including whether such use is of a commercial nature or is for nonprofit educational purposes; (2) the nature of the copyrighted work; (3) the amount and substantiality of the portion used in relation to the copyrighted work as a whole; and (4) the effect of the use upon the potential market for or value of the copyrighted work" (Copyright Act, U.S. Code, vol. 17, sec. 107).

When the use is for commercial purposes, the presumption is often that the use is not fair use. In scientific, educational, and research contexts, the concept of fair use is given broad latitude. When the work is factual, the concept of fair use also is given broad interpretation. If the work is unpublished, the concept of fair use is given a narrower interpretation; that is, only a limited use of the work will be deemed to be fair. If a substantial portion or the core of a copyrighted work is copied, the use generally will not be deemed fair.[12] The fourth factor, effect on the market, has been said to be the most important factor (*Harper & Row Publishers v. Nation Enter.,* 471 U.S. 539, 566 [1985]; 105 S. Ct. 2218, 2233 [1985]).

As noted earlier, most publishing researchers do not possess the copyright for their published work and thus cannot bring an action for copyright infringement. In general, then, prosecution for copyright infringement remains at the discretion of the publisher holding the copyright. Whoever possesses the copyright can bring an action for a variety of damages even if the copying was unintentional. Such damages include injunctions; impoundment or destruction of the infringing copies; recovery of actual damages plus the defendant's profits attributable to the infringement, or statutory damages; and costs and attorneys' fees (Copyright Act, U.S. Code, vol. 17, secs. 502–5).

A publisher's liability for publishing a substantially copied work may be pursued as contributory infringement or vicarious infringement. A person who uses or authorizes the use of copyrighted works is a *direct infringer.* A person who knowingly induces, causes, or materially contributes to the infringing conduct of another is a *contributory infringer*. A person who has the right and ability to supervise the infringing activities of another is a *vicarious infringer*. The concept of *vicarious liability* is of greatest significance to a publisher. The crux of this liability is whether the publisher had a financial interest in the exploitation of the copyrighted work and had the right and authority to supervise the infringing activity. The liability of vicarious infringers is joint and several—that is, the party whose copyright was infringed may sue one or more of the parties liable for the infringement or may sue all of them together. Liability is imposed irrespective of the intent or knowledge of the vicarious infringer, although lack of intent or knowledge may mitigate damages.

It is important to distinguish the legal concept of copyright infringement, which is an action available only to protect the particular expression of an idea and does not require intent, from a scientific misconduct allegation of plagiarism, which is an action brought to protect both the idea and the words of the original source and requires intent. This distinction was illustrated in the case of *Weissmann v. Freeman* (868 F.2d 1313 [2d Cir. 1989]). In that case, two collaborators prepared a syllabus for a review course taught to medical students who were preparing to take a comprehensive examination. The syllabus was updated and revised by the collaborators as presentations were made. The two collaborators had a falling out, and Weissmann registered with the U.S. Copyright Office a version of the syllabus she had revised, which contained material developed jointly and material developed independently by Freeman. Continuing with their former practice, Freeman planned to use the most recent version of the syllabus in a review course and had 50 copies of the syllabus made. Weissmann brought a copyright infringement action and ultimately prevailed in her lawsuit. The institution, however, declined to make a finding of scientific misconduct. It noted the pattern of conduct between the collaborators and Freeman's reasonable belief that he could use the syllabus that essentially was an amalgam of material developed by both of them.

False Passing Off

Although many researchers are willing to relinquish the copyright of a manuscript in exchange for publication, most expect to be acknowledged as authors of the work.[13] Although a publisher may not be required to acknowledge the original author, the prohibition against *false passing off* precludes a publisher or secondary writer from representing the work as being generated by a person or entity other than the original author. The principle underlying the claim is that the false designation of origin not only perpetrates an insult against the original author but also deceives the purchasing public. Thus, many authors who cannot pursue a copyright claim because they failed to secure copyright protection or surrendered it to another person may file a cause of action based on a section of the Lanham Act (U.S. Code, vol. 15, secs. 1125[a] and 43[a]). The relevant section of the Lanham Act prohibits the false designation of origin for a product (e.g., labeling a product with a designer's name when it was made by another, typically inferior, individual or entity).

One form of false designation of origin prohibited by the relevant section of the Lanham Act prohibits *reverse passing off*. Reverse passing off occurs when party A sells party B's product under party A's name. When applied to a written product, the Lanham Act prohibits misrepresentation of credit belonging to the original creator of the written work (Nimmer 1963). To maintain such a claim, the goods (i.e., the writing) must be in interstate commerce; the person bringing the claim must believe that he is or is likely to be damaged by the conduct (i.e., believe that he will lose income he would have received from the sale or promotion of his written work); and there must be substantial similarity and a likelihood of confusion. There can be a Lanham Act claim if one co-author is listed but the others are not (*Lamothe v. Atlantic Recording Corp.,* 847 F. 2d 1403, 1407 [9th Cir. 1988]).[14]

Nonetheless, Lanham Act claims that have been brought in the academic setting have been treated hostilely by the courts. In general, courts focus on the likelihood of consumer confusion, not the substantial similarity of the works, in determining whether a Lanham Act violation occurred (*Smith v. Montoro,* 648 F.2d 602 [9th Cir. 1981]; *Litchfield v. Speilberg,* 736 F.2d 1352 [9th Cir. 1984], cert. denied, 470 U.S. 1052 [1985]; *Lamothe v. Atlantic Recording Corp.,* 847 F.2d 1403 [9th Cir. 1988]; *Shaw v. Lindheim,* 919 F.2d 1353 [9th Cir. 1990]). In the case of *Rosenfeld,* a third edition of a medical textbook failed to give credit to the author of the original treatise, and the plaintiff brought a Lanham Act claim. The preface to the work states that "a scientific book is only an extension of earlier publications. . . . Many of the authors, however, have used material from the previous editions" (*Rosenfeld v. W. B. Saunders,* 728 F. Supp. 236 [S.D.N.Y.] aff'd, 923 F.2d 845 [2d Cir. 1990]). Further, the book was dedicated to the previous author, who had died. The court found that the author of the third edition had given sufficient credit and that purchasers of medical books understood that they built upon previous works and therefore the purchasers were not deceived. This hostility was also seen in *Debs,* a case involving the verbatim copying of Professor Debs's class notes by another professor who did not indicate that Debs was the origin of, co-author of, or contributor to the class notes (*Debs v. Meliopoulos,* 1993 WL 566011 [N. D. Ga.]). However, because the verbatim copying was limited and scientific principles can be expressed in only so many ways, the court did not find a violation.

Tortious Interference and Unfair Competition

Several researchers who have been the victims of plagiarism of either ideas or words have brought legal actions on the premise that the plagiarizer's publication of the work impaired the original researcher's professional and financial opportunities. Such a claim is known as a *tortious interference* with prospective economic advantages or relationships. For example, suppose a mentor published as his own the work of a graduate student and did not acknowledge that the ideas and data were generated by the student.[15] Because the work had been published under the mentor's name and most journals are interested only in original ideas and data, the student probably would have difficulty publishing the same work under his or her own name. Thus, because publications contribute to a student's professional advancement, which often translates into greater financial rewards, the mentor's publication of the work may have impaired the student's professional and financial opportunities. Similarly, when two researchers are conducting, teaching, or publishing research in the same area, the misappropriation of the work of one by the other gives one a competitive advantage. Such a competitive advantage at the expense of the first party may serve as the basis for a claim of unfair competition.[16]

Publishers' Issues

If a person notifies a publisher that a dispute has arisen regarding the authorship of a particular piece, the publisher often will withhold publication until the authorship issues are resolved. If the article has already been published, the publisher and co-authors may face a host of issues during and after an investigation of the allegation of plagiarism. While an investigation of plagiarism is proceeding, the nonaccused co-authors in a multiauthor publication may wish immediate correction of the offending publication and may submit a letter to the publisher or editor requesting immediate action. A letter submitted by the nonaccused authors may attempt to distance themselves from the accused author and attempt to lessen their being stigmatized by a finding of misconduct. Such a letter may state that the nonaccused authors had no knowledge of the impropriety (Parrish 1999).

Some accused authors have threatened legal action against an editor for publishing a letter of correction or retraction before the investigation of scientific misconduct is complete. (This has been a significant problem in countries other than the United States where defamation laws are more liberal and such actions are more difficult to defend.) Because institutions have primary responsibility for investigating allegations of scientific misconduct, have established policies and procedures, and typically have access to the information necessary to conduct an investigation and because publishers and editors lack those resources and mechanisms, most publishers wait until the institutional investigation is complete before deciding to publish a correction or retraction. The individual, not the institution, is responsible for correcting the literature, although institutions have notified publishers when the accused individual declined to notify the publisher.

If ORI determines that an article was plagiarized, one of the sanctions that may be imposed after such a finding or as a condition of a VEA is that the publisher be notified of the plagiarism and that a letter of correction or retraction be sent to the publisher of the publication containing the plagiarism. ORI has not taken this action in plagiarism cases, presumably because correction was made, but it has taken this action in other scientific misconduct cases. The contents of letters of correction or retraction are often negotiated by ORI with the accused and nonaccused authors. Ideally, all the authors sign the letter, although such letters have been signed by all co-authors except the accused author, by only the accused author, or by institutional officials in conjunction with some of the authors (Parrish 1999). Whether the publisher chooses to publish the letter of correction or retraction in the form submitted is up to the publisher. A publisher may also craft the retraction notice after receiving information that an article should be retracted (Thoolen 1990; Anderson 1991).[17]

The International Committee of Medical Journal Editors (ICMJE) issued a statement about the obligation to retract papers associated with research fraud and the form of such retraction. The ICMJE noted that "it is not the task of editors to conduct a full investigation [of allegations of research fraud] or to make a determination; that responsibility lies with the institution where the work was done or with the funding agency" (ICMJE 1988, 304; 1997, 45). The ICMJE, however, recognized that "research fraud" investigations may not be done or may be impaired for a variety of reasons. Thus, the committee stated, "If this method of investigation does not result in a satisfactory conclusion, the editor may choose to publish an expression of concern with an explanation" (ICMJE 1997, 45). The recommended retraction or expression of concern should explain why the article is being retracted, should include a reference to the article, should appear in a prominent place in the journal, and should not simply appear as a letter to the editor. The vast majority of letters of correction and retraction associated with a finding of scientific misconduct do not indicate that the publication is being corrected or withdrawn because of a finding of scientific misconduct (Parrish 1999). At least in countries other than the United States, the reluctance to publicize a finding of misconduct may stem from liberal defamation laws that make such actions difficult to defend.

Whether or not the publisher publishes a letter of retraction or correction after an ORI finding of scientific misconduct, the U.S. National Library of Medicine (NLM) will tag the article so it can be identified as having been the subject of a scientific integrity review. The tag directs the reader to the *NIH Guide to Grants and Contracts* for a description of the problem and the person(s) responsible. NLM applies the scientific integrity review tag only if the article is identified in the *NIH Guide to Grants and Contracts* as having been connected with an ORI finding of scientific misconduct. NLM will not apply the tag at the request of ORI, the publisher of the original article, or the co-authors. NLM does not delete the relevant publications from its database; it simply tags them.

As noted earlier, conduct that would not support a finding of scientific misconduct may support an action for copyright infringement, false passing off, or tortious interference with economic relations (*Weissmann v. Freeman*, 868 F.2d 1313 [2d Cir. 1989]). Conversely, all findings of plagiarism do not give rise to a copyright violation or a case of false passing off. If the copying is so significant that it would give rise to a copyright violation, a case of false passing off, or tortious interference with economic relations, the publisher of the plagiarism should take immediate action to limit liability and complicity with the plagiarizer.

The Fabrication or Falsification of Research

Falsification and fabrication of research are deemed by both ORI and NSF to constitute scientific misconduct and are actionable under their processes as described. *Fabrication* is the creation of false research results. *Falsification* is the misrepresentation of research results in either quantity or quality. Cases are investigated under the process described earlier for plagiarism. Sequestering the data early in the process is a particular concern. Two important issues in these cases are correction of the literature and recoupment of the federal funds associated with the research.

The Correction of the Literature

In cases involving falsified or fabricated research, correction of the literature is particularly important because of the possibility that other researchers, using other funds and resources, will undertake futile work based on the falsified data or that the falsification or fabrication will affect the treatment of patients. Some journals have explicit policies that address this form of scientific misconduct. For example, the *International Journal of Radiation Oncology, Biology, and Physics* (Policy on scientific misconduct 1996) has adopted an explicit policy that addresses only falsified data. This policy states that if falsified data are determined to exist, the relevant paper in its entirety will be retracted. The journal has stated that it will retract articles containing falsified data after institutional review and investigation, execution of a VEA, or publication in the *Federal Register*.

If public-health issues are at stake, the relevant federal agency may take immediate action and not wait until the completion of its investigation to request immediate correction of the literature by the authors, institution, or editor. Although agencies have not exercised this option, they have considered it in certain cases. Such an action may put the publisher in the awkward position of being asked to take corrective action before final disposition of the case.

The Recoupment of Federal Funds

Federal agencies have occasionally demanded the return of federal funds granted for research that is determined to have been fabricated. Recovery of research funds associated with scientific misconduct has not been pursued in countries other than the United States, although it is being considered in countries such as Canada. Civil actions also have been brought by or on behalf of the federal government to recover such funds under the False Claims Act (U.S. Code, vol. 31, sec. 3729 and following). In addition to penalties for each false statement, the False Claims Act provides for treble damages. Accordingly, the federal government can seek to recoup from the institution three times the amount of funds awarded for the flawed research. Clearly, the recoupment of such funds is of primary concern to the institution that received the grant money and employed the researcher. Because grant funds are technically given to an institution employing the researcher and not individual researchers, the recovery of funds has been from the institution, not the individual researcher. Recoveries in such cases have exceeded one million dollars (*United States ex rel. Condi v. University of California*, No. C89-3550-FMS [N. D. Cal. filed Sept. 29, 1989]).

Abuse of the Peer-Review Process

Abuse of the peer-review process is a problem that plagues the scientific community and undermines the review and publication processes. The most common forms of abuse of the peer-review process in scientific publications include breach of confidentiality, theft of ideas and language (discussed above), and the malicious rating of manuscripts.

Breach of Confidentiality

During the peer-review process for publication, a publisher may require each reviewer to sign a statement of confidentiality indicating that the reviewer will not use the information or manuscript provided during peer review and will not share it with others. Breach of confidentiality by a reviewer typically occurs when the reviewer shares with others a manuscript sent to the reviewer for comment. Such breaches are difficult to detect. They may be discovered when the reviewer or one of the reviewer's colleagues decides to "borrow" words or ideas from a manuscript.

Before ORI's creation, the DAB, the body that decides scientific misconduct cases for PHS, deemed such a breach to constitute scientific misconduct. In the *Bridges* case (DAB 1991), the accused scientist was alleged to have used improperly information from a draft manuscript sent to him for peer review. Specifically, Bridges received a manuscript describing a series of experiments, which he then decided to conduct in his laboratory while delaying the return of the manuscript. After an extended period, Bridges declined to review the manuscript and returned it to the editor. Bridges also attempted to gain priority over the research presented in the manuscript, stating that he had begun the experiments before receiving the manuscript. NIH made a finding that the accused scientist had "misused the privileged information available to him . . . and he failed to acknowledge properly the source of that information" (DAB 1991, 8). In the decision of that case, the DAB stated that "Dr. Bridges did not adhere to certain accepted standards of conduct for scientific research for handling of a manuscript received for peer review. These standards are: . . . To treat information contained in a manuscript received for peer review as confidential and privileged" (DAB 1991, 74). For his conduct, Bridges ultimately was debarred from receiving federal funds.

ORI has deemed such breaches of peer-review confidentiality to be beyond the PHS definition of scientific misconduct, although such breaches are an aggravating factor in a scientific misconduct finding based on plagiarism. However, ORI has accepted institutional findings based on such conduct and has referenced it in a VEA.[18] In contrast, NSF, which has deemed the breach of the peer-review process a serious deviation of the norms of the scientific community, has decided scientific misconduct findings based on that conduct alone.[19]

Finally, legal actions have been based on breach of confidentiality in peer review, the most famous of which has been *Cistron Biotechnology Inc. v. Immunex Corp.* (No. C93-1742 [W. D. Wash. filed December 11, 1993 and settled November 7, 1996]; *Cistron Biotechnology Inc. v. Gillis,* No. C94-1515 [W. D. Wash. filed October 11, 1994, and settled November 7, 1996]). In that case, Cistron, a biotechnology company, alleged that researchers working for Immunex, a competitor company, used data from a manuscript sent to one of the Immunex researchers, Steven Gillis, for peer review. Cistron alleged that the use of the information in the manuscript constituted unfair competition and misappropriation of trade secrets. The case promised to bring an exploration of whether a legal requirement of confidentiality exists during peer review. Immunex attorneys argued that there were no standards for peer review and no confidential relationships among authors, publishers, and peer reviewers. Specifically, Immunex's attorneys argued that no rule prevents a reviewer from using information in a scientific manuscript referred to him for peer review. Immunex noted that the guidelines for handling manuscripts under review are so variable and vague that reviewers do not have a sense of what is and is not appropriate. Immunex's experts, which included a patent attorney, a laboratory chief, and a dean for research and sponsored programs, stated that no codes, standards, or rules governed peer review.

Cistron lined up an impressive array of experts, including former editors of prestigious journals and a Nobel laureate, who were prepared to testify that it is generally accepted in the biomedical community that peer review is confidential and that theft of ideas or data from a manuscript provided during peer review breaches that generally known norm. Like other cases in which breach of peer review was alleged, the case was settled before the trial; Immunex agreed to pay Cistron 21 million dollars and to assign some of its related patents to Cistron. The case prompted an exploration about expectations of confidentiality during peer review, causing some editors to revisit their confidentiality agreements with reviewers (Marshall 1995a, 1995b; Wilson 1996; Day 1996).

The Malicious Rating of Manuscripts

In an effort to ensure frank and rigorous reviews, most publishers do not reveal the identity of the reviewers. Clearly, a reviewer should have expertise in the relevant field to provide an in-depth critique of a manuscript. Thus, an article often will be sent to an investigator's research competitors. Some unscrupulous reviewers have taken the opportunity, through a malicious or delayed review of a manuscript, to preclude effectively the publication or primacy of a competitor's work.

Neither ORI nor NSF has deemed such conduct to constitute scientific misconduct, although it was examined by PHS in the cases of *Bridges* and *Robert C. Gallo*. As detailed above, Bridges received a manuscript to review in July 1986, but he did not "decline" to review it until September 2, 1986. The DAB (1991, 17) noted that "Dr. Bridges' failure to decline review promptly after reading the . . . manuscript had the potential to delay its publication." Although Bridges formally declined to review the manuscript, he provided some comments on the paper, stating that he was "concerned at the total lack of primary data" and that "the paper was messily written" (DAB 1991, 17). These comments were consistent with those of another reviewer. The DAB articulated standards of conduct for science and found that

> Dr. Bridges did not adhere to certain accepted standards of conduct for scientific research for handling of a manuscript received for peer review. These standards are:
>
> "To act promptly when declining to review a manuscript on the basis that the proposed reviewer's current research is closely related to that reported in the manuscript; . . . and
> To take no action that might delay publication of a competitive manuscript."
> (DAB 1991, 74)

As noted earlier, Bridges was debarred from receiving federal funds for these and other violations of standards within the scientific community.

In the *Gallo* case, ORI asserted that

Dr. Gallo inappropriately inserted changes into a paper written by scientists at the Pasteur Institute. . . . The paper had been forwarded to Dr. Gallo for his assistance in having it accepted for publication by *Science*. In the process of shepherding the paper, and eventually serving as its peer reviewer, Dr. Gallo authored an Abstract and made significant substantive modifications which advanced his own hypotheses rather than those of the Pasteur scientists. . . . These representations were not identified as comments by Dr. Gallo but rather added as gratuitous and self-serving changes purportedly representing the views and findings of the French authors.[20]

However, because the Pasteur scientists admitted that they may have seen the galley proofs for the article with Gallo's insertions and raised no objections to them, ORI declined to find that Gallo had committed scientific misconduct with respect to such conduct. Nonetheless, ORI found that such "actions reflect Dr. Gallo's propensity to misrepresent and mislead in favor of his own research findings or hypotheses" and asserted that such conduct warranted censure, although it did not rise to the level of scientific misconduct (ORI 1989, 53).[21]

The Violation of Human-Subjects Regulations

All U.S. institutions that receive federal funding to conduct research involving human subjects or that conduct research regulated by the Food and Drug Administration must comply with federal regulations protecting such subjects. Institutions file an assurance that they have a method for assuring the protection of research subjects, both human and animal, in DHHS-sponsored research. Federal regulations require that each research institution have an institutional review board (IRB). The IRB reviews the proposed research for scientific merit and ensures that all human subjects participating in such research are aware of and consent to the procedures they will undergo and, if they are patients, how those procedures differ from usual therapies and the risks and benefits of the proposed study. The PHS agency involved in cases involving human-subjects violations is the Office for Protection from Research Risks (OPRR).[22]

OPRR determines the applicability of the human-subjects regulations and oversees adherence to those regulations (U.S. Code of Federal Regulations, title 45, part 46). When allegations of noncompliance are made, the institution is directed to conduct an inquiry, investigate, report to OPRR, and provide OPRR with all information related to the allegations. OPRR reviews the institutional findings and makes its findings, and it may also conduct its own investigation. OPRR focuses on institutional responses and education during its review. When repeated violations are discovered, OPRR may suspend or restrict an institution's assurance and thereby preclude or limit the institution from conducting biomedical research involving human subjects.

ORI does not assert jurisdiction over cases involving solely violations of regulations governing human or animal protection and thus does not make a separate finding of scientific misconduct based solely on a breach of those regulations. Further, OPRR does not define violations of regulations governing human or animal subjects research to be scientific misconduct. However, NSF has deemed the violation of federal regulations involving human subjects a serious deviation under its definition of scientific misconduct and has made a finding of scientific misconduct based on such violations.[23] Further, violation of regulations for protection of human subjects may constitute scientific misconduct in the misconduct models used by other countries. For example, violations of human-subjects regulations would constitute scientific misconduct under the British, Canadian, and Danish models.

Publication provides recognition of the validity and importance of research and gives recognition to the researcher. Publishers have debated the propriety of publishing research conducted in violation of human-subjects regulations. For example, publishers have debated whether data collected from the Nazi hypothermia experiments should be published. The Helsinki Declaration (1964), which has served to guide many national laws and regulations on human-subjects research, states that "reports of experimentation not in accordance with the principles laid down in this Declaration should not be accepted for publication." However, OPRR does not notify publishers when it discovers that research has been conducted in violation of ethical standards. Thus, whether research conducted in violation of ethical standards should be published or corrected is left to the institution to address.

Conclusions

Misconduct in biomedical publication by a researcher, whether scientific misconduct or some other violation of research regulations or ethical principles, raises ethical and policy issues for the institution that employs the researcher, for co-authors, and for publishers. Moreover, such misconduct can initiate a variety of processes within the institution, courts, and federal agencies. Despite the existence of federal schemes, because of limitations in the definition of research misconduct, jurisdiction, resources, and the judicial and administrative processes used, it is apparent that federal governments will play an extremely limited role in establishing and enforcing ethical norms within the scientific community. For example, although the U.S. federal definitions of research misconduct capture many more ethical breaches than the definitions used in other countries, they do not address repetitive publication, conflicts of interest, and often research conducted in violation of international guidelines on human subjects. Federal schemes may still sensitize and educate institutions and professional societies about ethical breaches in the scientific community and may encourage the development of policies and procedures. Ultimately, it seems that it will be left to institutions and professional societies to create an environment that encourages ethical practices in biomedical research and publication.

Editors' note: While this book was in press, a proposal for a new U.S. policy on research misconduct was under consideration. Part of that proposal called for shifting the authority to conduct investigations of scientific misconduct from ORI to OIG. In October 1999, the DHHS Secretary accepted this recommendation, but the change had not been formalized in regulations. See note on p. xiv for more information about the proposed policy.

Notes

1. Registration and notice are required for federal statutory protection of works created before 1978, although common-law copyright protection (i.e., protection accorded by state statutes) existed in such works until they were published (i.e., placed on sale, sold, or publicly distributed).

2. For example, copyright registration creates a presumption of copyright validity, entitles one to bring suit in federal court for copyright infringement, and entitles an author to reap certain statutory damages and attorneys' fees in a subsequent action that must be brought. Further, although notice of copyright protection is not required, if such notice is affixed to a work, the defense of innocent infringement is not available to a person infringing on the work.

3. As of November 1996, 119 "States," as understood in the international sense, were parties to the Berne Convention. Many intellectual property treaties are administered by the World Intellectual Property Organization (WIPO), an intergovernmental organization that is responsible for the promotion of the protection of intellectual property throughout the world and the administration of multilateral treaties addressing the legal and administrative aspects of intellectual property.

4. See the British response to research misconduct which, because no inspectorate exists and because industry has had most of the cases thus far, has been based

on referrals by the Association of the British Pharmaceutical Industry to the General Medical Council (Lock and Wells 1996).

5. Federal responses to the problem have been developed in the United States, Denmark, Australia, Norway, and Finland. The Danish system is administered by the Danish Committee on Scientific Dishonesty and Good Scientific Practice (DCSD). The Norwegian Research Council has established a national committee. Finland has a decentralized system under which the Finnish National Research Ethics Committee serves as an appellate body. In 1990, the Australian National Health and Medical Research Council passed a set of guidelines and procedures that had to be implemented by 1992 by all institutions applying for grants. In Canada, the Tri-Council, comprising the Medical Research Council of Canada, the Natural Sciences and Engineering Research Council of Canada, and the Social Sciences and Humanities Research Council of Canada, has encouraged universities and institutions to develop specific guidelines that address "research integrity issues." See Korst and Axelsen (1996) for a discussion of scientific misconduct experiences and developments in other countries.

6. Parrish (1994) explored the effects of different agency definitions on scientific misconduct cases and reviewed plagiarism cases that resulted in agency findings of scientific misconduct.

7. ORI was established in 1992. Before 1989 scientific misconduct cases were investigated by individual PHS agencies. In 1989, the Office of Scientific Integrity (OSI), organizationally located in the National Institutes of Health (NIH), and the Office of Scientific Integrity Review (OSIR), organizationally located in the Office of the Assistant Secretary of Health, were created to address PHS scientific misconduct cases. In 1992, OSI and OSIR were abolished and merged into ORI.

8. A similar sanction has been imposed against researchers in the United Kingdom. Of the 16 cases resulting in a finding of research fraud in the United Kingdom, nine of the doctors were removed from the medical register and thereby debarred from practice, three were suspended for a period between six and 12 months, and four were admonished (Lock and Wells 1996).

9. As of the publication of this book, NSF has not had a scientific misconduct hearing, although such hearings are available under the NSF model.

10. The VEA executed by G. Yuan, for example, states that the agreement was entered "based on allegations of Fox Chase Cancer Center." This document is available from the U.S. Department of Health and Human Services (DHHS) through the Freedom of Information Act.

11. The panel is created in accordance with the Research Integrity Adjudications Panel Guidelines. Under those guidelines, a three-person panel generally is drawn from a group of attorneys at the DAB. A scientist may be appointed to the three-person panel if one is requested by ORI or the accused scientist. See Parrish (1997) for a more detailed discussion of the nature of this panel. Under the Danish system, a similar panel, which has three members and three substitutes, is estab-

lished, with a significant distinction being that two of the members and two of the substitutes must be active researchers.

12. The copyright owner is the individual or entity who, with respect to a copyrighted work, generally has the exclusive right to make copies and distribute the work. Thus, simply providing attribution is not sufficient to preclude a copyright infringement action.

13. This claim becomes complicated if the work generated was a *work for hire* (i.e., the work was generated by an employee or contractor within the scope of his or her employment or contract). In the work-for-hire situation, the employer or body commissioning the work is deemed the author.

14. See also *Dodd v. Fort Smith Special School Dist. No. 100,* 666 F. Supp. 1278 (W. D. Ark. 1987), a case involving a work prepared by a teacher and her students, which was edited by another, with substantial new material included. The editor did not note the contribution of the teacher and students, and the court found a Lanham Act violation, noting that false attribution of even partial authorship is actionable.

15. For a discussion of the incidence of such practice and whether dental researchers considered such conduct scientific misconduct, see Bebeau and Davis (1996).

16. Such a claim was unsuccessfully asserted in *United States ex rel. Berge v. University of Alabama,* 104 F.3d 1453 (4th Cir., 1997), cert. denied 118 S. Ct. 301.

17. The *Journal of Histochemistry and Cytochemistry* published the accusation of plagiarism, the rebuttal, and an editorial, leaving it to the readers to make their own determinations regarding whether plagiarism had occurred (Thoolen 1990; Anderson 1991).

18. For example, see the Voluntary Settlement Agreement of Dr. G. August. This document is available from DHHS through the Freedom of Information Act.

19. See NSF OIG Semiannual Report 15 (OIG 1996, 37, 42) and NSF cases 91-04 and 93-06. Documents pertaining to these cases are available from NSF through the Freedom of Information Act.

20. Offer of Proof of the Office of Research Integrity, filed *In re R. C. Gallo, M.D.,* DAB Docket No. A-93-91, at 3. This document is available from DAB through the Freedom of Information Act.

21. ORI had made a scientific misconduct finding based on other conduct by Gallo, but ultimately retracted that finding after procedural rulings by the DAB. This document is available from the DAB through the Freedom of Information Act.

22. In cases involving abuse of human subjects in PHS-funded research, ORI defers to OPRR, although concurrent jurisdiction may exist (e.g., if an individual sponsored by PHS funds fabricated consent forms). However, because the foci of the agencies differ, each agency's final report and required corrective action may differ.

23. For example, see NSF case 92-05, finding scientific misconduct based on a

researcher's failure to obtain informed consent and pay study participants. This case is available from NSF through the Freedom of Information Act. In fact, until May 1991, the NSF definition of scientific misconduct explicitly included material failure to comply with federal requirements for protection of human subjects. That portion of the NSF definition was dropped because it was deemed unnecessary in light of the *other serious deviation* prong of the NSF definition.

References

Anderson, P. J. 1991. The road to publication is sometimes paved with bad intentions. *Journal of Histochemistry and Cytochemistry* 39:379.

Association of American Medical Colleges (AAMC), Ad Hoc Committee on Misconduct and Conflict of Interest in Research. 1992. *Beyond the "framework": Institutional considerations in managing allegations of misconduct in research.* Washington, D.C.: Association of American Medical Colleges.

Bebeau, M. J., and E. L. Davis. 1996. Survey of ethical issues in dental research. *Journal of Dental Research* 75:845–55.

Bersoff, D. N. 1996. Process and procedures for dealing with misconduct: A necessity or a nightmare? *Journal of Dental Research* 75:836–40.

Danish Committee on Scientific Dishonesty (DCSD). 1996. Appendix 1: Statutes. In *The Danish Committee on Scientific Dishonesty: Annual report 1995.* Copenhagen: Danish Research Councils. See also http://www.forskraad.dk/publ/rap-uk/kap12.html. Site accessed 31 March 1999.

Day, K. 1996. Patents and peer pressures: Two firms' legal fight may shake a mainstay of scientific research. *Washington Post,* 19 April.

Departmental Appeals Board (DAB), Department of Health and Human Services. 1991. Decision No. 1232 (7 March). http://waisgate/hhs.gov/cgi-bin/waisgate?WAISdocID=965343858+0+0+0&WAISaction=retrieve. Site accessed 17 March 1999.

Hallum, J. V., and S. W. Hadley. 1991. Rights to due process in instances of possible scientific misconduct. *Endocrinology* 128:643–44.

Helsinki Declaration. 1964. (Adopted by the 18th World Medical Assembly in 1964 and amended by the 29th World Medical Assembly in 1975, the 35th World Medical Assembly in 1983, and the 41st World Medical Assembly in 1989.) http://ethics.cwru.edu/research_ethics/helsinki.html. Site accessed 31 March 1999.

International Committee of Medical Journal Editors (ICMJE). 1988. Retraction of research findings. *Annals of Internal Medicine* 108:304.

——. 1997. Uniform requirements for manuscripts submitted to biomedical journals. *Annals of Internal Medicine* 126:36–47. See also http://www.acponline.org/journals/resource.unifreqr.htm. Site accessed 5 February 1999.

Korst, M., and N. Axelsen. 1996. International developments. Chap. 6 in *The*

Danish Committee on Scientific Dishonesty: Annual report 1995. Copenhagen: Danish Research Councils. See also http://www.forskraad.dk/publ/rap-uk/kap09.html. Site accessed 17 February 1999.

Lock, S., and F. Wells, eds. 1996. *Fraud and misconduct in medical research.* 2d ed. London: BMJ Publishing Group.

Marshall, E. 1995a. Peer review: Written and unwritten rules. *Science* 270:1912.

——. 1995b. Suit alleges misuse of peer review. *Science* 270:1912–14.

National Health and Medical Research Council (NHMRC). 1997. Joint NHMRC/AVCC statement and guidelines on research practice. http://www.health.gov.au/nhmrc/research/nhmrcavc.htm. Site accessed 31 March 1999.

Nimmer, M. B. 1963. *Nimmer on copyright.* New York: Matthew Bender.

Office of Inspector General (OIG), National Science Foundation. 1994. Semiannual report to the Congress. No. 10. October 1, 1993–March 31, 1994. http://www.nsf.gov/cgi-bin/getpub?oig10. Site accessed 13 July 1999.

——. 1996. Semiannual report to the Congress. No. 15. April 1, 1996–September 30, 1996. http://www.nsf.gov/cgi-bin/getpub?oig15. Site accessed 13 July 1999.

Office of Research Integrity (ORI). 1989. Final report National Cancer Institute, ORI 89–67. To obtain a copy of this report, contact the Office of Research Integrity, 5515 Security Lane, Suite 700, Rockville, MD 20852. Telephone 301–443–5300; fax 301–443–5351.

——. 1994. *ORI Newsletter* 3(December):3. See also http://ori.dhhs.gov/newsltrs.htm. Site accessed 11 July 1999.

Olswang, S. G., and B. A. Lee. 1984. Scientific misconduct: Institutional procedures and due process considerations. *Journal of College and University Law* 11:51–63.

Parrish, D. 1994. Scientific misconduct and the plagiarism cases. *Journal of College and University Law* 21:517–54.

——. 1997. Improving the scientific misconduct hearing process. *JAMA* 277:1315–19.

——. 1999. Scientific misconduct and correcting the scientific literature. *Academic Medicine* 74:221–30.

Policy on scientific misconduct. 1996. *International Journal of Radiation Oncology, Biology, Physics* 35:4.

Royal College of Physicians (RCP). 1991. *Fraud and misconduct in medical research: Causes, investigation, and prevention.* London: Royal College of Physicians.

Thoolen, B. 1990. BrdUrd labeling of S-phase cells in testes and small intestine of mice, using microwave irradiation for immunogold-silver staining: An immunocytochemical study. *Journal of Histochemistry and Cytochemistry* 38:267–73.

U.S. Code. http://www4.law.cornell.edu/uscode. Site accessed 31 March 1999.

Wilson, W. 1996. Immunex agrees to settle suit on patent issues. *Seattle Post Intelligencer,* 31 October, B5.

Scientific Misconduct

9

Policy Issues

C. K. Gunsalus

> Questions of ethics almost invariably involve the publishing process,
> directly or indirectly.
>
> Preface to *Ethics and Policy in Scientific Publication* (*CBE* 1990)

It is hard to find a scholar who has not experienced some violation at the hands of others with respect to publication, whether through outright plagiarism, unauthorized addition to or omission from a list of authors, omission of acknowledgment or attribution, or unfair treatment at the hands of anonymous peer reviewers. Given the importance of these issues to careers and reputations, feelings about these incidents run strong and deep. If unresolved, disputes can become acrimonious and divisive.

The tools to resolve these problems are disparate: minor breaches of professional etiquette may call for mediation or sensitive complaint handling, whereas major transgressions require strong procedures for responding to allegations of misconduct. In all of these situations, the fundamental value at stake is whether the information presented through the peer-reviewed literature accurately represents results from work performed and is correctly credited. Underlying this idea are some central issues, including the standards of conduct community members expect of themselves and each other. Are there any such standards, whether written or unwritten? Should there be? How should the academic community respond to breaches of commonly understood norms of behavior? What response should be given to actions that erode trust in the foundation of the research enterprise, the archival literature?

Despite their apparent prevalence, their centrality to the integrity of the scientific literature, and the strength of feelings they generate, the scientific community does not seem much inclined to address publication improprieties in an organized way. Proposed standards generate reactions ranging from distaste to outright rejection. Further, because there is no one place to find the policies that govern good practice or the rules that apply when an individual scientist has a question or problem, multiple sources must be consulted. These include the policies of each of the many institutional participants in the research system: the sponsors of research, scholarly journals, professional societies, and the universities and other institutions where research is conducted.

One of the most common publication problems involves collaborators who have differing ideas about authorship credit and priority. Problems of this nature often first come to attention within the institution where the work was performed and are voiced by a junior member of the research team.

> Tim Prentice, a graduate student in the laboratory of Dr. Important, stops in to see the graduate studies advisor in his department, Dr. Wise, asking questions about authorship. Prentice is worried that Important is planning to take first authorship on a manuscript Prentice is developing from a chapter in his thesis. He has heard from other students in the laboratory that without consultation Important has been known to change the order of authors on manuscripts—and sometimes to add or delete names—between development of the final draft and publication. Because Prentice is on track to receive his doctorate at the end of the semester and has been interviewing for postdoctoral positions, he is anxious to get full credit for his work, which he plans to submit to the most prestigious journal in his field.
>
> Wise should have a variety of materials at her disposal if the university and Wise have both done their jobs: the authorship statements put out by the major journals in the field, including those of the International Committee of Medical Journal Editors (ICMJE) (1997); the ethics statement from the primary disciplinary society of most members of Prentice's department (Friedman 1993); a statement on responsible authorship practices adopted or developed by the university; a statement on relationships between graduate students and advisors (including how students may seek mediation of disputes before lodging grievances); and a bibliography on the ethics of authorship and publication.

In pursuing this conversation, Wise knows that, aside from the questions of who can be an author and who makes this decision, there are other core issues here:

- How are priority and order of authorship established? By whom?
- When can a participant in a project be removed from or demoted in authorship credit (that is, dropped from the list of authors entirely or moved later in the list)? When may a name be added?

- How are the applicable rules in a given situation discerned and communicated?
- How are disciplinary standards developed and communicated? How much idiosyncrasy is or should be tolerated in deviations from such standards?
- Where can a participant go for guidance or redress when he or she is concerned that publication practices are unfair or improper?

Before examining how this case unfolds, consider the purpose of the various policies we hope Wise has collected to use as the basis for her response to Prentice's questions.

The Purpose of Policy: Consider the Source
The Sponsor of Research

A government agency or private organization that sponsors research has one overriding interest when it issues a policy on scientific misconduct: assuring accountability. Recent debate over accountability for research mirrors in some important ways the historical development of regulations governing the use of human subjects in research in the United States. In 1968, congressional hearings were convened to decide whether to establish a national commission on human experimentation and medical ethics. The scientific community protested this governmental intrusion, one witness going so far as to predict that the proposed step would so impede research progress that the American biomedical research community would fall far behind its peers and "never catch up" (U.S. Senate 1968, 70).[1] Nevertheless, Congress persisted, and the resulting commissions—the National Commission for the Protection of Human Subjects of Biomedical and Behavioral Research (1974) and the President's Commission for the Study of Ethical Problems in Medicine (1978)—eventually led to federal regulation of human subjects in research. However, issues surrounding the use of human subjects in research have continued to attract public attention, and the National Bioethics Advisory Commission has been formed to examine the evolution of standards and concepts of patient autonomy. These developments suggest that the rules will probably never be static and that continual reexamination may be more the norm than the exception.

The history of the regulations governing the protection of human subjects also suggests that the disinclination of a profession to regulate itself in the face of violations leads to external intervention. The debate on scientific misconduct echoes the earlier debate and shows a reluctance of the scientific community to police itself. When concerns about scientific misconduct began to be aired in the media, scientists argued that only they knew enough to make decisions about the responsible conduct of research; lawmakers, however, disagreed. Thus, in 1985, Congress mandated that federal regulations be developed to address allegations of scientific misconduct. The research community is often still resistant to regulations concerning research misconduct, and arguments persist over federal jurisdiction, the definition of scientific misconduct, and investigative procedures.

The Commission on Research Integrity (CRI) was mandated by Congress in the annual process of reauthorizing National Institutes of Health (NIH) funding, in the NIH Revitalization Act of 1993. Known as the Ryan Commission, after its chair, Professor Kenneth J. Ryan of Harvard Medical School, it was directed to advise the secretary of the Department of Health and Human Services (DHHS) and the Congress about ways to improve the Public Health Service (PHS) response to misconduct in biomedical and behavioral research receiving PHS funding. The Ryan Commission (CRI 1995, sec. B.1.a.) described carefully what it saw as the government's interest in this area:

> The Federal Government's interest in research misconduct stems from its funding of research and, in the biomedical sphere, its interest in the collective health of the citizenry. . . .
>
> A federal research agency must refuse to fund researchers who have engaged in certain actions, or deny them participation as reviewers, or place conditions on their applying for or using its funds. A research misconduct regulation enables the Federal Government to take such actions when research-related misconduct occurs in connection with proposals and awards.

Almost four years later, the Office of Science and Technology Policy (OSTP) released a new proposed federal definition of research misconduct. It defined the scope of the federal interest much more restrictively as "the accuracy and reliability of the research record and the processes involved in its development" (OSTP 1999).

Just as no sponsor can assure that a grant or contract will yield discoveries or a specific desired outcome, but only that the effort is expended as promised, neither can a policy on misconduct prevent a problem from arising. What a well-conceived policy can do is to provide a framework for accountability by defining the misconduct it will take action against and stating how allegations are to be assessed and investigated and the results reported. In this way, the sponsor puts on notice all those who supply—and receive—its funding that it takes seriously its role in the creation and dissemination of new knowledge. Because a sponsor's interest is largely in accountability for its funding and the validity of work performed with its funding, few maintain policies on relatively minor transgressions. Those they leave to the other institutional participants, journals, professional societies, and universities.

Some research sponsors maintain their own investigative functions for responding to the most serious transgressions. For example, some of the science agencies of the U.S. government have such large budgets and scope that they maintain in-house staff to perform investigations. Although these agencies have the force of law behind them, they still cannot directly investigate every allegation of scientific wrongdoing they receive. They are usually distant from the site of the research and, even with their large budgets, do not have sufficient resources for that purpose. Thus, their policies must describe when they take direct responsibility for investigating allegations and when instead they refer problems to the home institutions of the researchers for investigation and response back to the agency. For those circumstances, the policy must define how the agency will assess those responses, the procedures it expects (and will follow itself), and the standard of proof against which evidence is to be assessed when cases are judged.

Outside the United States, the Danish Committee on Scientific Dishonesty (DCSD), established by the Danish Medical Research Council, has the most far-reaching statement (Riis and Anderson 1996). That committee focuses on scientific dishonesty, which it defines relatively broadly compared to the definitions in use in the United States (Andersen and Brydensholt 1996). It currently has few, if any, counterparts elsewhere in the world.

Prentice consults the "Instructions for Authors" of the journal to which he plans to submit his manuscript. The standards of the ICMJE have been adopted by the journal, and they require an author to have contributed substantially to the following phases of article development: "conception and design, or analysis and interpretation of data; drafting the article or revising it critically for important intellectual content; and final approval of the version to be published." When he reads this, Prentice feels that he is right to be uneasy. Important has not had much time for him; in fact, Prentice and Important have not met to discuss the results in some months. Most of Prentice's meetings have been with the senior postdoc in the laboratory.

Journals

Journals work at the other end of the spectrum from sponsors of research, after at least some portion of the research project is complete. Because their concerns center on the importance and rigor of work submitted for publication, journals have little choice but to address—at least at some level—the less serious problems sponsors prefer to avoid.

A journal's policies must inform authors of its standards and expectations, set out what it seeks from reviewers, and inform readers about what they may expect from the journal and its editors. Thus, a sensible scientific journal adopts policies on authorship (defining which contributions merit authorship status); disclosure of potential conflicts of interest by reviewers and authors (so authors know what to expect from the review process and readers have a context in which to evaluate articles); rebuttals (defining under what conditions and with what evidence they are published); retractions (delineating whether they must be made by an original author or by all authors and what to do if the results of an institutional investigation discredit the research but the researcher persists in defending it); and how it responds to complaints about authorship and allegations of serious misconduct (whether it takes any action at all, declines to publish work by the author under some circumstances, or refers the matter to the home institution of the researcher). As a condition of submission of a manuscript, some journals also require authors to agree to make their data available for review if questions about them arise (Instructions for authors 1998).[2]

Journal editors are not well placed to resolve authorship disputes or to investigate allegations of scientific misconduct because reviewers and authors usually do not have an employment relationship with the journal, the contractual relationship that does exist may be quite limited in scope, and few if any journals have the resources to perform investigations at distant sites. Thus, journals and most sponsors of research are dependent upon the institutions where research is conducted to perform investigations. However, the journal may have significant leverage over the institution, which it should not hesitate to use. Further, the policies of journals in which scientists hope to publish their work—especially the most selective and prestigious journals—have enormous influence over ethical standards of conduct.

To determine whether specific conduct is ethical or has perhaps crossed a line, consultation with the ethical standards of the individual's discipline is essential. The most straightforward way to discern those standards is in a code of ethics from a disciplinary society or association.

When Prentice reads his professional society's code of ethics, he finds good news and bad news. His society is one of the majority (according to a 1994 study [Jorgensen

1995], 58% of scientific societies had adopted codes of ethics) that has developed an ethical code. But when he read the section on the ethics of authorship, he found it somewhat dissatisfying. It merely said that, to qualify for authorship, a researcher must have contributed "significantly and meaningfully" to the work in question. No further guidance is available. Prentice does not know whether providing the financial support for his work—his perception of Important's contribution—meets this standard or how he can find out whether it does.

Professional Societies

Academicians commonly belong to a community of scholars who study similar problems or use similar tools. Professional societies, if they have policies or a code of ethics for members, usually intend them to be aspirational statements of correct ethical conduct in that discipline, unless the field is one where professional licensure or certification is required. The vast majority of scientific disciplines do not require licensure, however, and enforcement of aspirational codes of ethics has proven problematic for a variety of reasons, including fear of legal liabilities and the absence of a contractual or employment relationship with members. As a result, professional societies rarely consider or take action on even the most serious charges against their members, let alone violations of professional etiquette or good practice (Gardner 1996).

Yet there is great value in the development and promulgation of codes of ethics by professional societies because they provide clear standards both for encouraging appropriate professional conduct and for judging deviations from accepted ethical standards. Their value is only amplified by the diversity of the research community and the absence of widely applicable standards. Broad ethical maxims apply across the range of scientific specialties, but particulars of ethical conduct vary (sometimes widely), depending upon the nature of the discipline. Thus, a statement of the parameters of responsible conduct within the professional community carries great weight.

Wise gives Prentice sensible advice about how to pursue a professional conflict from a position of relatively little power (Gunsalus 1998a). Wise sends Prentice to consult with Dr. Grand, the most senior person available who is approachable, known to keep confidences, and knowledgeable in Important's area of specialization. Grand points out that Prentice's concerns are premature; thus far, he doesn't know how—or even if—the authorship will be changed. He also talks with Prentice about Important's related lines of research, his designation of the problem, and his total funding of Prentice's work.

Prentice acknowledges these factors but insists that the ideas in the final research are largely his own and that he performed all of the work. Grand advises Prentice to assemble documentation as to the originality of his work and his sense that Important has not been much involved in it. Meanwhile, Grand promises to convene, with the assistance of the departmental librarian and a faculty member with expertise in publication and research ethics, a department-wide symposium on the discipline's authorship standards. He tells Prentice he had been meaning to do this anyway, and it may help in the present situation. After reflection, Grand decides to ask Important to make a few remarks at the event. Prentice accepts Grand's advice and adopts a wait-and-see attitude.

The Research Institution

A university or institution where research is performed (whether or not the research is externally sponsored) has broader interests than the sponsor, the publisher of research, or the professional society of the researcher. The university is the employer of professionals for whom it must set and enforce standards of conduct. This alone confers responsibility above and beyond that derived from financial support or publication of research. More importantly, the university is responsible for the education of its students, including ethical grounding for their future careers. Where students are participating in the research as part of their education, scientific misconduct can damage not only the institution's reputation and those depending on the results of research, but also those students. Thus, while a university must have a policy on responding to allegations of misconduct and must take disciplinary action for proven violations, even more fundamental are policies and educational programs that promote integrity in research.

These policies should set high standards for ethical conduct, higher than the bare minimum standard of avoiding charges of misconduct. They should include ways to respond when the conduct of individuals within the university's community does not meet those standards. Topics addressed should include guidelines for recording and retaining data, mentoring and authorship practices, compliance with research regulations (including the ethical treatment of human and animal subjects), and, most of all, the responsibilities conferred by and corollary to the rights of academic freedom.

Prentice soon learns from the departmental secretary (whom he dates) that the chapter from his thesis, now a single-authored publication by Important, has been submitted to the journal and has come back with reviewers' comments. Prentice returns immediately to Grand, who, after a review of all the materials Prentice has assembled, agrees that sections of the manuscript are taken virtually verbatim from the thesis and that this raises serious questions about the proposed authorship. He suggests that he and Prentice meet jointly with Important to discuss the situation. Prentice, with some trepidation but driven by his concern for credit for his work, agrees.

For responding to the problems that will arise, the university should have a system for training those who receive complaints and questions about conduct (including advisers like Wise) (Gunsalus 1998b), well-crafted grievance procedures, and a carefully drawn policy for responding to allegations of misconduct. Those interested in the details of institutional procedures for responding to allegations of misconduct are referred to other sources, including the guidance documents issued by the Association of American Universities (1988), the Association of American Medical Colleges (1992), the American Association for the Advancement of Science (Gunsalus 1997), the Office of Research Integrity (ORI) (1995), and other reports of the U.S. government (Gunsalus 1993; CRI 1995). The most critical elements of such procedures are provisions for protecting the rights of both complainant and accused while assuring a rigorous analysis based upon relevant facts. With respect to the complainant, the procedure must include prohibitions against retaliation, and the institution must enforce these prohibitions. For the accused (often referred to as the respondent to avoid the overtones of criminal law), the provisions must ensure an opportunity to examine all evidence and an opportunity to respond to it. Other important features are protections against conflicts of interest that could bias the outcome and separation of the investigation from decision making so that different parties conduct the investigation and then act upon it after reaching a decision (Gunsalus 1993).

In their meeting, Important tells Grand and Prentice that he feels his single authorship is justified. He feels that he did the work represented by the thesis chapter and just "let" Prentice use it in his thesis; that there are other chapters Prentice can use for his own publications; that this is an accepted practice in the field; and, besides that, Important feels that he needs a single-authored publication on this topic right now to shore up his prospects of winning an award for which he knows he is under consideration.

Questions about allocation of credit, especially those between senior and junior members of a research team, are questions most properly handled in the work environment of the scientists, preferably at the lowest possible level. However, juniors are often reluctant to raise the questions for fear of the consequences they may suffer, and peers and colleagues may be disinclined to deal with problems when presented because of a combination of uncertainty as to the correct response and distaste for unpleasant confrontations.

The problems resulting from collaboration are many. Some common scenarios include the following:

- As in the case here, a student wonders whether his major professor can publish a chapter from the student's dissertation as a single-author publication by the professor.
- Two researchers collaborated on a research proposal to an agency that did not result in an award, and one now wonders about the rules governing his resubmission of sections of that proposal to a different agency, without the involvement of the other.
- A project was finished but never written up, and the researcher who did the work has left the institution and cannot be located; the remaining collaborators want to publish the results and wonder how the authorship should be assigned.
- Two collaborators have a falling out and will no longer work together; who has the right to publish what from their collaboration?
- A researcher receives a reprint with a nice note from a former postdoc saying, "Thank you for the wonderful experience." The researcher is listed as an author on the reprint but was never involved in any aspect of the published work.

Allocation of credit is especially problematic when there are significant imbalances of power among the participants, exemplified in collaborations between senior researchers and their subordinates. During the intense period of graduate study, students focused on their own assigned research projects are not always aware of the magnitude of the effort required to sustain a laboratory and its flow of projects. Further, in relationships with an uneven distribution of power and information, misunderstandings are sometimes slow to be addressed and resolved. This is particularly the case when expectations are high and competition is fierce. Current constraints in funding and the very tight job market may exacerbate such problems.

If practices for allocating authorship are not clearly understood, students may come to feel that their contributions are improperly subsumed or inadequately credited. And although students may be slow to raise their concerns, especially if they feel the environment is inhospitable to such questions, the issues are so fundamental and the stakes so high that the problems tend to surface eventually, even if through no other mechanism than the departmental grapevine or rumor mill.

Ombudspersons, department heads, research integrity officers, and grievance deans see many such cases. One difficulty in resolving these cases is that students often do not have a sufficiently broad base of experience and knowledge to differentiate between an exploitative situation and the discomfort of being asked to achieve at a standard higher than their previous work. Tact, finesse, and open discussion are required ingredients for differentiating research misconduct from the many difficult questions that complicate daily interactions, causing friction and malaise.

> After their meeting with Important, Prentice and Grand discuss the matter at length, including the costs to Prentice for pursuing the matter as opposed to letting it go. With permission from Prentice, Grand privately calls the editor of the journal, whom he knows well, for advice. The editor confirms that this is a very serious matter and adds that, not only should it be resolved before publication, but she cannot let publication proceed without assurances that the attribution of authorship conforms to the journal's policies. She is grateful to be alerted before publication that there might be a question, as she mostly receives such concerns after the fact. The editor, while stressing that an examination must occur, has little direct assistance to offer. Although she can (and will, if asked) use her position as leverage to get the institution to initiate a process of examination, she advises that Grand and Prentice may first wish to raise the issue inside the university. Grand and Prentice decide to seek further advice and possible assistance from the campus research integrity officer. There they discuss the most constructive way to proceed. The main choices seem to be making additional efforts to persuade Important to reexamine the authorship of the paper or to file formal charges of plagiarism. At this point, Prentice has not yet brought any charges. His concerns fall into one of the grayest areas of publication ethics: relations between students and their mentors.

Publications that grow out of dissertations represent a special category. Although the dissertation must always be singly authored, the mentor's role in the student's work may be sufficient to support co-authorship of excerpts that are published individually. This practice, however, can lead to serious misunderstandings (and allegations of misconduct) if the principles being applied to authorship decisions are not first sufficiently discussed and understood. Careful reflection upon the standard for these and other assignments of authorship in faculty-student collaboration is always merited.[3]

In the case described here, Prentice is concerned about when Important can or should become the first author on a manuscript being adapted from a chapter of Prentice's thesis. In Prentice's view, Important has not played a very central role in the research, inasmuch as Prentice asserts that Important has not been in the laboratory or discussed data with Prentice in a number of months. Prentice's perception may or may not mirror the reality of his situation accurately. But in a culture that values integrity, there should be some mechanism through which knowledge of the elements of publication can be obtained and advice received when questions arise.

Allegations of Plagiarism: Pitfalls, Problems, and Defenses

Some concerns about attribution of credit become allegations of plagiarism. Despite the central importance of originality in publication for academic environments, responses to these allegations are not always consistent or clear-sighted. As with other issues in the area of publication ethics, one of the fundamental problems is a lack of consensus as to what constitutes plagiarism.

> Before meeting with the campus research integrity officer, Prentice considers whether Important's actions constitute plagiarism. The prevailing applicable U.S. standard for judging conduct stems from the regulations adopted by the National Science Foundation (NSF) and NIH that encompass FFP—falsification or fabrication of data and plagiarism. In this case, plagiarism is the only possible category that will apply, and as we will see, there are significant drawbacks in resorting to this regulation for someone in Prentice's situation.

Although there is no systematic collection of this information, anecdotal evidence suggests that queries about authorship and credit attribution constitute a major portion of the caseload of American university officials who handle research integrity questions. For example, Price (1994) cited annual reports submitted to ORI by research institutions, which indicate the high percentage of formal caseloads devoted to plagiarism. In my personal experience, 70% of the questions brought to me as research standards officer involved attribution of credit. The definition of research misconduct in the United States (that found in the federal regulations for the first decade) did not define plagiarism (DHHS 1989; NSF 1991). Neither did it stipulate whether intent was required or a professional standard of care applied. That is, it did not address whether serious errors of attribution were sanctionable only when the offender omitted the attribution on purpose, meaning to take credit for the work of another, or whether serious carelessness leading to the same result was sufficient cause for a penalty. The Danish Committee on Scientific Dishonesty stands essentially alone in endorsing a standard that equates "deliberate or grossly negligent" acts with intent (Andersen and Brydensholt 1996).

The Ryan Commission recommended that a unified definition for all U.S. government-supported research be embraced, that universities adopt higher standards than those of the government, and that the term *plagiarism* in the current U.S. federal definition of research misconduct be dropped in favor of the broader term *misappropriation*, with a clarifying internal definition, including breach of the confidentiality of the peer-review process. The 1999 OSTP proposal retrieved the use of the word *plagiarism* but provided a definition of it much like that in the Ryan Commission report, including the breach of the peer-review process.

In addition to providing a fuller internal definition of plagiarism, the commission's proposed definition explicitly addressed two issues upon which faculty review panels repeatedly stumble. First, it incorporated within its scope misconduct in reviewing manuscripts or grant applications. Second, it proposed that deviation from a defined standard of professional care in authorship should be sanctionable. Thus, in common with the approach of the DCSD, the proposed definition encompasses both intentional and reckless conduct in authorship to serve as a warning that the carelessness or sloppiness defense for a lack of attribution or citation is not acceptable.

Although the entire Ryan Commission report was controversial, one of its most contentious aspects was the commission's proposed new definition for research misconduct. The National Academy of Sciences (NAS) Council was specifically disapproving of the commission's "expansion of the concept of plagiarism into 'misappropriation'" (Alberts et al. 1996, 3). The Council reendorsed a previous report by the Committee on Science, Engineering, and Public Policy (COSEPUP), based on virtually the same standard. The 1999 OSTP proposal adopted the broader standard, in keeping with the Ryan Commission and COSEPUP reports: "Plagiarism is the appropriation of another person's ideas, processes, results, or words without giving appropriate credit, including those obtained through confidential review of others' research proposals and manuscripts."

Within universities, the situation is equally disparate. In the United States, *student* codes of conduct are often explicit about standards for quotation, attribution, and paraphrasing.[4] *Faculty* codes of conduct (following current definitions of research misconduct) are much less clear. In common with the U.S. governmental agency regulations, they often contain no explanation of plagiarism at all. This lack of clarity leads to constant reconceptualization, as each misconduct committee thus develops its own definition of plagiarism, sometimes citing dictionary definitions or the personal experiences of each panel member. The definitions some committees develop are quite expansive; others are very narrow.

Institutional Responses to Questions of Publication Impropriety

Grand and Prentice's meeting with the university's research integrity officer, Dr. Perry, has some bumpy moments. Perry's first response is one of shock and dismay: "There must be a mistake: I'm sure Dr. Important would never do such a thing!" Prentice asks Perry to examine the documentation, and Perry reluctantly concedes that either Important has improperly approved the chapter of Prentice's thesis (by permitting the inclusion within it of work not done by Prentice) or that he has improperly appropriated sole authorship of the article accepted for publication. Grand explains that the journal editor is prepared to insist that the university examine the question of authorship. Perry agrees that an internal examination is better than official involvement by the journal and offers to talk to Important and then get back to Grand and Prentice.

Perry has a very candid discussion with Important, in which she points out the obvious similarities in the documents and the very serious ramifications of the situation. Emphasizing that Prentice has chosen the most professional way of raising his concerns and that he has not filed formal charges (but could), Perry persuades Important to restore Prentice as a co-author on the article. Perry spends a considerable portion of her interview with Important talking through Important's anger with Prentice and cautioning Important against actions that might be viewed as retaliation against Prentice. When Important retorts that Prentice has not been a very satisfactory student, Perry asks him to explain his own writings extolling Prentice's achievements, including several commendations Important wrote for Prentice, from recommendations for prestigious fellowships to nominations for student accomplishment awards. Important has no reply and instead tells Perry how very busy, overwhelmed, and stressed he has been in recent months.

Perry's job is made significantly easier than it might otherwise be by several factors: involvement by Grand, a respected senior faculty member, which has moderated Prentice's reactions and lent weight to the questions

Prentice is raising; the explicit definition of authorship provided by the journal to which the manuscript was submitted; Perry's own homework into Prentice's file revealing Important's unequivocal statements about the quality of Prentice's work on multiple occasions; and the university's own very clear guidelines about attribution of authorship and about how mentors and their students should interact. This may represent an idealized situation, as there remain many journals and universities that either have no written policies for how to respond to such a situation or do not consider it their problem. As problems accumulate and the value of these tools reveals itself, however, the number of institutions moving in this direction increases.

Preventing or Solving Problems of Publication Impropriety

The old saying has it that an ounce of prevention is worth a pound of cure. Its enduring wisdom is demonstrated in situations of research misconduct, especially in cases of proper conduct in publication. Experience suggests that many authorship or attribution disputes arise from misunderstandings, which emphasizes that early and frequent communication about the basic issues is good practice. Raising questions of credit and attributions before conflicting assumptions have an opportunity to collide represents the colloquial ounce of prevention.

Contrary to some advice, it is not necessarily useful to devise in advance a written contract among collaborators to delineate the nature of contributions and resulting authorship priority. Aside from the difficulties of predicting how the research will proceed and thus who may make the seminal contributions, circumstances over the life of a project may dictate changes that could not be anticipated at the outset. What is more useful is to develop a shared understanding of the applicable principles for the collaboration, particularly among those who have not worked together before. As with many awkward topics, addressing this issue before participants are too deeply committed can forestall many hard feelings later. At the end, another open and candid discussion should be held to allocate contributor credit. Rennie, Yank, and Emanuel (1997, 584) responded to the concern that this process will be too complex by observing that "with practice researchers should become more used to openly discussing and resolving what their contributions have been. The benefits of a better system will outweigh the effort required for such discussions."

Individual Action and Responsibility

When a researcher seeks to assure that his or her conduct in publication is proper, the concept of the *compact with the reader* is key. In scholarly publication, there is a well-understood set of agreements between the reader and the author, with the journal editor in a mediating and reinforcing role. Correct conduct in most, if not all, matters concerning publication can be discerned by consulting the compact with the reader and honoring it.

The core set of understandings forming the compact with the reader in a scientific journal (whatever further disciplinary idiosyncrasies may arise) are that the material presented is original to the authors, it represents work actually performed by the authors, and it was performed as described. The rule is that, wherever the specific publication at issue will deviate from this implicit compact, the reader should be signaled. A short note suffices, however presented.

There are nuances to the compact. For example, the reader brings a different set of expectations to the methods section of a paper than to the presentation of findings and discussion. Thus can be discerned the answer to the self-plagiarism dilemma raised so plaintively: "But I always use the same methods. Must I write the methods section each time from scratch for fear of being accused of self-plagiarism?" The expectation of the reader that the methods section is novel is usually quite low, especially when it is clear from context that the research presented is part of a continuing series of explorations using the same or similar methods. However, in a situation in which there are no other signals to the reader, adding such a signal costs little in words or space and puts the author on solid ground with editors and readers.

Similarly, the compact with the reader can resolve the dilemma of the missing primary author who cannot be located, has become disabled, or has developed personal differences leading to a refusal to communicate or collaborate. This situation can be addressed through a short note (negotiated as appropriate among the funding officer, other authors, and the editor) indicating that the publication is based upon work performed by Dr. John Doe, who was unavailable to participate in preparing or reviewing the manuscript. Alternatively, in some circumstances where primary authorship is warranted and seems desirable despite an inability to secure the individual's permission (e.g., death of the primary author), such authorship can still be awarded, so long as a clarifying note explains the situation. In this case, the footnote reveals that the manuscript was completed posthumously by the named individuals and that the publication occurs with the permission of the heirs.

The compact with the reader can also cut through issues of multidisciplinary collaboration. As a rule, the key to authorship responsibility is the ICMJE statement that "each author should have participated sufficiently in the work to take public responsibility for the content" (ICMJE 1997, 38). For those who protest that they are collaborating with others and that taking responsibility for the entire work is impractical, what is probably indicated is taking note of the compact with the reader and adding a signal to that effect in the publication. In some journals, specifying contributions provides this signal.

Recommendations for Institutions and Journals

The report of the Ryan Commission explored many of the policy issues surrounding publication questions in scientific research. The controversy over those recommendations is one indication that there is little or no consensus in the research community about these issues. The fact is that external standards of accountability are changing. As with medical practice and human-subjects regulations, these standards are moving in a direction that reduces the autonomy of the affected professional community. The transition is painful.

The main question is whether the research community will respond by developing meaningful self-regulation to give external observers confidence that the community is accountable to the public that funds research and to those who rely upon its results. Whether greater consensus will lead to such self-regulation is yet to be seen. Seven specific areas in which leaders of the scientific community, academic institutions, and journal editors might act are education, the formulation of guidelines for responsible conduct, the definition of misconduct, institutional and individual responses to problems, institutional incentives for responsible conduct in publication, confidentiality and university research, and journal policies.

Education

As scientists move through their careers, they develop from being consumers of knowledge as undergraduate students to being producers of knowledge as graduate students and professional researchers. It is the rare student who arrives at college knowing the standards of professional conduct, much less how they apply in an array of circumstances. Unless these standards are addressed explicitly in the course of students' education, how will they acquire that information? The cultural traditions of science have it that students receive this guidance from their mentors in the process of graduate education. The need for increased formality of such training is rooted in the explosive growth of the graduate education system across the United States over the last several decades and is emphasized by recurring questions about the quality of the education students receive on the structure and conduct of research (see chap. 10).

The requirement introduced by NIH in 1992 that institutions holding training grants offer programs in research integrity has spawned a tremendous diversity of materials to support such training efforts. The Ryan Commission recommended that this training requirement be extended to all individuals supported by PHS research funding. Educational efforts are discussed in chapter 10.

Guidelines for Responsible Conduct

A key element of creating a positive environment for research integrity is providing information to the well-intentioned on how to resolve dilemmas relating to professional conduct. Biomedical researchers in corporate settings are subject to many requirements within their research practices, starting with those imposed by lawyers wanting to protect corporate intellectual property. Those involved in businesses that submit data to government agencies for drug or product approval must conform to federal Good Laboratory Practice regulations. Although a similarly elaborate set of regulations for academic research is not advisable or desirable, simple guidelines that provide information about responsible professional practices can be helpful for educational purposes, for establishing a climate of research integrity, and for resolving questions when they arise.

Guidelines might include such topics as the recording and retention of data, authorship and publication practices, and other professional conduct. Whether such guidelines are established institutionally or by professional societies, it makes a great deal of sense to have in place standards to which all conscientious professionals should aspire and to provide positive guidance to researchers who seek such information.

The Definition of Misconduct

A workable definition of research misconduct is required for both the federal government and research institutions. Components of a workable definition include sufficient clarity that peer researchers can apply the definition in institutionally conducted misconduct proceedings and sufficient legal validity that well-based misconduct findings will hold up when challenged in court. Despite the intense controversy and effort expended within the research community since the late 1980s, the evidence suggests that we have not yet arrived at a definition of research misconduct that meets these two standards and the needs of the community.

Institutional and Individual Responses to Problems

Much has been written about institutional responses to allegations of misconduct. The continuing legalization of these processes (as with our society as a whole) is having a profound effect upon institutional regulation of and responses to allegations of scientific misconduct, and this trend is likely to continue. Where it is taking us is not yet clear.

Improved Institutional Responses to Problems. The goal is not to eradicate allegations of misconduct (not a feasible goal in any event), but to assure sufficient expertise and competence in response that public confidence in the conduct of research can be maintained. That is, if the response to an incident of alleged research misconduct is prompt and effective—and if the end result is disclosed when misconduct is found—the public is remarkably accepting. For example, in the unfortunate 1996 incident in the laboratories of Dr. Francis Collins, where a promising junior researcher fabricated results, most of the publicity praised the response of Collins and the University of Michigan for taking the situation seriously, for expeditiously alerting the research community, and for investigating the entire matter thoroughly. Very little of the publicity condemned the laboratory or the university, although questions were raised about why a reviewer would catch an error not caught by supervisors and collaborators. Most of the publicity instead focused upon the betrayal of trust by one from within. In fact, there was significant sympathy for the position in which Collins found himself and regard for his response to the situation.

For the validity and credibility of findings on allegations of scientific misconduct, substantive decisions must be made by scientists of high repute and standing. However, just as scientists must serve in this capacity because they are the experts on scientific matters, they should at all times have access to and support from those with legal and procedural expertise when involved in one of these cases. The training of academic research scientists, however rigorous, cannot fully prepare them for such service. Several national associations and societies have collaborated in developing materials to support procedural rigor, and they should be consulted for assistance in approaching allegations of research misconduct. Too much of the history in this field involves one university after another making the same understandable, but serious, mistakes in administering a misconduct investigation.

Public Disclosure of Findings of Misconduct. Just as we seek expressions of remorse and pledges to do better from rule-breakers in other sectors of our society, so do we want our institutions to behave in a straightforward and forthright manner. In the 1970s and 1980s, universities, often out of fear of legal liability, were known to accept a resignation quietly and allow an individual found to have committed research misconduct to move on. Mallon (1989, 144–93) and Broad and Wade (1982, 38–59) described how recidivist plagiarists moved from institution to institution with impunity, with scant interruption in their prodigious (stolen) output. Dan Greenberg (1988, 4–5), a Washington science journalist and experienced observer of science, observed in commenting upon the harshness of the penalty suffered by one researcher in a celebrated case at Harvard that, "in similar circumstances in past years, violators of scholarly propriety were tolerated or were permitted to go quietly. . . . The misfortune of Harvard's [researcher] was that his derelictions were revealed at a time when the issue of scientific fraud has become politically volatile. It is a safe assumption that in quieter times, the episode would have remained a little secret within the Harvard family."

Whatever the disciplinary disposition within an institution, there is an obligation to correct the archival literature when misconduct in publication has been established. There should be a similar obligation to sister hiring institutions.

Institutional Incentives for Responsible Conduct in Publication

Universities must pay attention to how their own practices affect the conduct of those who perform research under their auspices. This should include the climate created for students and the messages they are receiving about how to succeed as professionals. If the institution provides education about the responsible conduct of research but is conspicuously uninterested in reports of concerns—or, worse, is perceived to punish whistleblowers—perhaps more damage has been done than if the topics were not addressed at all.

Institutions should also attend to the messages that they send through their personnel practices. Is quantity in publication and research rewarded over quality? Do internal mechanisms for quality control function well? Are standards of behavior consistent across the institution? Or are exceptions made for powerful (and well-funded) researchers? Students and other junior researchers will be acutely sensitive to these issues and aware of institutional realities.

Confidentiality and University Research

One of the missions of universities is to create and disseminate knowledge. It follows that the practices adopted by technology transfer offices may have broad ramifications. For example, if implementation of the university's intellectual property policies emphasizes the generation of income through research support or royalties to the detriment of other values (such as peer review or collegial interaction), then the long-term effects may be damaging. If scientific discoveries are announced through press conferences rather than the peer-reviewed literature or if a university routinely accepts prohibitions on publication as a condition of access to materials, then the values of the university are undermined. In the most egregious cases, attempts were made to suppress research results not to the liking of a corporate sponsor (Rennie 1997; Dong et al. 1997). The research community will need to confront these issues directly and take a group stand restricting individual actions that will, in the long run, undermine our system of basic research.

Journal Policies

Good policy in one sector is often similarly good policy in another. Just as it is a positive development for institutions and disciplines to articulate responsible conduct guidelines, so is it for journals. Although some journals have followed the lead of the ICMJE and developed written guidelines for authorship and publication practices, not all have done so. (Of course, even among those that have, not all authors read or comply with the requirements. It is not uncommon, for example, for researchers to acknowledge cheerfully that they forged the signature of collaborators to expedite submission.)

To resolve problems that do arise, journals must have guidelines by which they will respond to allegations and to proven misconduct. The Council of Biology Editors has taken a leadership role in this regard, but further training and consciousness raising seems to be required. Perhaps groups of editors can establish procedures by which journals establish a standard framework for responding to allegations of misconduct, much as universities in the United States have already done. Elements of such procedures might include information on and steps to

- review the facts when they are available to the editors. An example would be to compare manuscripts when plagiarism is alleged to determine at least whether there is an obvious problem on the face of the matter.
- establish a protocol in which the editor's role is clarified. Minimal steps might include a standard practice for referring questions to the home institution of the author, requesting feedback from the institution within a stipulated period, and following up if it is not received.
- ensure that the problems are not compounded by proceeding with publication while questions are unresolved.
- understand differences between plagiarism and copyright.
- be proactive about obligations, having ethical guidelines, codes of conduct, guidelines for authorship, and so forth.
- be prepared to deal with problems through established mechanisms and networks for referral and advice.

One serious policy issue requiring attention from journal editors is running (and indexing) retractions. For example, if an institutional investigation establishes that data do not exist or have been fabricated, the author (especially if advised by an attorney) may refuse to participate in the retraction. Regrettably, authors and institutional officers continue to report that some journals are reluctant to run retractions when submitted by only a subset of authors, by the institution itself, or even at all.

Conclusions

The challenge for those responsible for settings in which research is conducted is to create and maintain an environment that supports ethical choices and makes researchers comfortable with asking questions about those choices. If the well-intentioned have ways to raise their questions and do not feel they will be attacked as ignorant (or worse) for having them, miscommunications will be reduced and goodwill (usually) generated. If permission to explore ethical issues is granted, either implicitly through the culture of the research group or explicitly through direct statements, the myriad disputes that arise in daily life will be more easily resolved and will less frequently grow into larger disputes. Even where conflict over an issue is unavoidable because the participants have irreconcilable views, it is more likely in such settings that the dispute will be resolved without undue damage and hardship.

An open environment—however competitive—in which professional differences can be aired and explored without being made or taken personally is more likely to produce rigorous results. Although it is probably not possible to eradicate disputes when working in heterogeneous settings with multiple participants, it is certainly possible to provide an environment in which differences can be addressed with a minimum of venom and procedural intervention. Further, the skill, compassion, and common sense with which such concerns are met will reverberate in many quarters, underscoring the importance of good procedures and training for the many individuals who may be asked to handle complaints about ethical issues.

Notes

1. "If I am in competition with my colleagues of this country, which I am not . . . then I would welcome such a commission, because it would put the doctors [in the United States] . . . so far behind me, and hamper the group of doctors so much that I will go so far ahead that they will never catch up with me" (U.S. Senate 1968, 70).

2. "All persons listed as authors must meet *all* the following criteria for authorship.

—'I certify that I have participated sufficiently in the work to take public responsibility for the content.

—I certify that (1) I have made substantial contributions to the conception and design or analysis and interpretation of data; and (2) I have made substantial contributions to drafting the article or revising it critically for important intellectual content; and (3) I have given final approval of the version of the article to be published.

—I certify that the manuscript represents valid work and that neither this manuscript nor one with substantially similar content under my authorship has been published or is being considered for publication elsewhere, except as described in an attachment.

—I attest that, if requested by the editors, I will provide the data or will cooperate fully in obtaining and providing the data on which the manuscript is based for examination by the editors or their assignees.'" (Instructions for Authors 1998, 19)

3. For one discipline-specific example, see Fine and Kurdek (1993).

4. I am indebted to Walter Stewart of NIH for this observation. For example, the University of Illinois at Urbana-Champaign's *Code of Policies and Regulations Applying to All Students* (1998, sec. 33.I.D.) defines *plagiarism* as follows (reprinted with permission):

Plagiarism
Representing the words or ideas of another as one's own in any academic endeavor.

Comments:
1. Direct Quotation: Every direct quotation must be identified by quotation marks or by appropriate indentation and must be promptly cited in a citation. Proper citation style for many academic departments is outlined in such manuals as the *MLA Handbook* or K. L. Turabian's *A Manual for Writers of Term Papers, Theses and Dissertations*. These and similar publications are available in the University bookstore or library.

Example: The following is an example of an uncited direct quotation from a case in which the student in question was found guilty of plagiarism.

Original Source: To push the comparison with popular tale and popular romance a bit further, we may note that the measure of artistic triviality of works such as "Sir Degare" or even "Havelok the Dean" is their casualness, their indifference to all but the simplest elements of literary substance. The point is that high genre does not certify art and low genre does not preclude it. (From Robert M. Jordan, *Chaucer and the Shape of Creation*, Howard University Press, 1967, page 187.)

Student Paper: To push the comparison with popular tale and popular romance a bit further, you can note that the measure of artistic triviality in some works of Chaucer's time period is their casualness. Their indifference to all but the simplest elements of literary substance. The point is that high genre does not certify art and low genre does not preclude it.

2. Paraphrase: Prompt acknowledgment is required when material from another source is paraphrased or summarized in whole or in part. This is true even if the student's words differ substantially from those of the source. To acknowledge a paraphrase properly, one might introduce it with a statement such as "To paraphrase Locke's comment . . . " and conclude it with a citation identifying the exact reference. Or the concluding citation might say, "The last paragraph (two paragraphs, etc.) paraphrases statements by . . . " and then give the exact reference. A citation acknowledging only a directly quoted statement does not suffice as an acknowledgment of any preceding or succeeding paraphrased material.

Example: The following is an example of unacknowledged paraphrase that could warrant a charge of plagiarism.

> Original Source: The era in question included three formally declared wars. The decision to enter the War of 1812 was made by Congress after extended debate. Madison made no recommendation in favor of hostilities, though he did marshal a "telling case against England" in his message to Congress of June 1, 1812. The primary impetus to battle, however, seems to have come from a group of "War Hawks" in the legislature. (From W. Taylor Reveley III, "Presidential War-Making: Constitutional Prerogative or Usurpation?" *University of Virginia Law Review,* November 1969, footnotes omitted.)

> Student Paper: During this period three wars were actually declared by Congress. For instance, in 1812 a vehemently pro-war group of legislators persuaded Congress, after much discussion, to make such a declaration, despite the fact that Madison had not asked for it, though, to be sure, he had openly condemned England in his message to Congress of June 1, 1812.

3. Borrowed Facts or Information: Information obtained in one's reading or research that is not common knowledge should be acknowledged. Examples of common knowledge might include the names of leaders of prominent nations, basic scientific laws, etc. Materials that contribute only to one's general understanding of the subject may be acknowledged in the bibliography and need not be immediately cited. One citation is usually sufficient to acknowledge indebtedness when a number of connected sentences in the paper draw their special information from one source.

References

Alberts, B., J. Halpern, P. H. Raven, D. D. Brown, J. E. Dowling, I. M. Singer, and M. F. Dresselhaus, for the Council of the National Academy of Sciences. 1996. Letter to William Raub (March 15). Released by the National Academy of Sciences.

Andersen, D., and H. H. Brydensholt. 1996. The DCSD's opinion of actions which are at variance with good scientific practice and the definition of the DCSD's order of business. Chap. 3 in *The Danish Committee on Scientific Dishonesty: Annual report 1995.* Copenhagen: Danish Research Councils. See also http://www.forskraad.dk:80/publ/rap-uk/kap06.html. Site accessed 17 February 1999.

Association of American Medical Colleges (AAMC), Ad Hoc Committee on Misconduct and Conflict of Interest in Research. 1992. *Beyond the "framework": Institutional considerations in managing allegations of misconduct in research.* Washington, D.C.: Association of American Medical Colleges.

Association of American Universities. 1988. *Framework for institutional policies and procedures to deal with fraud in research*. No. 4. Washington, D.C.: Association of American Universities, National Association of State University and Land-Grant Colleges, Council of Graduate Schools. Reissued 10 November 1989.

Broad, W., and N. Wade. 1982. *Betrayers of the truth: Fraud and deceit in the halls of science*. New York: Simon & Schuster.

Commission on Research Integrity (CRI), Ryan Commission. 1995. *Integrity and misconduct in research: Report of the Commission on Research Integrity to the Secretary of Health and Human Services, the House Committee on Commerce, and the Senate Committee on Labor and Human Resources*. Washington, D.C.: Department of Health and Human Services, Public Health Service. See also http://www.faseb.org/opar/cri.html. Site accessed 17 February 1999.

Council of Biology Editors (CBE), Editorial Policy Committee. 1990. *Ethics and policy in scientific publication*. Bethesda, Md.: Council of Biology Editors.

Dong, B. J., W. W. Hauck, J. G. Gambertoglio, L. Gee, J. R. White, J. L. Bubp, and F. S. Greenspan. 1997. Bioequivalence of generic and brand-name levothyroxine products in the treatment of hypothyroidism. *JAMA* 277:1205–13.

Fine, M. A., and L. A. Kurdek. 1993. Reflections on determining authorship credit and authorship order on faculty-student collaborations. *American Psychologist* 48:1141–47.

Friedman, P. J. 1993. Standards for authorship and publication in academic radiology. Association of University Radiologists' Ad Hoc Committee on Standards for the Responsible Conduct of Research. *Radiology* 189:33–34; *Investigative Radiology* 28:879–81; *AJR American Journal of Roentgenology* 161:899–900.

Gardner, W. 1996. The enforcement of professional ethics by scientific societies. *Professional Ethics* 5:125–38.

Greenberg, D. S. 1988. Panicked about misconduct, Harvard bashes a professor. *Science and Government Report,* 15 December, 4–5.

Gunsalus, C. K. 1993. Institutional structure to ensure research integrity. *Academic Medicine* 68 (suppl to issue 9):S33–38.

———. 1997. Inquiry outline; Investigation outline; Document and data control procedures; Inquiry [casebook]; Investigation [casebook]. In Responding to allegations of research misconduct: Inquiry and investigation, a practicum, sec. III and IV. Presentations at a symposium sponsored by the American Association for the Advancement of Science, 26-28 January, Le Meridien Coronado, San Diego. Duplicated.

———. 1998a. How to blow the whistle and still have a career afterwards. *Science and Engineering Ethics* 4:51–64.

———. 1998b. Preventing the need for whistleblowing: Practical advice for university administrators. *Science and Engineering Ethics* 4:75–94.

Instructions for authors. 1998. *JAMA* 280:19.

International Committee of Medical Journal Editors (ICMJE). 1997. Uniform requirements for manuscripts submitted to biomedical journals. *Annals of Internal Medicine* 126:36–47. See also http://www.acponline.org/journals/resource/unifreqr.htm. Site accessed 17 February 1999.

Jorgensen, A. 1995. *Society policies on ethics issues.* Washington, D.C.: Council of Scientific Society Presidents.

Mallon, T. 1989. *Stolen words: Forays into the origins and ravages of plagiarism.* New York: Ticknor & Fields.

National Science Foundation (NSF). 1991. Misconduct in science and engineering: Final rule. *Federal Register* 56:22286–90.

Office of Research Integrity (ORI). 1995. ORI model policy and procedures for responding to allegations of scientific misconduct. http://ori.dhhs.gov/models.htm. Site accessed 12 July 1999.

Office of Science and Technology Policy (OSTP). 1999. Proposed federal policy on research misconduct to protect the integrity of the research record. http://www.whitehouse.gov/WH/EOP/OSTP/html/9910_20_3.html. Site accessed 19 November 1999.

Price, A. R. 1994. The 1993 ORI/AAAS conference on plagiarism and theft of ideas. *Journal of Information Ethics,* fall, 54–63.

Rennie, D. 1997. Thyroid storm. *JAMA* 277:1238–43.

Rennie, D., V. Yank, and L. Emanuel. 1997. When authorship fails: A proposal to make contributors accountable. *JAMA* 278:579–85.

Riis, P., and D. Andersen. 1996. Authorship and co-authorship. Chap. 2 in *The Danish Committee on Scientific Dishonesty: Annual report 1995.* Copenhagen: Danish Research Councils. See also http://www.forskraad.dk:80/publ/rap-uk/kap05.html. Site accessed 17 February 1999.

University of Illinois at Urbana-Champaign. 1998. Code of policies and regulations applying to all students. http://www.uiuc.edu/admin_manual/code/. Site accessed 17 February 1999.

U.S. Department of Health and Human Services (DHHS). 1989. Responsibility of PHS awardee and applicant institutions for dealing with and reporting possible misconduct in science. 42 CFR part 50: subpart A. http://ori.dhhs.gov/89rule.htm. Site accessed 5 March 1999.

U.S. Senate. 1968. Hearings before the Subcommittee on Government Research of the Committee on Government Operations. *National Commission on Health Science and Society: Hearings on S.J. Res. 145.* 90th Cong., 2d sess. Washington, D.C.: Government Printing Office.

Susan Eastwood

Publication documents the precedence of ideas. It documents the stewardship of research funds. It documents the productivity of scientists, justifies our salaries and our reputations, and allows the cultivation of our egos. But most importantly, it liberates information and knowledge from the imprisonment of chaos and file cabinets to the free access of other scientists and for the betterment of mankind.

Sojka and Mayland (1993)

When reports of misconduct in biomedical science began to reach disturbing numbers during the 1980s, it was still taken for granted that young researchers learned their craft from mentors who guided them in the ethics and complexities of the scientific endeavor. Some scientists denied the existence of a rift in the ethical practice of science (Koshland 1988). Others acknowledged that research institutions had grown so large and diverse that often trainees' relationships with their mentors had become frail, tangential, or even exploitative (Bebeau and Davis 1996; Bloom 1995; Friedman 1990; Namenwirth 1986; National Academy of Sciences [NAS] 1992; Petersdorf 1986; Singer et al. 1993; Watson 1993). A Nobel laureate (Schwartz 1993, 12) noted that most scientists become administrators as they mature and, while they are still called scientists, to a greater or lesser extent they tend to lose touch with research and the people doing it. Few scientists were as bluntly honest as the professor who deplored that his "chief contribution to [his] research is to raise money for it" (Leon Lederman's quest 1991, 153), but that condition was typical of many institutions, and the situation has not changed substantially since.

Compounding senior scientists' administrative responsibilities are swelling demands of regulatory paperwork and increasingly severe competition to find funding for their laboratories. Practicing clinicians who lead investigations have still less time to dedicate to mentoring. There is no doubt that these responsibilities are authentic and necessary to the prog-ress of research, and there is no doubt that they legitimately may stand in the way of senior scientists' fulfilling their role as mentors. Nonetheless, the conviction that a scientific education is best gained in a one-to-one relationship with a mentor (Conley 1993; Larson 1992; Swazey 1993) has been shared persistently by faculty and trainees, even as many such rela-tionships have deteriorated to the extent that faculty regard responsibili-ties such as peer review and the writing of book chapters as independent study opportunities for trainees. Over several generations, research fellows whose mentors were seldom available simply trained one another, at times inadvertently exchanging ignorance and falling into careless research prac-tices. Cumulatively, it may be that more damage is done to science by such ignorance and neglect than by fraud (Bloom 1995; Eastwood et al. 1996; Hamilton 1990; Institute of Medicine [IOM] 1989; Sabine 1985).

In 1989, the Institute of Medicine in the United States observed that trainees gain greater "awareness of the ethical and professional dimensions of research work" when mentoring is supplemented with formal instruc-tion (IOM 1989, 185; Krulwich and Friedman 1993). Shortly afterward, the National Institutes of Health (NIH) responded to U.S. policy makers inves-tigating misconduct in science by requiring institutions that receive Na-tional Research Service Award training grants to provide trainees with in-struction in the responsible conduct of research (NIH 1992). In 1993, NIH recommended that such instruction include all trainees regardless of their source of support (Office of Research Integrity [ORI] 1993). Although there was no mention of a decline in mentorship, a reproach to faculty could be inferred.

The task of infusing ethics into scientific training could have been ap-proached by inducing systemic change, by policing the scientific commu-nity, or through education. Of these, modifying or policing a system as multifaceted as the research enterprise presented formidable obstacles. Only education could afford a realistic potential for sustainable change (Cohen 1995). Of the many approaches research institutions have taken to this task (Alberts and Shine 1994; Bloom 1995; Glazer 1997; Hoshiko 1993; Pollock, Curley, and Lotzová 1995; Taubes 1995a–e; University of Califor-nia, San Francisco [UCSF] 1996), the Survival Skills and Ethics Program at the University of Pittsburgh (Taubes 1995d) is the most comprehensive, pervading the trainee's scientific education.[1] Most institutions have devel-oped less extensive programs that maintain a tight scientific focus, relating research ethics in the context of general guidance about developing and implementing a research proposal. The practice and ethics of scientific writing and publication may occupy as little as one hour in such programs. The focus is usually on publishing your results with an accent on the pressures to publish or perish, peer review, conflict of interest, authorship, and plagiarism. Despite the acknowledged need for lucid written communication in science (Avery 1996; In pursuit of comprehension 1996) and its importance to a successful career, few such programs emphasize the critical reading and writing of research reports, and few speak in detail to the ethical aspects of scientific reporting and publishing that can have professional, ethical, and legal consequences (Taubes 1995c).

The reason for this neglect of such an essential element of professional training lies in the assumption that trainees would not have attained their postdoctoral status without an education in which the development of critical reading and writing skills had the highest priority. Science is a culture with its own conventions and dialects, however, which trainees learn in substantial part from the language spoken during their day-to-day interactions with faculty and the information, messages, and predilections they infer from faculty during informal conversations, at professional meetings, and at social gatherings. This invisible curriculum is as critical to trainees' professional development as is the formal curriculum, particularly in learning to adapt their critical reading and writing skills to the demands of the literature and in learning the rules governing research and publication. To restore the information trainees learned when young researchers served as close apprentices to a mentor, those lessons from the invisible curriculum must somehow be formalized.

If it were possible to restructure graduate education for trainees, courses could be instituted to complement their scientific curriculum with education in the elements of scientific writing, critical reading of the literature, and responsible, ethical research publication. Pragmatically, however, there is little time in a basic-science graduate curriculum and none in a medical school curriculum to provide such courses. Although some postdoctoral training programs in academic institutions have offered such courses, they have tended to wane with reductions in funding and the demands of managed care. Ironically, it is the restrictions those events have placed on institutions that make it all the more crucial for young faculty to be efficient in producing clear, accurate, publishable reports of their work. Without refined development of their reporting skills and knowledge about the publication process, it will be increasingly difficult for current trainees to be promoted and successful in an academic career and correspondingly difficult to encourage them to remain in academic medicine.

This chapter offers a practical, accessible curriculum for postdoctoral trainees who want to publish in English-language journals. The proposed curriculum is intended for trainees who plan to pursue an academic career, whether as clinical or as basic-science investigators. Its purpose is to provide trainees with the tools they need to be ethical investigators who are capable of communicating their work and its importance effectively in writing. The curriculum has two goals:

1. to develop trainees' abilities as skeptical readers, skilled in rapidly making lucid and accurate critical assessments of both published reports and their own written drafts (Bailar 1986; Barry and Rudinow 1990; Cassel and Congleton 1993; Medawar 1981, 62–68); and
2. to permit trainees to sharpen their writing and reporting skills while assimilating information and ethical principles that will serve them in reporting and publishing their work.

A program like that at the University of Pittsburgh may provide an ideal environment for such a curriculum, permitting it to be integrated into the trainees' curriculum and laboratory experience with discussions of ethical issues undertaken whenever applicable (Taubes 1995d). However, the curriculum can readily be adapted to less structured programs in responsible research or can supplement a traditional academic training program.

A Curriculum in Biomedical Reporting and Publication

A curriculum to educate trainees in effective and ethical scientific reporting and publishing must meet particular educational and ethical objectives (table 10.1). For the purposes of this chapter, assume an institution in which this curriculum has been instituted.

The Faculty

The core faculty of the curriculum are scientific and medical educators who teach scientific writing, academic editors who teach in one-to-one consultation with physicians and scientists, and teachers of English as a second language who have specialized in English for scientific or medical purposes. These faculty are experienced in teaching scientific writing and collateral language skills, they are familiar with adult education techniques, and they keep up to date with the conventions and process of

Table 10.1. Objectives of the Curriculum in Effective and Ethical Scientific Reporting and Publishing

Offer the curriculum in such a way that its content is immediately useful to the trainee and is presented in a pragmatically satisfying context when it has the greatest empiric weight.	Foster discussion of the extent to which those values are actually practiced and elicit possible responses trainees may make to ethical choices they may encounter.
Advance the skills trainees require in critical thinking and communication based to the maximum extent possible on trainees' current level of accomplishment.	Address ethical dilemmas and ambiguities that may arise in reporting and publishing.
Convey the values that are conventionally held in the scientific culture.	Provide information and case discussions on aspects of reporting and publishing that have potential ethical, professional, personal, social, legal, or financial consequences for the trainee and others.

publication.[2] To succeed in engaging trainees, the core faculty enlist the frequent participation of junior and senior biomedical faculty, biostatisticians, librarians, and other specialists to provide a curriculum that projects a realistic and integrated experience of the place that writing and publication hold in an academic career (Taubes 1995d). Journal editors on the faculty of the institution promote optimum standards of reporting and publication by participating actively in the curriculum as well.

Principal investigators (PIs) are primarily responsible for assuring that their postdoctoral trainees are equipped to meet the standards required by the institution. They may encourage their trainees to participate in the curriculum and may participate themselves, but participation is voluntary.

The core faculty work collaboratively with PIs to develop an effective critical-reading journal club in their laboratories and to schedule their trainees for writing consultation when the trainees' research papers are prepared. PIs may choose to take a training session in critical reading, which the core faculty offer, and lead the journal club themselves, or they may enlist a member of the core faculty to lead the journal club either permanently or occasionally. Similarly, PIs may participate in the writing tutorials, or they may review the paper when the trainee feels the paper is ready for the PI's scrutiny.

The Curriculum

The curriculum begins with an introductory session during postdoctoral trainees' orientation to the institution (table 10.2). It consists of quarterly panel and discussion sessions with faculty and a series of workshops that combine didactic and interactive learning. The quarterly panel ses-

Table 10.2. Postdoctoral Curriculum in Scientific Reporting and Publication

Program	Topics	Duration
Orientation	Introduction to the Curriculum in Scientific Reporting and Publication	1.5 hours; held during postdoctoral trainees' orientation to the institution
Faculty panel and case discussions on issues related to publication	Successful collaborative authorship	1–3 hours; 1 held each quarter annually
	Conflict of interest	
	Duplicate or repetitive publication	
	Peer review	
Critical-reading journal club		1–1.5-hour sessions held twice monthly
Workshops	Information management and bibliographic databases	1–3 hours each; held monthly or as needed
	Visual presentation of data	
Reporting of research	Reporting basic science research	
	Reporting clinical research, including trials	
	Writing review articles and meta-analyses	
Biomedical publication	Conventions and requirements of biomedical publication	
	The biomedical publication process	
	How to peer review a paper and respond to peer review	
English language	English for basic-science trainees	1–3 hours each; held monthly
	English for clinical trainees	1–3 hours each; held monthly
	English as a second language for scientific purposes	1–2-hour sessions; held twice weekly
Critical-writing tutorials		By appointment

sions include faculty and journal editors from the institution who speak to issues related to publication ethics, such as authorship, conflict of interest, repetitive publication, and peer review. These sessions also include small-group discussions of cases illustrating ethical aspects of the issues addressed. Comprehensive, advanced workshops on topics crucial to trainees' optimum career development are given several times each year.

The panel and discussion sessions and most of the workshops are designed to be relevant to the training of both medical and basic-science postdoctoral trainees. Where their needs differ, specialty workshops are available as well. Trainees are encouraged to attend all workshops irrespective of their apparent relevance to the type of research path they intend to pursue. As research becomes increasingly multidisciplinary and collaborative, the understanding gained from a cross-fertilization of ideas and experience between academic physicians and basic-science researchers can foster innovative translational research. Workshops in the English language are integral to the curriculum. These workshops may be useful to native speakers of English, and they are essential to enfranchise foreign trainees who are invited to work in biomedical laboratories (Committee on Science, Engineering, and Public Policy 1995).

The central features of the curriculum are the adaptation of the journal club, which expressly promotes critical reading in the trainee's discipline, and writing tutorials, which take place while trainees are producing their first papers for submission to a peer-reviewed journal. Although they do not compare with a full curriculum of relevant course work and experience, these in-depth training programs are effective and efficient because they focus finely on trainees' individual problems and specific pitfalls in their critical reading and writing skills. They elicit trainees' interest because they offer sophistication in the process of developing and submitting a paper, and they promote trainees' success at a time when trainees have an urgent personal stake in seeing their papers accepted for publication.

Orientation

Because each institution has a unique character, postdoctoral trainees attend an orientation that reviews the responsibilities, conventions, regulations, and legal obligations governing research and publication by which the institution operates. The orientation acquaints trainees with the institution's standards, policies, procedures, and resources. Postdoctoral trainees are openly told what they can expect of the institution and what the institution expects of them. Equally, the institution acknowledges its responsibility to ensure that each trainee has the knowledge, information, and skills necessary to meet its expectations (Eastwood et al. 1989; NAS 1993).

Trainees are introduced to the curriculum in reporting and publication as a component of the institution's orientation. Highly regarded senior physicians, scientists, and journal editors on the faculty participate in the introduction to project the institution's regard for the importance of this aspect of training (Taubes 1995e). After the concept and design of the curriculum are described, faculty members focus on the research report, first asking, Why write and publish a paper at all? They emphasize that writing the report of research findings is as integral to the research process as are the analysis and interpretation of data because writing the report is instrumental to interpretation of the data, because the report justifies the funding that permitted the work and its continuation, and because scientific convention dictates that the work is not complete until the results are published in the peer-reviewed literature. The faculty articulate the view that investigators who publish their research findings strike a covenant with the reader of their report (see chaps. 1 and 2, on authorship). Where issues related to publication merge with interests related to the institution's policies, as in authorship disputes and conflicts of interest, those issues are discussed to emphasize their gravity. To the maximum extent possible, the introduction is interwoven with references to the history, philosophy, and sociology of science to convey to trainees a sense of the context of their career.

The introduction finally conveys that one goal of the proposed curriculum is to provide a learning milieu in which trainees can come to regard writing their research articles not as a chore, but rather as a contribution needed for science to progress, a step in the evolution of their next study, and a rewarding aspect of the research process. Another goal is to lead trainees to realize that, although the course of peer review and publishing may be difficult and sometimes frustrating, it is a process that usually improves the report of their findings and thereby promotes their continued learning and heightens their professional reputation. The introduction concludes with small-group discussions, in which the senior faculty participate, appraising cases that portray ethical elements of biomedical reporting (Fischbach 1994; Korenman and Shipp 1994).

Faculty Panel and Case Discussions

The faculty panel and case discussions that are held quarterly throughout the year follow a pattern similar to the introduction to the curriculum but focus on one issue or on closely related issues. Each session ends with small-group discussions of cases related to the focal issue, in which senior and junior biomedical faculty participate.

Critical Reading in Biomedical Science

The critical-reading facet of this curriculum consists of one-hour sessions held twice monthly throughout postdoctoral training. Critical reading is the precursor of good writing. The journal club, as modified by Bailar (Taubes 1995c) to promote critical assessment of published papers, is an effective venue for encouraging logical reasoning while developing scientific knowledge and critical reading and writing skills. It is all the more effective for being a familiar component of research training. By adding a focus on skeptical assessment of the paper, the journal club fosters critical and scientific thought and also permits the faculty to address ethical issues related to conducting and reporting research. By reinforcing the principles that distinguish scientific thinking from nonscientific thinking, the faculty help trainees make choices that avoid biased conclusions (Glazer 1997). By adding critical examination of the completeness, accuracy, and effectiveness with which the study and findings are reported, as well as questions regarding rhetorical components, the faculty emphasize the elements of excellence in scientific reporting. By projecting familiar concepts from an oblique perspective, the faculty help trainees realize that ethical dilemmas are frequently covert or ambiguous and alert them to pitfalls in complacent thinking. This learner-centered approach encourages intellectual excitement and promotes the development of logical thought and critical skills more effectively than an inductive method (Brookfield 1987; King and Kitchener 1994). In transmitting ethical concepts it also avoids the pitfalls of a purely case-discussion approach (Hoshiko 1993).

As much as possible, the content of the papers considered during this journal club relates to the trainee's discipline. Each trainee is assigned to draft a critical dissection of one published research report, reviewing articles cited in the report as necessary. Trainees are asked to evaluate the paper in terms of the logical development of a hypothesis or scientific question and a strategy for investigating it, including the appropriateness of the methods to the study design and the rational development of thought in interpreting the data and formulating conclusions. They dissect the paper as a lucid, logically presented communication of scientific findings, a contribution to science, and an ethical construct. They assess the organization of ideas and identify errors, inconsistencies, lapses into sloppiness, hyperbole or other forms of misrepresentation, and even inadvertent humor. They also evaluate whether the visual presentation of data is appropriate, effective, ethical, and sufficiently informative to permit another researcher in the field fully to comprehend the study. Trainees' written critiques are discussed during the journal club. They are also assessed individually by curriculum faculty for all of those elements as well as for the trainees' perception, logical development of the critique, critical assessment skills, and language skills. Those faculty discuss the results of the assessment in a meeting with each trainee.

Workshops

By arrangement among faculty, the workshops in this curriculum intersect as nearly as possible with training related to the responsible conduct of research (NIH 1992). Facets of the curriculum that in particular should intercross the training in responsible research are those related to developing a research protocol and the stages of research synthesis (Cooper and Hedges 1994, 399–409)—problem formulation, study design, and the collection, management, evaluation, analysis, and interpretation of data—as they relate to developing the research report.

Information Management and Bibliographic Databases. This workshop gives specific information about the institution's resources. It also conveys that references are a key to the integrity of any scientific work because they provide for fair and accurate attribution of ideas, support statements or positions that may be considered controversial, and permit readers to consult the original source of ideas and data (Ordway, Eastwood, and Derish 1994). The workshop reviews literature-search strategies, retrieval, and the bibliographic and other information resources available. It also raises ethical issues involving searching and citing the literature, which are similar for original studies, meta-analyses, and reviews. These, for example, are from Sipe and Curlette (1995):

- establishing perimeters of a search (e.g., inclusive years and whether to include primary studies, secondary studies, published work, or unpublished sources)
- selecting key words
- deciding on the language(s) of articles to be searched (e.g., implications of searching English-language articles only)
- selecting sources of references (computerized and prior paper databases; by ancestry, in which new citations are identified from reference lists of documents obtained primarily; personal readings; readings from the "invisible college"; theses; government reports)

- deciding whether a manual search of journals, technical reports, books, and dissertations is conducted
- establishing criteria for inclusion and exclusion of studies from citation

The ethical cornerstones of literature searching include reading original sources in their entirety, respecting the proper attribution of ideas, recognizing the signs of missing or misleading attribution and citation, verifying quotations and derived methods against the original sources, and also verifying accurate citations from the original sources (de Lacey, Record, and Wade 1985; Eichorn and Yankauer 1987; Feinstein and Spitzer 1988; Mundy and Shugar 1992). In some instances, the extent of the search may have an ethical component. An investigator whose search does not include articles indexed in the paper indexes that predate electronic databases may risk repeating research that previously proved futile, wasting resources and even lives (Clark 1988).

Training in techniques for retrieving and evaluating references and the ethics and etiquette of citation can spare young researchers delays in the publication of their work and also embarrassment or a compromised reputation. Readers and journal editors may consider inaccurate references a sufficient reason to question other aspects of a biomedical report. Questions of inadvertent plagiarism aside, inaccurate citations can earn the wrath of colleagues whose work is not cited correctly and the contempt of those whose time is wasted in attempting to retrieve inaccurately cited references or those who find that a cited reference is irrelevant.

Visual Presentation of Data. This workshop is based on the view that tables, charts, and figures are at the heart of a biomedical paper and, after data selection, their construction is the first step in reporting biomedical results (Woodford 1986). The work of Tufte (1983, 1990) provides a valuable foundation for instruction, which includes information and practice in constructing effective tables and graphs, selecting illustrations, evaluating the quality of illustrations, and developing poster presentations. It details the varied and comparatively effective uses of schematic diagrams, line drawings, half-tones, and color photographs or drawings. It emphasizes criteria for illustrations prepared for publication. It addresses the use of digital figures and their manipulation. Among the ethical and practical facets of this seminar are questions of bias, intentional or unintentional deceit, and respect for people's dignity and privacy.

Tables provide background information and experimental or clinical data, especially numerical data, and are constructed so they can be fully comprehended without reference to the text. Figures, including illustrations, charts, and graphs, are used for evidence, emphasis, and efficiency. Tables, figures, and legends must agree with findings reported in the text and must represent the data without bias. Questions a trainee must consider include whether data are adequately represented in a figure or whether, instead, a table provides a more complete picture of the results; whether the type of graph used is appropriate to the data reported; whether the proportions and scale of a graph visually misrepresent some aspect of the findings; and whether an illustration reflects or could create bias. Visual displays must also be evaluated for accuracy and attribution of credit if they contain data from other studies and for originality in papers based on previous work (Ordway, Eastwood, and Derish 1994).

Although clinical scientists may know that the identity of human subjects must remain confidential in a publication, many do not realize the extent of this requirement. Some journals require patients' written consent to publish any information that arises from the physician-patient relationship (Advice to contributors 1998). In every publication, human subjects must be identified by a case number, not by actual or fictitious initials. Every potentially identifying factor must be removed from the text, tables, and figures (e.g., radiographic scans), including names, initials, dates, and hospital numbers. Information not directly relevant to the case, such as race or occupation when it entails no risk factors, must be excluded, as must any factors that could compromise privacy. When publishing photographs of a person's face or any part of the body that may identify him or her, researchers must protect the person's privacy. This is often accomplished by masking the eyes and any other uniquely identifying feature, but many editors and publishers consider masking insufficient protection. To ensure the person confidentiality and the investigator freedom from potential legal repercussions, it is a good idea—whenever photographs of a person are taken for medical, educational, or research purposes—to ask the person (or legal guardian) to sign a consent form, just in case it is needed later. The form should document permission to take the picture as well as to publish it (Ordway, Eastwood, and Derish 1994).

Reporting Research. Three workshops introduce trainees to fundamental principles of writing reports of basic-science research, reports of clinical research including clinical trials, and review articles and meta-analyses. In-depth instruction is reserved for individual tutorials when trainees write their first papers for publication. These workshops reinforce the view that writing the report of original research findings is integral to the research process. Underlying each workshop is the intent that trainees realize how writing their report leads them from one stage to the next in the progression of their thoughts, forcing them to draw relationships among concepts and ideas and explore implications of their results in a way that is unique to the writing process (Woodford 1986). The approach to statistical reporting and guidelines for producing a comprehensive report include principles applicable to both basic-science and clinical research (Altman et al. 1983; Asilomar Working Group 1996; Begg et al. 1996; Glantz 1992).

Data-Selection File. Writing an original research paper involves the selection of specific experimental data from the investigator's experimental notebook. Establishing a habit of creating a data-selection file when a paper is being planned fosters a link between the research and writing aspects of biomedical investigation, and such a file is invaluable in the event of later scrutiny of the reported work. In the proposed curriculum, for each paper resulting from a study that is to be submitted for publication, a separate data-selection file is created to contain the data selected for publication and documents related to publication (Eastwood et al. 1989, 10). This file consists of the following:

- the data selected for reporting and their analyses (including graphic presentations and statistical manipulations), which are photocopied from the original experimental notebook and, unless the cross-reference is evident, cross-referenced to it page by page
- the rationale for selecting the specific data used in that particular paper, recorded narratively (e.g., "I selected this datum on the basis of X; I excluded this datum on the basis of Y"), including justification for the selection of specific data to make a curve or other statistical representation
- a document naming the investigators and detailing their specific contribution(s)
- a document naming the persons to be cited in the acknowledgments and detailing their specific contribution(s) to the study or paper
- any other material considered pertinent to selection of data, to authorship, or to any substantial related matter arising during the development of the paper

At the completion of a research project, the PI reviews and evaluates the trainee's data-selection file for each paper before writing begins. After the paper is published, the file is archived together with the experimental and methodology notebooks for the project.

Abstracts. The point that an abstract should be complete and understandable on its own is reinforced by reminding trainees that the abstract may be the only part of their paper that many readers will read. A well-constructed abstract is always structured (Ad Hoc Working Group 1987; Haynes et al. 1990), whether or not a structured format is specified. It provides a précis of the paper (Medawar 1981, 62–68), a concise but essentially complete statement of the background needed to understand why the study was performed, its purpose, and the methods, results, conclusions, and implications of the study. Abstracts submitted for meetings resemble abstracts for publication, often with the difference that the conclusions of the study have not yet been confirmed. Trainees should know that this is the only piece of biomedical writing in which they may hedge without misgivings. Phrases like "these findings may suggest" permit them to propose conclusions while leaving room to change them later when they make their presentation. However, reporting "anticipatory research" (Watson 1993, 5) in the hope of being awarded a platform presentation is unethical and also, from the viewpoint of enlightened self-interest, risks embarrassment and even professional repercussions. Abstracts for lay readers entail a social responsibility to communicate the essence of the research, its importance to science, and, if relevant, its importance to society, without exaggeration or understatement.

Research Reports. Introducing trainees to the classic IMRAD format (Introduction, Methods, Results, and Discussion) and the variations used in journals, the workshops on writing clinical and basic-science research reports describe the structure and organization of the IMRAD format, delineating the specific purpose of each section and the types of information each should include. Although IMRAD is an artificial construct that does not represent the process of research or thought, it does serve to focus the report and averts, to some extent, the discursions, distortion, and hyperbole that can edge in when the methods, results, and discussion are combined (Medawar 1981, 62–68). Key elements of a responsibly written research report are detailed in several excellent resources that are recommended to trainees (Booth 1993; Day 1998; Greenhalgh 1997; Huth 1999; Woodford 1986; Zeiger 1991).

The focus of these workshops is on writing an ethical paper—that is, a report that fulfills the researcher's covenant with the reader. For example, trainees no doubt recognize that misstatement of fact constitutes misconduct, but they may not realize that an investigator who does not report everything that another investigator needs to know to evaluate the data also breaks the covenant by misleading the reader (Glazer 1997). The workshops emphasize Bailar's view—that it is wrong to mislead readers about the strength of the evidence, to make the results appear more substantial than they are, or to ferret out a statistically significant result when the result may be spurious (Taubes 1995c). While affirming that science itself is often ambiguous and that a study altogether lacking in ambiguity could be regarded with suspicion, the workshops also convey that a report that is ambiguous or misinforms a reader wishing to interpret or replicate the work is unethical because it wastes intellectual resources, time, money, materiel, and sometimes lives, and it delays the progress of science. Aspects of the research and findings reported may have facets open to interpretation, and decisions made in selecting and omitting data may have been laden with ambiguity, but the ethical paper is a report that candidly acknowledges those ambiguities. It is shaped to define precisely the hypothesis tested or the question asked as the basis for the study, to convey sufficient information sufficiently clearly that colleagues can replicate the findings, to detail the conclusions, and to tell how the findings relate to the existing body of knowledge.

Scholarly Scientific Reviews of the Literature and Book Chapters. Although systematic reviews including meta-analyses may replace many review articles in the future, there will remain a place for scholarly scientific reviews. These reviews, often book chapters, examine the accumulated literature since the last definitive review, categorize areas of increased understanding, and assess all reports critically. It is a criterion of an adequate review, but also of ethical importance, that the critical assessment classify the articles and findings on the basis of their contribution to science, distinguishing better from less optimal study designs and determining whether the methods are sound for evaluating the hypothesis, whether the results can be obtained with those methods, and whether the interpretation of both the data and the results is sound (Ordway, Eastwood, and Derish 1994). There is also an ethical component in the responsibility to synthesize the ideas that have been generated in the field from a perspective that puts the research in a new light (Ordway, Eastwood, and Derish 1994). As a critical assessment does not permit verbatim repetition of reported findings accompanied by a litany of authors' names, the review article or chapter that meets these criteria averts the most common ethical problem with this type of paper, the issue of plagiarism.

Biomedical Publication. The workshops on the publication process concern conventions and requirements of publication, the publication process, and how to peer review a paper and respond to peer review. In these workshops, a point is made of advising trainees that—in addition to useful information about the types of articles a journal will accept and limitations on the length of papers—a journal's instructions to authors gives guidance about ethical and legal obligations involved in publishing a paper. Among the vast number of points related to publishing ethics and etiquette that may be crucial to trainees' making responsible decisions are the following:

- Determining the point at which findings are important enough and adequately developed for publication has several facets with ethical impact. When findings are published too early—whether in enthusiasm or in fear for establishing priority (Namenwirth 1986)—the results may not be confirmed later. The premature misinformation may influence other researchers to build their work on a false assumption. Trainees need to know that timing in communicating research results can have professional consequences because the retraction or withdrawal of mistaken, published conclusions can taint a career (Korenman and Shipp 1994). That consideration must be tempered, however, by the understanding that retraction—should it be necessary—is preferable to leaving flawed work unacknowledged.
- When a study produces more than one interesting or even important finding, investigators have a choice of submitting the study for publication as one complete report or slicing it into several separate papers submitted to several journals. The issues this choice entails are discussed in chapter 5, on repetitive publication.
- Trainees may know that authors initially own the copyright to their papers but may not know that they are almost always required to assign copyright to the publisher on acceptance of the paper for publication (except as noted in the journal). Copyright issues are reviewed carefully so that trainees are aware of copyright law, definitions of pla-

giarism, and the accepted conventions of scientific authorship, acknowledgment, attribution of credit or ownership, and conflict of interest, as discussed in chapter 8.

- Even trainees who are aware of copyright law do not always think of it in relation to republication of their own or others' published work. In a new paper being submitted for publication, written permission of the copyright holder (usually the publisher) is often needed to quote or adapt and almost always required to reproduce any substantial areas of text and any tables, figures, or illustrations that have been published before—even if the material is the investigator's own work.

- Unlike a grant application, which often may be submitted simultaneously to various granting agencies, an article may not be submitted to more than one peer-reviewed scientific journal at a time.

- While trainees may realize the value of publishing first in a peer-reviewed journal, many are not aware that most peer-reviewed journals do not want to consider papers on data or essential findings that have been submitted to another journal or those that have already been accepted or published by another journal (ICMJE 1997a, 1997b). Most are not aware that they may jeopardize their opportunity to publish in a peer-reviewed journal or be in violation of copyright law if they publish details of their work in publications with very different readerships, in a publication in a different language, or in the proceedings of a meeting. They also may not know that publications in a proceedings can make their findings irretrievable because even many peer-reviewed proceedings are not purchased by libraries and are not included in some citation databases. Whenever they wish to republish a paper in any form, trainees must know that they have an obligation to let the editor know about the earlier publication.

- Investigators may want to submit their paper to a second journal rather than respond when a journal returns their paper for revision after peer review. As a matter of etiquette if not ethics, the cost the journal has incurred in considering the paper and the time the journal's reviewers have spent on the paper should be a factor in making this decision. Also to be considered is that the quality of the report and the chances of a successful submission to a second journal are often improved if the manuscript is revised according to constructive criticisms received from the first journal's reviewers.

- Journal editors usually ask that a report state that institutional research approvals were obtained, and occasionally they may ask to review approval documentation before they accept a paper. Before a study is submitted for publication, all this documentation must be in place in the data-selection file, including approval for human or animal experimentation, radioisotope use, signed consent forms, and any other necessary approvals.

- The peer-review system is based on respect for colleagues and confidentiality in reviewing their work. A PI asked to review a paper for a journal is obliged to keep the content of the paper in strictest confidence and may obtain the opinion of a colleague or trainee only with the express permission of the journal editor who requested the review, unless the journal specifies otherwise. In the proposed program, biomedical and curriculum faculty collaborate to integrate the content of the critical reading and reporting aspects of the curriculum so they reinforce one another and provide reciprocal opportunities to address ethical issues of peer review.

It is not known how frequently an incident construed as misconduct may be simply a matter of ignorance. Often trainees and even more experienced physicians and scientists do not realize that they may, and should, write or call the journal's editor about their concerns and questions and about reporting and publishing conventions.

Individual Critical-Writing Tutorials

The individual tutorial program may be implemented in different ways, with curriculum core faculty tutors based institution wide, in research centers, or in departments and laboratories. Essential, however, is that it be convenient for each trainee to receive one-to-one consultation from a tutor throughout the development, writing, submission, peer review, and publication of at least one research report submitted to a peer-reviewed journal and one review article or chapter. During the first consultation, the core faculty tutor introduces each trainee to learning styles and techniques and elicits the information necessary to determine how best to conduct the tutorials. In discussing with trainees how to shape a report of original research, the tutors again focus on writing an ethical paper that reflects the covenant with the reader. Through a tutor's attentive reflection on their work, trainees learn to comprehend their own individual style of thought and expression, becoming aware of biases and habits of expression they need to watch for when writing reports of their research. With this understanding they then quickly learn how to write more precisely, express what they mean more accurately, and increase their awareness about facets of effective and ethical biomedical writing. Examples used in outlining the structure and organization of trainees' papers and in showing them ways to use language with precision also provide opportunities to illustrate the ethical writing practices introduced during the workshops on reporting research.

The Effect of the Research Environment

The most influential factor in fostering responsible research practices is providing trainees with an ethical training experience (Krulwich and Friedman 1993). In an institution where trainees perceive too wide a gap between the practices represented in the curriculum and practices in the real world of their research environment, the most well-designed effort is likely to fail (Bebeau and Davis 1996; Kalichman and Friedman 1992; Eastwood et al. 1996).

In one study of faculty perceptions, most faculty believed that inappropriate assignment of authorship was moderately inappropriate, but there was no clear consensus that publishing a student's work without acknowledging its source constituted inappropriate behavior (Bebeau and Davis 1996). In another study surveying postdoctoral trainees (Eastwood et al. 1996), a significant proportion who felt they had been denied authorship they deserved or had been pressured to list an undeserving author on a paper said that they would grant gift authorship in the future if doing so would benefit their career ($p < .001$). Despite the stature of scientists who have objected that at least 25% of authors named on scientific papers have not contributed substantially to the work reported (IOM 1989; Shapiro, Wenger, and Shapiro 1994) and that current authorship practices in science contribute to the corruption of trainees' values (Goodman 1994; Relman 1990), the lessons of the invisible curriculum prevail. Perhaps more disturbing is that, in the survey of postdoctoral trainees (Eastwood et al. 1996), 41% of those who would grant gift authorship were also willing to select or omit or fabricate data for a grant application or paper if it would benefit their career.

Trainees subjected to unethical or irresponsible professional behavior are at risk of developing a cynical view that affects their own professional conduct (Alberts 1985; Eastwood et al. 1996; Sigma Xi 1986) because their career is controlled by others who are in a position to approve or deny their success and livelihood. The success of the proposed curriculum depends on its place in the institution's invisible curriculum. When the proposed curriculum is compatible with the trainees' research experience, its benefits extend beyond the goal of fostering responsible science to that of improving the extent and quality of trainees' scientific productivity.

The Criteria for Success

Taught about scientific writing, publication, and ethics in the manner described here, trainees have an opportunity to adopt high standards in the context of a challenging experience that provides them with useful information, improves their chances of success, and increases their productivity. Because this curriculum relates ethical principles to the trainees' immediate experience, it sustains their interest and, of necessity, proceeds in a straightforward manner at a pace that permits trainees to absorb the information without becoming bored. Among features that, in combination, are also effective in making a successful curriculum are these (Eastwood et al. 1996):

- enthusiastic participation of well-regarded senior faculty, mentors, and other role models in endorsing and teaching the curriculum (Bird 1993; Conley 1993; Korenman and Shipp 1994; Lee, Yalow, and Weinberg 1993; Lo 1993; NAS 1992; Taubes 1995e)
- enthusiastic participation of junior faculty to ensure its relation to the perspective of the trainee and bridge the gap between the experience of trainees and their mentors
- explicit acknowledgment of the sociocultural context in which research is conducted and discussion of its influence on the practice of science
- components that highlight the ethical facets of biomedical reporting and publication; explore questions of the bias, selection, interpretation, and ambiguities that arise in research; and provide trainees with tools to help them make ethical decisions in resolving moral ambiguities
- a regularly scheduled, informal, case-history component to give trainees virtual experience of diverse ethical dilemmas and a forum for their own experiences
- enthusiastic and dedicated participation by faculty who foster an ethical research environment reflecting the values taught in the curriculum and who provide trainees with the information, skills, supervision, and support necessary to meet high ethical and scientific standards in fulfilling their responsibilities (Bird 1993; Conley 1993; Korenman and Shipp 1994; Lo 1993; NAS 1992; Taubes 1995e)

- consistent updating of information, issues, and cases provided to trainees
- frequent and unbiased evaluations of the curriculum's reception by trainees and effectiveness as assessed over both the short and long terms
- earnest support by the institution in making the curriculum and the values it conveys integral to the institution's educational mission

Science has always been a demanding and aggressive profession, attracting some people willing to bend the rules to benefit their career. As scientists have made astonishing discoveries at an exponentially increasing rate, the profession has become a competitive fellowship of highly independent people. The satisfaction in a competitive fellowship is lost, however, when a sizable proportion of the people competing are confused about the rules of play. Research institutions are absorbing increasing numbers of postdoctoral trainees from outside the European and Anglo-American communities, when even many trainees raised within these communities have not assimilated the skills so important to success in a scientific career, let alone the lessons of the invisible curriculum (Minorities in science 1993). With a knowledgeable curriculum faculty, the participation of respected biomedical faculty, and a supportive administration, the proposed curriculum can contribute substantially to making the keys to a successful and productive career more accessible to all trainees. Within its objectives the curriculum augments mentorship rather than replacing it, enabling faculty to fulfill their responsibilities while enhancing the training of the young researchers who will carry on their work in the future.

Acknowledgments

Many people have influenced the content of this chapter. The author is indebted in particular to Pamela Derish, Evangeline Leash, Faith McLellan, Stephen Ordway, Aviva Abosch, Stephanie Bird, Dennis Deen, John Fike, Philip Cogen, and with special gratitude to Raymond Berry and Charles Wilson.

Some text is adapted with permission from Eastwood et al. (1996).

Notes

1. Survival Skills and Ethics Program, University of Pittsburgh, 4K26 Forbes Quadrangle, Pittsburgh, PA 15260; 412–624–7098; fax 412–648–7081; survival+@pitt.edu; http://www.pitt.edu/~survival/.

2. Few university degree programs in scientific writing and publication exist. Resources for qualified tutorial faculty include the international certifying organization, Board of Editors in the Life Sciences (BELS: PO Box 8133, Radnor, PA 19087-8133; 610–687–4796; fax 610–995–0835; petesm@op.net; http://www.bels.org/), and professional organizations such as the Council of Biology Editors (CBE: 11250 Roger Bacon Drive, Suite 8, Reston, VA 20190; 703–437–4377; fax 703–435–4390; CBEHDQTS@aol.com; http://www.cbe.org/cbe), European Association of Science Editors (EASE: PO Box 426, Guildford, GU4 7ZH, UK; tel/fax +44 (0)1483–211056; secretary@ease.org.uk; http://www.ease.org.uk/), Teachers of English to Speakers of Other Languages (TESOL: 1600 Cameron Street, Suite 300, Alexandria, VA 22314–2751; 703–836–0774; fax 703–836–7864; tesol@tesol.edu; http://www.tesol.edu/), and American Medical Writers Association (AMWA Advanced Core Curriculum: 40 West Gude Drive, Suite 101, Rockville, MD 20850–1192; 301–294–5303; fax 301–294–9006; amwa@amwa.org; http://www.amwa.org.

References

Ad Hoc Working Group for Critical Appraisal of the Medical Literature. 1987. A proposal for more informative abstracts of clinical articles. *Annals of Internal Medicine* 106:598–604.

Advice to contributors. 1998. *BMJ.* http://www.bmj.com/guides/advice.shtml. Site accessed 27 June 1999.

Alberts, B. M. 1985. Limits to growth: In biology, small science is good science. *Cell* 41:337–38.

Alberts, B., and K. Shine. 1994. Scientists and the integrity of research. *Science* 266:1660–61.

Altman, D. G., S. M. Gore, M. J. Gardner, and S. J. Pocock. 1983. Statistical guidelines for contributors to medical journals. *British Medical Journal* 286:1489–93.

Asilomar Working Group on Recommendations for Reporting of Clinical Trials in the Biomedical Literature. 1996. Checklist of information for inclusion in reports of clinical trials. *Annals of Internal Medicine* 124:741–43.

Avery, L. 1996. Write to reply. *Nature* 379:293.

Bailar, J. C. 1986. Science, statistics, and deception. *Annals of Internal Medicine* 104:259–60.

Barry, V. E., and J. Rudinow. 1990. *Invitation to critical thinking.* 2d ed. Fort Worth: Holt, Rinehart, & Winston.

Bebeau, M. J., and E. L. Davis. 1996. Survey of ethical issues in dental research. *Journal of Dental Research* 75:845–55.

Begg, C., M. Cho, S. Eastwood, R. Horton, D. Moher, I. Olkin, R. Pitkin, D. Rennie, K. F. Schulz, D. Simel, and D. F. Stroup. 1996. Improving the quality of reporting of randomized controlled trials: The CONSORT statement. *JAMA* 276:637–39.

Bird, S. J. 1993. Teaching ethics in the sciences: Why, how, and what. In *Ethics, values, and the promise of science,* 228–32. Research Triangle Park, N.C.: Sigma Xi.

Bloom, F. E. 1995. Scientific conduct: Contrasts on a gray scale. *Science* 268:1679.

Booth, V. 1993. *Communicating in science.* 2d ed. New York: Cambridge University Press.

Brookfield, S. 1987. *Developing critical thinkers: Challenging adults to explore alternative ways of thinking and acting.* San Francisco: Jossey-Bass.

Cassel, J. F., and R. J. Congleton. 1993. *Critical thinking: An annotated bibliography.* Metuchen, N.J.: Scarecrow Press.

Clark, S. B. 1988. Computer searches: Effect on animal research. *Science* 240:587.

Cohen, J. 1995. Conduct in science: The culture of credit. *Science* 268:1706–11.

Committee on Science, Engineering, and Public Policy. 1995. *Reshaping the graduate education of scientists and engineers.* Washington, D.C.: National Academy Press.

Conley, F. K. 1993. Toward a more perfect world: Eliminating sexual discrimination in academic medicine. *New England Journal of Medicine* 328:351–52.

Cooper, H., and L. V. Hedges, eds. 1994. *The handbook of research synthesis.* New York: Russell Sage.

Day, R. A. 1998. *How to write and publish a scientific paper.* 3d ed. Phoenix: Oryx Press.

de Lacey, G., C. Record, and J. Wade. 1985. How accurate are quotations and references in medical journals? *British Medical Journal* 291:884–86.

Eastwood, S., P. H. Cogen, J. R. Fike, H. Rosegay, and M. Berens. 1989. BTRC guidelines on research data and manuscripts. San Francisco: Brain Tumor Research Center, University of California, San Francisco. Reprinted in *Responsible science: Ensuring the integrity of the research process,* National Academy of Sciences, Panel on Scientific Responsibility and the Conduct of Research, 2:206–22. Washington, D.C.: National Academy Press, 1993.

Eastwood, S., P. A. Derish, E. Leash, and S. B. Ordway. 1996. Ethical issues in biomedical research: Perceptions and practices of postdoctoral research fellows responding to a survey. *Science and Engineering Ethics* 2:89–114.

Eichorn, P., and A. Yankauer. 1987. Do authors check their references? A survey of accuracy of references in three public health journals. *American Journal of Public Health* 77:1011–12.

Feinstein, A. R., and W. O. Spitzer. 1988. Who checks what in the divided responsibilities of editors and authors. *Journal of Clinical Epidemiology* 41:945–48.

Fischbach, R., ed. 1994. *Educating for the responsible conduct of research.* NIH Policy and Other Mandates. Boston: PRIM&R.

Friedman, P. J. 1990. Research ethics: A teaching agenda for academic medicine. *Academic Medicine* 65:32–33.

Glantz, S. A. 1992. *Primer of biostatistics.* 3d ed. New York: McGraw-Hill.

Glazer, S. 1997. Combating scientific misconduct. *CQ Researcher* 7:3–20.

Goodman, N. W. 1994. Survey of fulfillment of criteria for authorship in published medical research. *BMJ* 309:1482.

Greenhalgh, T. 1997. *How to read a paper: The basics of evidence based medicine.* London: BMJ Publishing Group.

Hamilton, D. P. 1990. Publishing by—and for?—the numbers. *Science* 250:1331–32.

Haynes, R. B., C. D. Mulrow, E. J. Huth, D. G. Altman, and M. J. Gardner. 1990. More informative abstracts revisited. *Annals of Internal Medicine* 113:69–76.

Hoshiko, T. 1993. Responsible conduct of scientific research: A one-semester course for graduate students. *American Journal of Physiology* 264:S8–10.

Huth, E. J. 1999. *Writing and publishing in medicine.* 3d ed. Baltimore: Williams & Wilkins.

In pursuit of comprehension. 1996. *Nature* 384:497.

Institute of Medicine (IOM), Committee on the Responsible Conduct of Research. 1989. *The responsible conduct of research in the health sciences.* Washington, D.C.: National Academy Press. See also IOM report of a study on the responsible conduct of research in the health sciences. 1989. *Clinical Research* 37:179–91.

International Committee of Medical Journal Editors (ICMJE). 1997a. Uniform requirements for manuscripts submitted to biomedical journals. *Annals of Internal Medicine* 126:36–47. See also http://www.acponline.org/journals/resource/unifreqr.htm. Site accessed 27 June 1999.

——. 1997b. Uniform requirements for manuscripts submitted to biomedical journals. *JAMA* 277:927–34.

Kalichman, M. W., and P. J. Friedman. 1992. A pilot study of biomedical trainees' perceptions concerning research ethics. *Academic Medicine* 67:769–75.

King, P. M., and K. S. Kitchener. 1994. *Developing reflective judgment: Understanding and promoting intellectual growth and critical thinking in adolescents and adults.* San Francisco: Jossey-Bass.

Korenman, S. G., and A. C. Shipp. 1994. *Teaching the responsible conduct of research through a case study approach: A handbook for instructors.* Washington, D.C.: Association of American Medical Colleges.

Koshland, D. E., Jr. 1988. Science, journalism, and whistle-blowing. *Science* 240:585.

Krulwich, T. A., and P. J. Friedman. 1993. Integrity in the education of researchers. *Academic Medicine* 68 (suppl to issue 9): S14–18.

Larson, E. B. 1992. Academic mentorship: An important ingredient for our survival. *Journal of General Internal Medicine* 7:255.

Lee, Y. T., R. Yalow, and S. Weinberg. 1993. Ethical research: Principles and practices. In *Ethics, values, and the promise of science: Forum proceedings,* 21–24. Research Triangle Park, N.C.: Sigma Xi.

Leon Lederman's quest: Double science funding. 1991. *Science* 251:153.

Lo, B. 1993. Skepticism about teaching ethics. In *Ethics, values, and the promise of science: Forum proceedings,* 151–56. Research Triangle Park, N.C.: Sigma Xi.

Medawar, P. B. 1981. *Advice to a young scientist.* New York: Harper & Row.

Minorities in science '93: Trying to change the face of science. 1993. *Science* 262:1089–1135.

Mundy, D., and C. Shugar. 1992. Copyright review at one institution's editorial office. *CBE Views* 15:126.

Namenwirth, M. 1986. Science seen through a feminist prism. In *Feminist approaches to science,* ed. R. Bleier, 18–41. New York: Pergamon Press.

National Academy of Sciences (NAS), Panel on Scientific Responsibility and the Conduct of Research. 1992. *Responsible science: Ensuring the integrity of the research process,* vol. 1. Washington, D.C.: National Academy Press.

———. 1993. *Responsible science: Ensuring the integrity of the research process,* vol. 2. Washington, D.C.: National Academy Press.

National Institutes of Health (NIH). 1992. Reminder and update: Requirement for instruction in the responsible conduct of research in National Research Service Award institutional training grants. *NIH Guide for Grants and Contracts* 21:2–3.

Office of Research Integrity (ORI), U.S. Public Health Service. 1993. NIH strengthens responsible conduct of research requirement in training grant applications. *ORI Newsletter* 1(April):2. See also http://ori.dhhs.gov/newsltrs.htm. Site accessed 11 July 1999.

Ordway, S., S. Eastwood, and P. Derish. 1994. *A guide to publishing biomedical research.* San Francisco: Department of Neurological Surgery, University of California, San Francisco.

Petersdorf, R. G. 1986. The pathogenesis of fraud in medical science. *Annals of Internal Medicine* 104:252–54.

Pollock, R. E., S. A. Curley, and E. Lotzová. 1995. Ethics of research training for NIH T32 surgical investigators. *Journal of Surgical Research* 58:247–51.

Relman, A. S. 1990. Responsible science—responsible authorship: Discussion. In Council of Biology Editors, Editorial Policy Committee, *Ethics and policy in scientific publication,* 199. Bethesda, Md.: Council of Biology Editors.

Sabine, J. R. 1985. The error rate in biological publication: A preliminary survey. *Bioscience* 35:358–63.

Schwartz, M. 1993. Lecture presented at the Sixth International Conference of the International Federation of Science Editors (IFSE), Marine Biology Laboratory, Woods Hole, Mass., October 1991. In Eastwood, S. Summary: Science editing in the age of global communication. *International Federation of Science Editors,* July, 4–14.

Shapiro, D. W., N. S. Wenger, and M. F. Shapiro. 1994. The contributions of authors to multiauthored biomedical research papers. *JAMA* 271:438–42.

Sigma Xi. 1986. *Honor in science.* Research Triangle Park, N.C.: Sigma Xi.

Singer, A. L., Jr., G. Jones, J. Gurley, L. Backus, and T. Meyer. 1993. Postdoctoral researchers: A panel. In *Ethics, values, and the promise of science: Forum proceedings,* 47–59. Research Triangle Park, N.C.: Sigma Xi.

Sipe, T. A., and W. L. Curlette. 1995. A meta-meta-analysis: Methodological aspects of meta-analyses related to educational achievement. Paper presented at the Analytic Methods Forum, Centers for Disease Control and Prevention, Department of Health and Human Services, 21 June 1996. Part of a larger study: Sipe, T. A. 1995. A meta-synthesis of educational achievement: A methodological approach to summarization and synthesis of meta-analyses. Ph.D. diss., Georgia State University.

Sojka, R. E., and H. F. Mayland. 1993. Driving science with one eye on the peer review mirror. In *Ethics, values, and the promise of science: Forum proceedings,* 202–6. Research Triangle Park, N.C.: Sigma Xi.

Swazey, J. P. 1993. Teaching ethics: Needs, opportunities, and obstacles. In *Ethics, values, and the promise of science: Forum proceedings,* 233–42. Research Triangle Park, N.C.: Sigma Xi.

Taubes, G. 1995a. Indiana: Wrong answers—but no right ones. *Science* 268:1707.

———. 1995b. ITT: Serving ethics up for lunch. *Science* 268:1716.

———. 1995c. McGill: Analyzing the data. *Science* 268:1714.

———. 1995d. Pittsburgh: Interwoven with the fabric of learning. *Science* 268:1709.

———. 1995e. Stanford: Bringing in the big guns. *Science* 268:1711.

Tufte, E. R. 1983. *The visual display of quantitative information.* Cheshire, Conn.: Graphics Press.

———. 1990. *Envisioning information.* Cheshire, Conn.: Graphics Press.

University of California, San Francisco (UCSF). 1996. UCSF postdocs form new organization: Survey will provide demographic data. *Synapse* 40:1, 4.

Watson, J. D. 1993. Lecture presented at Sixth International Conference of the International Federation of Science Editors (IFSE), Marine Biology Laboratory, Woods Hole, Mass., October 1991. In Eastwood, S. 1993. Summary: Science editing in the age of global communication. *International Federation of Science Editors,* July, 4–14.

Woodford, F. P., ed. 1986. *Scientific writing for graduate students.* Bethesda, Md.: Council of Biology Editors.

Zeiger, M. 1991. *Essentials of writing biomedical research papers.* New York: McGraw-Hill.

Educating the Leaders

11

Toward Systemic Change

Addeane S. Caelleigh

Members of the scientific community may feel dismay, anger, even cynicism when they come face to face with fellow members' misconduct in conducting and publishing research. They usually see their errant colleagues, however, as a corrupted few who fall outside the normal world of science, and the accepted solution is to exile these colleagues from the community and move on with the important work at hand. This approach has the satisfying elements of good drama, including villains and renewed dedication to right principles, but it creates a false picture of the community, the workings of science, and the work of scientists.

A clearer and ultimately more useful approach is to consider that the scientific community actually works like a *community*, that it shares important features and dynamics with a neighborhood or a small town. Sociologists have given considerable thought to how communities function, to what holds them together and what endangers them. The scientific community can gain useful insights into how to deal with ethical problems in scientific publication by considering analogies from the sociology of communities and neighborhoods. The basic insights of the social sciences about how people in neighborhoods live, and how they misbehave, can translate well into our thinking about how scientific communities act. By incorporating these concepts into their thinking, the leaders of scientific communities would be better able to deal with the unethical behavior of their members and, more importantly, to see the social framework within which to approach the problems of publication ethics. The leaders include the editors of smaller specialty journals as well as the editors of large general journals and administrators of academic institutions and scientific organizations.

Communities and Behavior
Deviancy

We cannot create an academic publishing system that is immune to the emotions and motives that move human beings in their personal and professional lives. World-famous clinical researchers may cut corners, break laws, and lie, cheat, and steal; so may research fellows in obscure posts. This tells us nothing except that our colleagues have the usual human frailties and need the same careful monitoring as do the country's airline pilots, politicians, food manufacturers, and police officers. We need to understand that dishonesty and cheating are normal, even if undesirable, behaviors, and consequently we need to develop systems for our professional activities that take these human tendencies into account. We can construct monitoring systems that reveal these actions whenever possible without unduly burdening or penalizing the honest majority. Further, we must treat the problems that arise as normal aberrations rather than as ethical catastrophes (Douglas 1993). That is, they are the usual small amount of deviancy that turns up in any human activity—the equivalent of the engineer's "normal accidents."

Much of the conduct that editors, institutional monitors, and the public deplore has developed as responses to a system of rewards. "Gaming the system" is what humans do when faced with sets of incentives and disincentives; we try to garner as many benefits and as few punishments as possible. The present patterns of unethical conduct in scientific publication arose not because researchers are more depraved than the rest of the population but because their leaders did not teach, monitor, and enforce ethical standards properly. Violations went unchecked, often undetected, and often hushed up. In that vacuum grew the practices that trouble us today (Hackett 1993).

A useful by-product of having leaders and others speak in many settings about publication ethics is that research communities will begin to see these problems, however regrettable, as an infrequent but unavoidable part of the academic life. The open discussions, combined with careful and consistent monitoring by editors and institutional leaders, would eventually make these problems a part of normal science, to be handled in normal (rather than extraordinary) ways. When principal investigators, department chairs, deans, and CEOs talk as freely and openly in the hallway, the cafeteria, and the conference room about publication ethics and its problems as they now talk about grants and institutional politics and when the conversations take for granted that publication ethics is an essential part of their work, scientists will have truly integrated publication ethics into the fabric of their community.

Broken Windows and Fare Jumpers

Another fruitful idea from psychology and sociology is the *broken windows* concept of urban breakdown and crime (Kelling and Coles 1996; Wilson 1985; Wilson and Kelling 1982). It has insights for editors, who are the gatekeepers of scientific publishing. The idea of *broken windows,* usually associated with George Kelling and James Q. Wilson, has to do with repeated observations by police and other neighborhood regulars that, if a window in a building is broken and left unrepaired, all the other windows will soon be broken—and that this is true in good neighborhoods as well as bad ones.

An experiment based on that observation was conducted by Philip Zimbardo, a professor at Stanford University, and is a staple in recent psychology textbooks. It involved abandoning cars and filming what happened to them. One car was abandoned in the Bronx, where it was attacked within ten minutes, completely stripped within 24 hours, and destroyed soon afterward. Most of the vandals were well dressed and apparently respectable. A second car was abandoned in Palo Alto, California, where nothing happened to it for a week. After Zimbardo smashed the car's window with a sledgehammer, however, it was attacked by passersby and completely destroyed within a few hours. Again, the vandals appeared to be respectable members of the community. (The researchers were careful to point out, given the highly polarizing issue of race in thinking about crime, that in both cases, in the blue-collar Bronx and in middle-class Palo Alto, all of the vandals were white.)

This finding and related work have led to the idea that the appearance of disorder (abandonment, lack of repair, lack of ownership, absence of caring) elicits vandalism, destruction, and other law breaking, which starts a widening cycle of crime and decay in a neighborhood. Repairing the window is a sign that the neighborhood is intact, functioning, and monitoring what goes on in its streets and what happens to its members, and that sign alone seems to be a powerful social deterrent to some types of antisocial and unlawful behavior. A recent application of this idea involved fare jumpers in the New York City subway system (Pooley 1996; DiIulio 1995). The subways for years have had a major problem with *fare jumpers—* people, usually men, who jump the turnstiles and thereby avoid paying their subway fares. When the Transit Police made a major effort to stop fare jumping, they accomplished a great deal more than they had expected. Fare jumpers, it turned out, were likely to carry illegal weapons, to be fugitives, and to be wanted on outstanding warrants. The act of fare jumping, in itself a minor law breaking, was an indicator of much more serious social pathology. By stopping fare jumping, the Transit Police made a significant contribution to lowering crime. Also, the majority of honest riders saw that the authorities enforced the rules.

Editors can readily see loose parallels to their work as monitors and gatekeepers of journals, and senior academic administrators equally can see the relevance to their responsibilities. The past 20 years have shown what happens when it appears that the community's leaders do not care about issues of authorship, duplicate publication, and salami science. Scientific authors—and those responsible for teaching the new generations of researchers—must *see* that the editor is watching, as is the one in the next neighborhood and in the neighborhood across town. And department chairs, senior deans, and promotion committees must also be watching.

As with the fare jumpers, it may be that the authors who intentionally break one of the smaller commandments may be breaking far larger ones that are harder to see. A hypothetical example can show how this might happen. Many editors now require authors to sign a formal statement declaring that all of a paper's authors meet the journal's stated criteria for authorship. Sometimes, when all authors must sign a formal declaration that they meet the criteria, the declaration form is returned with a revised list of authors. It is sometimes easy to tell that a senior faculty member had claimed authorship inappropriately or that a junior colleague had been left off the initial author list. In such cases, the editorial staff might subsequently learn during the editing process that the authors cannot properly back up their data and analysis. For example, in examining and untangling editing problems, the editorial staff might learn that some of the authors do not seem to understand the paper, cannot account for apparent mistakes in the data, and cannot produce the work upon which the report is based. This hypothetical case may seem unlikely or farfetched. A simpler one, however, might be more convincing: an editor might conclude from experience that authors who inflate references to their own prior work are also likely to inflate the findings in papers under review.

A department chair or research administrator who properly monitored researchers' writing and publication would probably have similar experiences. A senior administrator who does not have systems to screen faculty and staff members' manuscripts being submitted for publication is sending a strong signal that publication ethics is not important. After all, leaders keep their eyes on the important things—that's part of their job. By the same measure, therefore, the reverse is true: if the leaders do not pay attention to it, it is not important.

Integrity

The concept of integrity lies at the heart of the publication ethics issues that concern editors and should concern all leaders of science institutions. The personal integrity of faculty members as researchers, authors, and teachers (and of editors as judges and managers) creates the integrity of their institutions (Pritchard 1993). The leaders set standards of conduct and ensure that members meet the standards. The concept of integrity as involving both awareness and action, as presented in a book for the reading public by Stephen Carter of Yale University, is one that helps us see what we are asking authors and their superiors to do and be (Carter 1996). In Carter's concept, integrity requires three steps: to discern right and wrong; to act on that discernment by choosing right over wrong, even at a cost to oneself; and to say openly that the action is based on an understanding of right and wrong.

Senior faculty need to have integrity in their professional publishing and to demonstrate and teach it to their students and junior colleagues. Editors want them to understand what is right and what is wrong in writing and publishing articles and want this to be a full rather than a superficial understanding—to know the consequences for the biomedical literature if unethical practices are allowed to operate unchecked. Also, faculty members should act on what they recognize as right and wrong. These actions must go beyond their own writing. The leaders must speak up in group discussions, counsel co-authors or colleagues who are doing wrong, and support the work of investigative and disciplinary committees. They should do right even at cost to themselves. If they have published incorrect information that affects a reader's understanding of their research and findings, for example, they must step forward to correct it, even if no one else knows about the error. Or they must give proper credit for work reported in an article, even if it means that a junior colleague is first author at an important time when the paper will be cited in a crucial grant proposal. Further, they should say publicly to all involved that their actions, reactions, and advice are based on issues of right and wrong—rather than expediency, for example—and that right must be both done and seen to be done.

A Hidden Curriculum

The medical education community has a useful insight about ethics and about assuring that trainees and junior colleagues understand their responsibilities. This insight concerns the "hidden curriculum," also called the "informal curriculum" (Hundert, Hafferty, and Christakis 1996, 624; Hafferty and Franks 1994, 861). For many years, medical schools (and to some extent, residency programs) have been increasingly concerned about the gap between what the medical curriculum teaches about being a humane, compassionate physician and how medical students and residents act with patients. National task forces, university committees, and respected leaders have again and again urged medical schools to emphasize and inculcate the humane aspects of doctoring, and curriculum committees and faculty have added major elements to students' education to close the gap. Faculty have watched with dismay, however, as the gap remained and sometimes even seemed to widen.

About ten years ago, a few people in the different parts of medical education, operating independently, began to recognize why the changes were not having the desired effect. They began to see that the students were getting mixed signals. The formal curriculum of syllabi, course work, and reading assignments said one thing, but the informal curriculum demonstrated daily by residents and faculty members taught far different values. The students watched their teachers to learn what really mattered, as opposed to what the curriculum said was important. Being bright and motivated, the students quickly learned which curriculum mattered more in terms of grades, recommendations, and entry into prestigious projects, and they modeled themselves according to the standards of the informal curriculum.

The application of this concept to publication ethics in science is, perhaps, even more readily apparent than that of the other concepts already presented. Trainees and junior colleagues watch senior researchers and faculty to learn what is expected and how to behave. They model their professional behavior, to a large extent, on what the leaders do, not what they say.

This is not surprising, but it reinforces one of the concept's applications to other parts of the academic enterprise and to other parts of the scientific community. Even though we know that we all model our behavior to some extent on the behavior of our leaders, we often nonetheless rely on pronouncements, mission statements, and handouts to foster and maintain ethical behavior. It is not that we do not know better, but we continue to hope—in a kind of magical thinking—that small, simple changes can produce large, complex results in behavior.

The lesson for publication ethics is that pronouncements and lecture handouts are not enough, just as they are not enough in molding the professional behavior of physicians. Scientists and their leaders need to know and act upon the ethical standards that the community expects its members to meet. Further, they need to internalize the standards, see personally and directly why they matter, and understand the ill effects of abandoning them.

Convincing the Whole Community

All the partners in publishing peer-reviewed scientific journals need to cooperate in undertaking long-term, concerted efforts to set out high ethical standards in publication (Korenman et al. 1998; Wenger et al. 1998; Reiser 1993). Editors of peer-reviewed journals, leaders and administrators of institutions, senior faculty, government funding agencies, and foundations must work together to assure that publication ethics is taken as seriously as are research design and funding. This work will be more successful if the core of concerned editors and administrators undertakes parallel and coordinated efforts with all editors in science and all heads of science institutions.

First, newly appointed and novice editors must understand the ethical ramifications of their role as editor-in-chief of a peer-reviewed journal. Senior, experienced editors must undertake concerted, long-term projects to raise the issues of publication ethics with the entire community of science editors and to move the novices progressively through stages of awareness, concern, and action. Second, senior editors need to undertake similar programs for the senior faculty who train and guide the new generations of researcher-scholars as they begin writing for peer-reviewed publication. Neither of these efforts has traditionally been considered part of the editor's job, nor are they spelled out by the oversight boards, publishers, or sponsoring societies that choose, oversee, and dismiss the editor. Third, senior editors and senior faculty must convince their institutional leaders that high ethical standards in publication are crucial to the health and reputation of the institution.

There is considerable overlap among these approaches, primarily because most editors of peer-reviewed journals are also faculty members or employees in research and education institutions. They form an existing and natural core of experts from which to teach and persuade both ends of the spectrum of their colleagues and associates to take publication ethics seriously. On the one hand, they interact daily with their research and teaching colleagues and are a bridge between the world of journal editors and the world of biomedical researchers, authors, and readers. Likewise, in their dealings with the leaders of their home institutions—who, coincidentally, are often leaders of scientific societies and national panels—they are a bridge between the highest leadership of their disciplines and the world of journal editorship. In each case, the dual role of serving as editor and serving in an academic or other scientific position means that experienced editors of peer-reviewed journals can successfully take the initiative for promulgating and enforcing high ethical standards in scientific publications.

Journal Editors

Senior editors' first obligation, and the most direct way to maintain high standards in publication, is to teach and counsel fellow editors (Caelleigh 1993; Parrish 1999). Most editors take up their positions with no specific preparation for the problems and issues that lie at the core of the standards and policies. Senior editors' counseling and service as mentors will directly affect the quality and standards of the journals with newly appointed editors. Indirectly, it can also eventually reach the leaders of scientific communities because the newly appointed editors are usually experienced, highly respected members of their disciplines, their professional organizations, and their home institutions. By helping them better understand the nature of their role as editor-in-chief and by helping them deal with the inevitable problems they will face as editors of peer-reviewed journals, senior editors will also add to the cadre of influential and visible editors who take seriously the ethical standards of publishing as they teach, sit on internal committees that set institutional policies, and serve on national committees and task forces (Peer Review Congress III 1998; Second International Congress on Peer Review 1994; Guarding the guardians 1990).

What We Do Now

Editorships are an interesting case of enormous power wielded behind a screen of secrecy, with the editor seldom, if ever, held accountable for decisions and actions. Editors who get into public or semipublic trouble usually have become involved in unethical or illegal handling of money. Smaller journals often consolidate greater power in fewer hands, with divided authority, and therefore secrecy can be greater; large journals have many senior editors and divided authority, and therefore secrecy may not be a problem but accountability may be.

Such a system of power might be safer if becoming an editor were similar to becoming a Jesuit priest or a Zen monk. In those systems, the newcomer knowingly enters a long, arduous training program, one developed over centuries and proven effective in molding a satisfactory member of the community. Becoming the editor of a peer-reviewed journal is, however, usually a case of receiving a prestigious job for which there is no direct experience and which, in most cases, must fit into an already demanding set of professional responsibilities. There are no degrees or certificates for becoming the editor of a peer-reviewed journal. Fellow editors can, if asked, give good general advice, but ultimately the new editor must learn on the job. (Earlier experience as an associate editor may help, depending on how the journal is organized, but in most cases that experience offers limited preparation for being editor-in-chief.) The biggest change is that the new editor must begin to see the familiar world from a new perspective that may share little with the viewpoints of previous roles.

Editors share an important characteristic of professionals in that they make independent judgments and do not have to justify them to outsiders (such as readers, librarians, fellow researchers, fellow editors). Unlike most professionals, however, editors have virtually no one monitoring their day-to-day work. They do not have to pass competency tests for licensure, they are not required to be certified for their new duties, and quality-review boards do not audit their files periodically to look for inappropriate behavior or to compare the editor's practices with those of other editors and with best-practice standards.

Most people do not think about this aspect of journal editorship. If pressed, thoughtful reader-researchers might speculate that the diversity of journals, sponsoring societies, and editors ensures that over time the editorial enterprise is self-correcting and that the unregulated actions of editors balance out overall to produce a sturdy, healthy scientific literature. And they could probably add that editors—who are, after all, part of their community—are basically good people, well intentioned, and smart. Readers would probably not, however, place equivalent faith in such a system if applied to patient care, financial management, or pharmaceutical research. This reaction reflects, perhaps, the researcher's feeling that being an editor is basically the same as being an author but from the other side, and therefore editorship can be learned readily by any member of the scientific community. They are right, of course, that the mechanics of running a journal system are easily learned, being a matter of consistency, discipline, and careful record keeping. The heart of editorship, however, lies not in these mechanics but in the application of intelligence, imagination, and integrity to daily decisions. These are aspects of character and personality, the very elements that we usually believe require training and monitoring.

If publication were not so important in the lives of academic scientists, these questions about ethics and editors would concern only a few ethicists and sociologists. But the reality is that editors make decisions every day that have sizable effects on the reputations, grant awards, and promotions of community members and that have even greater repercussions on the definition and credibility of the accumulated knowledge we sum up in the phrase *the literature.*

Editors do not, of course, operate completely without check. The relationship between editor and publisher is by definition touchy, but there is a generally recognized separation of powers and responsibilities. The publisher (the sponsoring society) owns the journal, and the editor captains it. In most cases each benefits from the prestige of the other. The publisher selects the editor, knowing that the editor must be allowed to be independent and autonomous in terms of the journal's content, while at the same time keeping to budget, deadlines, and publication standards. An editor accepts the job knowing that she serves only so long as the publisher has confidence in her editorial judgment and that she has an obligation to resign rather than let a publisher compromise her editorial independence. Obviously, this relationship rests on the integrity, good faith, and flexibility of the partners.

Usually, the mediator between the two is the editorial board, although the powers and duties of boards vary widely. (The publisher is responsible for setting the board's role, one of the most important factors when candidates decide whether to accept an editorship.) Some boards are filled by the publisher, some by the editor; some have a mandate to oversee the quality of the journal, others are purely advisory. When the editor and publisher disagree with each other—and their respective jobs virtually assure that they sometimes will—board members can mediate, present viewpoints, and in subtle and direct ways try to resolve the disagreements satisfactorily. A strong board can help protect an editor from a publisher who tries to meddle in publication decisions (keeping some articles or topics out of the journal; getting other articles or topics in), just as it can counsel an editor who is letting standards slide.

Editors can and do resign over principle, are pushed out by publishers, and are fired. Although the dispute and its fallout occasionally become public or semipublic, the editorial board and sponsoring society usually handle such a big problem discreetly, with the editor resigning quietly. The society would be concerned that an editor's missteps or malfeasance would bring the whole society into disrepute, and the editor's academic employer (usually a university or research institution) would not be eager to have the problem become public knowledge. The more public cases are likely to involve unethical or illegal handling of money.

Some editors come to be at loggerheads with the publisher over issues that are partly financial and partly editorial. A common area of dispute involves the relationship between editorial content and advertising in a journal heavily dependent on advertising revenue. An editor and sponsoring society might in good faith disagree about how to draw the line between the editor's perogative to make publication decisions without interference and the society's need to keep the journal financially healthy. (At some journals, angering a major advertiser by publishing an unfavorable article could make a journal financially ill.) This conflict deepened for the large biomedical journals in the past two decades as advertising declined while some editors became increasingly uncomfortable about the power of big advertisers (pharmaceuticals, for example). A related situation can occur when a sponsoring society wishes to broaden the business uses of its prestigious and money-making journal, such as the 1999 case of the Massachusetts Medical Society and the *New England Journal of Medicine*. The journal's editor-in-chief, Jerome P. Kassirer, was in effect fired after his disagreement with the society over the use of the journal's name in connection with the sale of the society's other publications, and the executive editor, Marcia Angell, agreed to stay only as long as needed for a new editor-in-chief to be hired (Kassirer 1999a; Angell 1999).

A clash between editor and publisher can also be caused by structural misalignments. The formal definitions of the editor's role and responsibilities, like those for the publisher, can inadvertently lead to problems. An invidious role is to be both editor of a journal and head of its business operations or perhaps of the sponsoring society's entire publications operations. A prestigious international medical journal and its U.S. sponsoring society learned this painfully in the early 1990s, when a long series of disagreements and tensions could be traced ultimately to an administrative structure that made the editor also the society's vice-president for publications and thereby the head of those business operations. Good intentions and integrity by all involved were not enough to overcome the problems.

Eventually the editor, widely recognized as innovative and principled, re-turned quietly to university research, and the society rewrote the job de-scription to cover editorship of the journal only. This was a case in which there was no villain—instead, the responsibilities assigned to the editor created deep, built-in conflicts with the publisher.

Occasionally, the breakup of the editor-publisher relationship is over editorial issues and is public. There were two big examples in the 1990s. The first, in Canada, caused an academic firestorm and wide media atten-tion; the second, in the United States, saw little outcry except among edi-tors. The first example involved an article in the *Canadian Journal of Physics,* a peer-reviewed journal published by the National Research Council of Canada (NRC), an agency of that country's federal government. The article was about the deleterious effects of mothers' participation in the work force on their children's ethical and social behavior as adolescents (Free-man 1990). The author was a chemistry professor who based his comments on his years of discussion with his students; in the article he described these discussions as social science research. Once the paper became known outside the journal's readership, the furor among social scientists led to petitions, position statements by leading Canadian academic societies, an academic conference, and formal apologies by the NRC (1993; Ethics of scholarly publishing 1993). It did not, however, lead to the immediate removal of the editor, although when he did not voluntarily turn over the editorship within a few months, the head of NRC journals asked for his resignation.

Leaving aside the question of whether the furor would have occurred if the author had expressed opinions more popular among academics, this was a case when an editor's publication decision had publicly embarrassing results that eventually cost him his editorship. The most disturbing out-come of the case was what the NRC learned when it inquired into the review procedures at the *Canadian Journal of Physics,* and it was this infor-mation, rather than the publication of the article per se, that led to the editor's being asked to resign. (The whole situation was muddled because the Freeman article appeared in a theme issue coordinated by a guest editor rather than in a regular issue of the journal.) The council did, however, begin to lay down criteria for peer review in its journals.

The other case occurred in the United States—the 1999 firing of George Lundberg as editor of *JAMA,* the *Journal of the American Medical Association.* Although ostensibly about his publication, during the impeachment trial of President Bill Clinton, of an article about undergraduate students' opinions about sexual behavior (an issue related by implication to the impeachment), the firing evidently reflected a wider disaffection between the publisher and the editor, in this case both strong-minded leaders of large and highly visible enterprises. The American Medical Association (AMA) executive vice-president, in announcing the firing, put the situation in those terms. The outcry among editors of biomedical journals was immediate. Individual editors and some academic societies wrote letters of protest to the AMA (Fletcher and Fletcher 1999; Horton 1999; Kassirer 1999b; Smith 1999), and organizations such as the Council of Biology Editors (CBE) and the World Association of Medical Editors (WAME) wrote protest letters or other formal statements condemning the firing (Firing of Dr Lundberg 1999). Outside this community, however, there seemed to be little public reaction. Even among the AMA membership, reaction was muted or minimal (Firing of Dr. Lundberg 1999). The other *JAMA* editors and editorial board members wrote an editorial acknowledging the publisher's right to remove the editor and presenting a strong defense of the intellectual integrity of the journal (*JAMA* editors et al. 1999). Only one member of *JAMA*'s editorial board resigned in protest (Tanne 1999).

The *JAMA* case highlights the difficult nature of the editor-publisher relationship, the extent to which the editor serves at the discretion of the publisher, and the importance of the publisher's making wise decisions. The first two are clear; the long-term effect of the firing on the AMA cannot be known yet, although it led to a new governance structure for *JAMA* (Editorial governance 1999). The AMA did not question the editor's right to publish whatever he chose; it did, however, question the editor's judgment. This will, presumably, be the position of the newly created Journal Oversight Committee because sound judgment is what a publisher hires an editor for. And it is in the eye of the beholder, who may be nearsighted or keenly perceptive.

What Else Needs to Be Done?

What obligations do experienced editors have to their newly appointed colleagues, who must now shift from being producers to being judges of the literature? What sort of outreach programs should editors organize for their academic colleagues who become editors?

Who Are the Editors? First, we need to know who is an editor now and, perhaps, who has been an editor within the past ten years. This alone is a major project because there are several thousand biomedical journals alone and thousands more in other sciences. Second, we need a mechanism for learning when new editors are appointed. Only then can we know the scope of what would be involved in giving new editors information and tutelage in the ethical standards that will be the core of their responsibilities.

It will be difficult to learn who the editors-in-chief are. A look at the biomedical community alone will highlight the difficulties of the task. There are approximately four thousand biomedical journals in MEDLINE. This total underestimates the number of peer-reviewed journals used by biomedical researchers because MEDLINE does not cover many of them, especially in social sciences, health outcomes research, and health policy research. Also, some excellent journals are not accepted into the MEDLINE index. Overall, there is no way to know how many are excluded. But, merely as a general illustration, the MEDLINE total of four thousand editors can be a starting point.

There is no way to know the average turnover rate for editorships, but we can arbitrarily use 10% per year. (It does not seem unreasonable that the average tenure might be ten years.) This would mean that approximately four hundred new editors-in-chief are appointed each year. If nine of each ten new appointees have not previously served as the editor-in-chief of another journal, the MEDLINE community might have as many as 360 neophyte editors each year. They must learn on the job, often unaided, to apply their education, experience, and judgment to the responsibilities of running a peer-reviewed journal. To understand the full dimensions of the need, we must then multiply the 360 new editors of the MEDLINE index by a factor of at least three or four to estimate the number for the scientific community overall. Those who become editors for the first time—as well as many of those who have served earlier terms—need to be introduced to issues of publication ethics, educated about the consensus standards that experienced editors have developed in the past 20 years, and engaged in the ongoing discussions of troublesome questions.

What Do New Editors Need? Newly appointed editors need substantial help to decrease their learning curve and establish publication policies that promote good science and the integrity of the biomedical literature.

General Information about Organizations and Resources. Newly appointed editors need to know about the societies and organizations that editors and publishers have created as meeting grounds for discussing the important issues in academic publishing. The three most prominent of these organizations are CBE, the European Association of Science Editors (EASE), and WAME. New editors need to know the focus and activities of each organization and the resources it makes available to them.

An Introduction to Being an Editor. Ten years ago there were no programs for newly appointed editors, and until recently there was only one, the Short Course for Journal Editors created by CBE. It is an excellent introduction, but most new editors never find out about it or do so only long after they most need it. Also, CBE does not have longer-term programs, such as follow-up meetings, or a mentoring program, or a confidential advisory group of senior or retired editors. In Europe, EASE began offering a similar course in 1996. WAME, the newest editors' organization (created in 1996), brings together editors-in-chief. One of its first acts was to create a Web site (WAME 1998) for shared information and a list serve for members where editors could seek advice and suggestions on difficult policies.

The organizers of the International Congress on Biomedical Peer Review and Global Communications (the continuation of the biennial international congresses on peer review begun in 1989) took a useful approach to its September 1997 meeting in Prague. They deliberately chose the meeting site in eastern Europe so that editors from the former Soviet Bloc could attend a special daylong workshop on peer review and the operation of peer-reviewed journals. The editors of prominent, international medical journals in the United Kingdom, Norway, the Netherlands, Australia, and the United States taught the workshop. During the additional days of the congress, editors from different regions discussed common problems and issues in peer review. The organizers used the approach suggested above to help new editors learn their jobs and thereby create a growing core of editors and faculty who can keep the issues prominent at their home institutions.

Continuing Editor Education. Editors need continuing editor education after they complete the early months of their tenure and have begun to understand firsthand the extent of the issues of publication ethics with which they deal. Such programs could offer more detailed examination and discussion of various ways to set and maintain appropriate standards for the review process, decision making, internal adjudication of disagreements, legal issues, and the like. These issues are covered at conferences organized by CBE or EASE, but as yet there are no higher-level education programs for editors.

Participation in Consensus Processes. Editors need to be brought into systematic efforts to collect information about editorial practices and policies, dissemination of cases or issues of special importance, and Adelphi-process querying about which issues are important in the day-to-day operation of journals and the relative importance of the broad issues affecting the biomedical literature (integrity of the literature, effect of different delivery formats, interaction of commercial and academic values in academic publishing and policy, etc.).

Science Leaders

All people with responsibilities for publication ethics must play major roles in the ethical education of the new generations of researchers. Although editors will necessarily need to be involved directly, much of the work will be done by other faculty members as they teach trainees and advise junior colleagues and by staff members responsible for developing and overseeing the curriculum and faculty development. Parallel to programs for new editors, there need to be long-term programs to teach young academics and researchers—and their supervising faculty and mentors—about publication ethics.

What Is Being Done Now?

Senior faculty should already be models of proper conduct in publication but often are not. The lack of ethics leadership in earlier decades gave rise to problems in research ethics that have aroused editors, legislators, and the public since the 1970s. Most of the problems have involved publication ethics at some stage.

Junior faculty should know the right conduct expected of them as they write and publish articles in peer-reviewed journals. The senior faculty responsible for their seven to ten years of postgraduate training should have ensured that they do. But the present generation of supervising faculty and researchers was usually not taught these publication standards, and the environment in which they worked often eroded the scruples they had brought with them into academic life. Regrettably, many of them today are practicing the corrupt or sloppy practices that they learned by default or example in their formative years in research.

The issue of authorship can illustrate this problem. Researchers trained during the 1960s and 1970s often worked in laboratories when the size of research teams was increasing and the publish-or-perish pressure was building. Postgraduates saw a system developing in which the head of the laboratory was the lead author or a prominent author of all papers published from the laboratory even when that person had not participated in the planning, execution, or analysis of the research. The point is not that the lab chief was the lead author, because chiefs had traditionally been active, hands-on members of research teams and therefore had naturally been authors of the resulting research reports. The important point is, rather, that when the lab became so large and differentiated that the lab chief no longer participated directly in many of the projects, the chief nonetheless retained authorship of reports written by team members.

As publication pressure mounted, researchers began to apply that example in inventive ways, such as honorary authorship; lab colleagues would put each other's names on research reports, so that all of them would have longer publications lists without incurring more work. Trainees in these labs learned how the system worked, and as they moved into higher positions they took these habits with them. A result was scandals such as those involving Robert Slutsky, who in his publication spree of 137 articles in seven years gave authorship to colleagues as favors and even to important strangers who had never seen the paper (see chap. 1). (Incidentally, some of the research being reported was fabricated, but that is a separate level of misconduct.) The same troublesome attitudes toward authorship are seen today when a junior colleague is pressured to add the department chair's name as an author or when a colleague across the hall expects authorship in return for reading a rough draft of a paper.

Most senior faculty are scrupulous in observing journals' guidelines for authorship, especially in the aftermath of scandals like the Slutsky case. Many, however, hold to the unethical standards they learned early in their training. They cannot, therefore, teach their students what they never learned and do not practice. Thus, for the next 20 years, both the teachers and the trainees must be trained (or retrained). After several years of consistent teaching and oversight by editors, scientific societies, and institutional leaders, today's trainees will know what is expected of them once they are in senior positions, and they will be able to apply proper standards to the exigencies of scientific publishing in 2020.

To use biomedicine again as an example, the experience of the Vancouver Group can be a cautionary tale (ICMJE 1997). The editors who met informally in 1978 as what came to be called the Vancouver Group (and later formally became the International Committee of Medical Journal Editors [ICMJE]) were straightforward. They thought, with understandable optimism, that it would be sufficient for them, the editors of a dozen leading international general medical journals, to develop consensus standards in publishing ethics; make the written standards widely available to their fellow editors, to authors, and by extension to faculty leaders; and to publish occasional editorials about publication ethics. They expected that within a few years the standards would have spread throughout the biomedical community and that the standards would be met through the editors' rules and the authors' compliance.

The ICMJE's consensus standards have made a considerable difference, but they have not spread as broadly or deeply as hoped. Although several hundred journals are signatories to the ICMJE standards, some journals made no changes in the face of these standards, some made a few, and a few made substantial changes. Still, many biomedical authors today know nothing about them. Worse, many new biomedical editors—who reflect faculty opinion—do not know about them. Active members of CBE, EASE, and similar groups often meet editors who have held their posts for months, even years, and who have never heard of the ICMJE and its standards. And it is rare to find biomedical trainees or their supervising faculty who know of these consensus standards, which affect the operation and policies of many of the journals to which they intend to submit articles. Neither the trainees nor their faculty advisers may know even the rudiments of how they are supposed to act in writing and publishing their articles and often have little or no understanding of why editors are making such a fuss about these matters.

What Needs to Be Done?

Aggressive action must be taken to get publication ethics into mainstream discussions within the research and teaching communities of science.

Get the Issues onto the Program at National and Regional Meetings. Editors need to maintain their perspective as editors when they participate in national scientific and specialty societies, and faculty should consider these issues to be an essential feature of educational and similar meetings.

Raise Appropriate Issues in Other Contexts. When editors and others serve on committees and advisory panels or as officers of their scientific societies, they should ensure that publication ethics is considered by the society as a major part of professional conduct. Some societies have written codes of conduct, and some of them cover publication ethics. The Association of

American Medical Colleges (AAMC), whose concerns are much broader than its name implies, has as one of its governing councils the Council of Academic Societies (CAS), which consists of representatives of more than 80 biomedical societies. CAS is working with all of its member societies to help them develop codes of conduct. Editors and other concerned faculty and administrators need to work with their specialty colleagues to incorporate publication ethics into the societies' codes and standards.

Work with Institutional Codes of Conduct. Editors and others who understand publication ethics need to step forward to serve on the committees that establish or oversee the codes of conduct drawn up by their universities, institutes, hospitals, and departments, so that publication ethics is appropriately covered by these internal codes. Faculty members who are also editors should sit on disciplinary committees because these committees often must render decisions on conduct that directly or indirectly has to do with publication.

Address Senior Colleagues. Editors may receive invitations to speak from their role as editor, but this happens mostly with the full-time editors of major international journals. Most editors hold full-time faculty positions, and speaking invitations are usually issued to them in their role as researchers and specialists. Editors of both types can use these occasions, when appropriate, to address their colleagues on important issues of publication ethics, particularly by serving as an honest broker between the community of editors and the mass of faculty members who are authors and reviewers but have not been editors. A candid discussion of publication ethics by a prominent member of a scientific society, who can speak as one of their own, can do more to raise awareness of the issues of publication ethics than can many learned articles, no matter how persuasive.

Address Junior Colleagues. Editors, faculty, and senior administrators need to create opportunities to speak about publication ethics with junior colleagues, both in formal presentations and in casual conversations. The words of the editor of a high-prestige journal (the small subspecialty journals as well as the international powerhouses) at an ethics seminar, a faculty development workshop, or a session for senior leaders carry great weight. Moreover, members of different divisions and parts of the hierarchy would hear the message at the same time, and the standards laid out by the editor would become part of an ongoing institutional discussion of the topic, which could be followed up effectively by faculty members and others. Further, the presence of the editor demonstrates in the most direct possible way the importance that editors place on ethics.

Write about the Issues. Editors and other leaders must write about publication ethics in a wide range of publications. The ethical issues are not part of an obscure adjunct to academic and research life. They are, instead, the issues that most directly affect the reputation of individuals and institutions: the public record of work, presented for the use of present and future researchers. The editorial is effective and keeps the issue alive among a journal's readers, but editors need to expand into other fields. Editors must join other concerned faculty in writing workbooks and manuals, computer-based self-study courses, reference documents, and Web documents. Faculty development specialists need to ensure that publication ethics is included with other ethical issues (human subjects research or patient confidentiality, for example) but, even more importantly, that it is covered at all proper points in the curriculum and that it is introduced in informal as well as formal teaching sessions. To do so, they may need to help write supportive documents and tools for the faculty.

Foundations and Funding Agencies

Foundations and funding agencies need to support, and even create, programs in publication ethics. Because of their flexibility, foundations will be especially important in developing the broad range of approaches, coalitions, and collaborations needed to convince science leaders of the importance of publication ethics. Government funding agencies can play a major role in commissioning studies, creating and maintaining bodies of information, and supporting nationwide programs that, for example, include publication ethics in courses on research ethics. Both groups, foundations and government agencies, can require ethical publication practices as a condition for receiving financial support, as they do now in terms of human-subjects research and other vital areas. The following preliminary list gives only a hint of the imaginative ways in which foundations could support this effort.

A Database on Editors. The basic building block for many of the programs and suggestions throughout this chapter is a database on editors of peer-reviewed journals. The community needs to know how many editors it has, where they are, and their basic characteristics. Because this is a large international project, it will need substantial underwriting. Only then could the different scientific communities know how to reach all their editors. Only with such a database could editors receive systematically the materials they need to run their journals well or to take part in editors' discussions of the issues of publication ethics. Also, such a database is the only way to identify editors who are available to help teach the next generation of researcher-authors. This database is also essential to involving as many editors as possible in surveys of editors' practices, policies, opinions, problems, and problem solving.

Print, Electronic, and Video Publication. Foundations should support the creation of workbooks, manuals, and other specialized documents for teaching and learning about publication ethics, and these materials should be designed for faculty and trainees. The materials should appear in several formats: print, CD-ROM, video, and online. For example, faculty and trainees need to practice role-playing exercises in handling various troublesome and difficult issues in publication ethics. Scenarios and other materials could be developed in different formats for individual study, small-group discussion, and lecture. Thus far, no one has developed "trigger tapes" or other videotapes for exercises that help faculty and trainees understand why salami science, repetitive publication, honorary authorship, and conflict of interest erode the usefulness of the scientific literature. Nor are teaching tools widely available for dealing with such commonplace disagreements as those over authorship.

Courses for Newly Appointed Editors. At a minimum, foundations could support programs that give information to new editors. More importantly, they could support cooperation among relevant organizations—EASE, CBE, the Association of Earth Science Editors, and WAME, as a beginning. These groups, acting perhaps through an executive committee representing all of them, could design and offer comprehensive introductory courses and follow-up programs. Also, special courses could be tailored for editors in specific scientific communities. With proper support the existing groups could create expanded workbooks and reference books based on their present courses (Korenman and Shipp 1994). These could be sold or (if properly subsidized) given to new editors even if they did not attend the course. The expanded materials could contain printed material, CD-ROMs, and well-annotated bibliographies of online sources.

Further, the course(s) could be offered to new editors two or more times each year in different parts of the country. One or two core faculty members—whose reputations alone would give credibility to the course, as is the case now with the CBE and EASE courses and was true for the Prague workshop—would travel to the site, where local faculty, editors, and other specialists would have been recruited as the rest of the course faculty. This approach offers several advantages. First, new editors would be more likely to participate if they did not have to travel far or greatly disrupt their schedules. Second, it would put the new editor in touch with nationally or internationally known editors of leading journals, as well as with a local or regional group of fellow novices and experienced editors. Each type of resource would be highly useful to new editors. Third, the course would instantly create a local or regional group that could work together on issues of publication ethics and related concerns.

Web Sites. A Web site could give or point to a wealth of information for those learning about or concerned with an issue in publication ethics. The site could also be linked to different journals' Web sites, which could give additional and specific information and advice. Another site could give information to editors about the policies, activities, and problems and solutions of fellow editors (as the WAME site is beginning to do) and could perhaps allow communication between experienced and newly appointed editors.

Government Agencies. Government granting agencies could expand the requirement that ethics teaching (including publication ethics) be part of research grants that involve trainees or their work. Some institutions have already expanded this required training to all graduate students in the sciences, for example. Further, granting agencies can continue to refine standards through well-focused task forces and working groups (National Academy of Sciences 1989a, 1989b), especially if they are focused on producing useful tools.

Conclusions

Editors are the members of the community most directly involved in publication, and because of their positions they see the broader issues of protecting the scientific literature. It is natural, therefore, that editors are leaders in setting ethical standards for scientific publication. The people most concerned about publication ethics are, naturally enough, talking primarily to each other. The discussions are lively and stimulating, and the

participants go away from the meetings with deeper, more complex understandings of issues of publication ethics and with more appropriate responses to them. The problem is that these hardy few are a tiny proportion
of their respective communities, and the people who most need to understand the issues are not even in the building, much less in the room. This is
not an unusual situation: tax specialists, religious leaders, and cultural critics face the same gap between the makeup of the people who are discussing
the important issues and the mass of others who are going about their daily
encounters with tax forms, sin, and MTV. Preaching to the choir is a natural stage of development when a group forms around a shared concern.

Now that the groups concerned with publication ethics are forming in
some parts of the scientific community—the biomedical community has
made considerable progress in this area—the groups need to take the message to those who are not in the room. We can choose among several
images for this active engagement, depending on our personalities and
vehemence: "moving to where the action is," "reaching out to the community," and "getting the word out" are some of the choices. Regardless of the
image, the scientific community must act on the issues of publication ethics—in the lab, the classroom, the department, the trainee-mentor meetings, the research team's working session, and the solitary office where the
author writes for publication.

References

Angell, M. 1999. The *Journal* and its owner—resolving the crisis. *New England Journal of Medicine* 341:752.

Caelleigh, A. S. 1993. Role of the journal editor in sustaining integrity in research.
Academic Medicine 68 (suppl to issue 9):S23–29.

Carter, S. L. 1996. *Integrity.* New York: Basic Books.

DiIulio, J. J., Jr. 1995. Arresting ideas: Tougher law enforcement is driving down urban crime. *Policy Review* 74:12–16.

Douglas, J. D. 1993. Deviance in the practice of science. *Academic Medicine* 68
(suppl to issue 9):S77–83.

Editorial governance for *JAMA*. 1999. *JAMA* 281:2240–42.

The ethics of scholarly publishing: A special issue. 1993. *Scholarly Publishing*
24:193–280.

The firing of Dr Lundberg [letters]. 1999. *JAMA* 281:1789–94.

Fletcher, S. W., and R. W. Fletcher. 1999. Medical editors, journal owners, and the
sacking of George Lundberg. *Journal of General Internal Medicine* 14:200–202.

Freeman, G. R. 1990. Kinetics of nonhomogeneous processes in human society:
Unethical behaviour and societal chaos. *Canadian Journal of Physics* 68:794–98.

Guarding the guardians: Research on editorial peer review. Selected proceedings from the First International Congress on Peer Review in Biomedical Publication, 1990. *JAMA* 263 (theme issue):1317–1441.

Hackett, E. J. 1993. A new perspective on scientific misconduct. *Academic Medicine* 68 (suppl to issue 9):S72–76.

Hafferty, F. W., and R. Franks. 1994. The hidden curriculum, ethics teaching, and the structure of medical education. *Academic Medicine* 69:861–71.

Horton, R. 1999. The sacking of *JAMA*. *Lancet* 353:252–53.

Hundert, E. M., F. Hafferty, and D. Christakis. 1996. Characteristics of the informal curriculum and trainees' ethical choices. *Academic Medicine* 71:624–33.

International Committee of Medical Journal Editors (ICMJE). 1997. Uniform requirements for manuscripts submitted to biomedical journals. *Annals of Internal Medicine* 126:36–47. See also http://www.acponline.org/journals/resource/unifreqr.htm. Site accessed 18 March 1999.

JAMA editors, AMA *Archives* journals editors, and *JAMA* editorial board members. 1999. *JAMA* and editorial independence. *JAMA* 281:460.

Kassirer, J. P. 1999a. Goodbye, for now. *New England Journal of Medicine* 341:686–7.

——. 1999b. Should medical journals try to influence political debates? *New England Journal of Medicine* 340:466–67.

Kelling, G. L., and C. M. Coles. 1996. *Fixing broken windows: Restoring order and reducing crime in our communities and cities.* New York: Free Press.

Korenman, S. G., R. Berk, N. S. Wenger, and V. Lew. 1998. Evaluation of the research norms of scientists and administrators responsible for academic research integrity. *JAMA* 279:41–47.

Korenman, S. G., and A. C. Shipp. 1994. *Teaching the responsible conduct of research through a case study approach: A handbook for instructors.* Washington, D.C.: Association of American Medical Colleges.

National Academy of Sciences (NAS), Committee on the Conduct of Science. 1989a. *On being a scientist.* Washington, D.C.: National Academy Press.

National Academy of Sciences (NAS), Institute of Medicine. 1989b. *Responsible conduct of research in the health sciences: Report of a study.* Washington, D.C.: National Academy of Sciences.

National Research Council of Canada. 1993. *Comments on the article* Kinetics of nonhomogeneous processes in human society: Unethical behaviour and societal chaos *by G. R. Freeman that appeared in the* Canadian Journal of Physics *68, 794–798 (1990).* Ottawa: National Research Council of Canada. See also *Canadian Journal of Physics* 71:181–203.

Parrish, D. M. 1999. Scientific misconduct and correcting the scientific literature. *Academic Medicine* 74:221–30.

Peer Review Congress III. 1998. *JAMA* 280 (theme issue):213–302.

Pooley, E., with E. Rivera. 1996. One good apple. *Time,* 15 January, 54–56.

Pritchard, I. A. 1993. Integrity versus misconduct: Learning the difference between right and wrong. *Academic Medicine* 68 (suppl to issue 9): S67–71.

Reiser, S. J. 1993. Overlooking ethics in the search for objectivity and misconduct in science. *Academic Medicine* 68 (suppl to issue 9): S84–87.

The Second International Congress on Peer Review in Biomedical Publication. 1994. *JAMA* 272 (theme issue):91–173.

Smith, R. 1999. The firing of Brother George. *BMJ* 318:210.

Tanne, J. H. 1999. U.S. medical association reaches agreement with sacked editor. *BMJ* 318:416.

Wenger, N. S., S. G. Korenman, R. Berk, and H. Liu. 1998. Punishment for unethical behavior in the conduct of research. *Academic Medicine* 73:1187–94.

Wilson, J. Q. 1985. *Thinking about crime.* Rev. ed. New York: Vintage Books.

Wilson, J. Q., and G. L. Kelling. 1982. Broken windows. *Atlantic Monthly,* March, 29–38.

World Association of Medical Editors (WAME). 1998. http://www.wame.org/. Site accessed 18 March 1999.

III

Commentaries and Epilogue

Research Misconduct and the Ethics of Scientific Publication

12

Paul J. Friedman

The ethics of scientific publication—the set of rules, often unwritten, that describes the proper actions of authors by today's standards—has received increasing attention in recent years because of the observation that an urge to be published motivates distasteful behavior in some scientists, a behavior that in the extreme is called *research misconduct*. In its broadest sense, research misconduct is deviation from the norms of good scientific practice (table 12.1). These deviations, which can range from recording results of experiments on paper towels in the laboratory to making up experimental results from whole cloth, lie along a wide spectrum of importance, from fairly trivial to very serious. Where to draw the line between trivial and serious and who should determine the seriousness of a particular deviation are matters of ongoing debate. Clearly, measures to reduce research misconduct by either punishment (see chaps. 8 and 9) or education (see chap. 10) must take into account both its range and causes. Inappropriate or deviant practices vary in cause, from ignorance or laziness to overconfidence, negligence, arrogance, recklessness, ambition, or a sociopathic (and unscientific) attitude toward the truth.

Misconduct, as I have learned in my career as a clinician, researcher, and adjudicator of a well-known case of scientific fraud (Engler et al. 1987; Friedman 1990), is not always black and white—it often comes in shades of gray. When, for example, is lack of citation an error, and when is it a culpable act? How serious must a breach of confidentiality or use of confidential information be to constitute misconduct? Is it misconduct to screen data with multiple statistical tests to find one that gives significance? When two scientists dispute which of them originated an idea or provided a key element of a grant application or research paper, is one of them guilty of plagiarism or misconduct? Why is the definition of good or bad publication practices even an issue?

Table 12.1. Violations of Good Research Practices: Gray and Black

Category	Examples
Data	Reusing old controls
	Ignoring the statistical need for replication
	Choosing incorrect statistical tests to favor a positive result
	Carelessly misinterpreting results
	Deliberately misinterpreting results
	Suppressing outliers or other unfavorable data
	Accepting collaborators' results uncritically
	Writing anticipated results in data notebooks
	Keeping records on paper scraps, in pencil, etc.
	Creating imaginary data to fit a graph, etc.
Methods	Changing the protocol between replications
	Failing to cite sources of methods
	Using new methods without validation
	Using others' unpublished methods without permission
	Using unqualified assistants without supervision
	Leaving out critical steps in published descriptions
	Claiming to have done steps that actually were not
	Describing experimental subjects or animals misleadingly
	Inflating numbers of experiments or subjects
	Failing to comply with Institutional Review Board requirements for the approval of human experimentation
	Violating the spirit or letter of informed consent requirements
	Changing research protocols after approval
	Ignoring institutional regulations for animal research
	Reusing animals for possibly conflicting experiments

Other chapters in this volume have examined the various prevailing definitions of misconduct and the broader topics usually associated with ethical considerations in publication. Here I highlight some less commonly discussed but critical areas of research practice, areas that may also play crucial roles in ethical scientific publication. Before examining specific practices, however, I want to step back and ask what causes these unethical behaviors. Motives are not hard to find, although they vary in the degree to which they earn our condemnation. Perhaps the most basic is an urgent

Table 12.1. continued

Category	Examples
Presentation	Presenting a biased selection of results
	Inflating claims of the significance of results
	Failing to qualify public statements about the work
	Misrepresenting the amount of work done
	Ignoring the work of predecessors
	Presenting the same work multiple times
	Dividing work into "least publishable units"
	Presenting methods or theories as original when they are not
	Presenting other's results as one's own
	Copying text or figures from prior writing without citation or permission; this includes methods sections
	Copying text from others' writing without attribution
Authorship	Granting gift, guest, or honorary (co)authorship, freely or in exchange for a favor
	Biased omitting of some workers as authors
	Failing to involve all authors in reviewing the manuscript
	Changing the order of authors without agreement
	Denying responsibility for the correctness of the work
	Excluding a trainee from deserved first authorship
	Denying a co-author use of the collaborative text or methods
Reviewing	Accepting a manuscript to review despite a conflict of interest
	Copying a confidential manuscript "for the file"
	Providing copies of a manuscript to one's students
	Showing a colleague a manuscript without consulting the editor
	Delaying review to gain a competitive advantage
	Using information from a confidential manuscript review
	Writing an unfair review to slow or prevent publication
	Copying and personally submitting another's manuscript
Retention and sharing of data and materials	Discarding primary data before they are reviewed
	Discarding research records after preparing the manuscript
	Sequestering research records away from co-workers
	Taking original data away from a laboratory
	Taking materials from a laboratory without agreement
	Refusing to share biological materials with qualified labs
	Exceeding reasonable delays in releasing detailed information or special biological materials

table continues

Table 12.1. continued

Category	Examples
Mentoring	Neglecting general as well as specific training for students
	Demanding all-consuming time commitments
	Providing speculative projects for thesis work
	Delaying trainees' completion of thesis requirements
	Setting students to work competitively on duplicate projects
	Requiring students to delay their own work to help others, without arranging for proper authorship credit
	Treating students or technicians with lack of respect
	Discriminating on the basis of gender or ethnicity
	Appropriating the ideas or work of a student without credit
	Setting a bad example with regard to research ethics
Managing misconduct	Ignoring deviations from acceptable behavior by colleagues
	Failing to report suspicions of serious misconduct
	Keeping knowledge of misconduct confined to the laboratory
	Covering up evidence of research fraud
	Ignoring institutional policies on misconduct or conflict of interest
	Breaking the confidentiality of an inquiry or investigation
	Failing to cooperate with institutional investigations
	Failing to disclose personal relationships or conflicts when serving on a misconduct committee
	Denying one's share of responsibility in collaborative work that proves incorrect or fraudulent
	Retaliating against a whistleblower who acted in good faith

desire to get papers published, driven in large part by the ethos of academia, which uses publications as a measure of merit and accomplishment, critical to advancement.

The Causes of Unethical Behavior

Scientific reputation has always been heavily dependent upon what appears in print, and even in the current era comparatively little weight is given to teaching or service. Many academic institutions act as if they were research institutions, or wish they were, and tailor their environment and advancement policies accordingly. It is not only the public notice, institutional prestige, and overhead dollars that lead to this thrust. It includes a realistic appraisal of what it takes to recruit, retain, and maintain the best academicians and a recognition that successful research has the greatest long-term effect on the accumulated store of knowledge and the well-being of society. Faculty reviewers are clearly more confident in assessing the value of research papers than that of lectures or courses, and they understand that success in research is what it takes to recruit the brightest students. And the measure of success in research is publication. One might counter that research grant support is a better measure of success, but it is clear that winning grants depends on showing published results. Therefore, the prospect of gaining or renewing financial support is as dependent as academic advancement is on research publication and authorship.

One of the first steps in assessing the merit of curriculum vitae is noting whether the papers are in first-rank peer-reviewed publications, secondary journals, or any of the multitude of commercial specialty journals or magazines. Reviews and chapters in books may be very useful to other scientists and students, but they are not valued as highly as original research articles. Even though reviewers are often criticized for counting or weighing papers (instead of doing a critical analysis), such discriminatory judgments *are* commonly made. This demand makes for tough competition among authors for the available pages in the top research journals, which puts a premium on getting exciting results that are new, not merely confirmatory, and surely not negative. Whether this point of view reflects reality or just authors' perceptions of reality does not make much difference in the outcome. In turn, the journals put a premium on space-saving articles, without too many words devoted to the intellectual progenitors of the project or the details of its methodology. Further, editors look more favorably on the work of a known leader or a manuscript on which such a figure is a co-author. These factors may have an effect on how research is conducted and authorship is decided.

Although it has always required a number of first-authored publications to earn promotion, it now takes a handful of papers even to get appointed. Gone are the days when a Ph.D. student graduated with a polished thesis and spent the first year or two as a faculty member publishing the results. Now it takes publications to get a postdoctoral position, and by the time the second postdoctoral term is over, the candidate for a regular position has about as many publications as it used to take to get promoted.

The academic emphasis on publication is not intrinsically bad, since it stems from the recognition that a meritorious publication is an excellent reflection of an individual's capabilities. And, the logical argument continues, surely someone whose name appears on 20 sound published papers is a stronger candidate than someone who has published only five papers. Promotion signifies a long-term investment by an institution and warrants careful scrutiny of credentials and clear demonstration of an individual's abilities as a productive investigator, prolific author, and successful grant writer. In other words, the stressful and overcompetitive system that keeps our faculty doing and publishing research is based on valid and worthwhile considerations. If the system can be criticized, it is for lack of balance.

Deceptive Manipulations

The pressure to publish felt by authors manifests itself in a variety of ways. These include rushing to complete a manuscript before the work is really finished in order to beat the known competition, ignoring the prior or current contributions of others to make the work seem more original, or improving the paper to make it more appealing to reviewers or editors. "Improvement" could consist of increasing the number of experiments reported, improving the significance levels of the statistical tests, adding a senior scientist as co-author, or doing elaborate analytical studies with a variety of controls. There's nothing wrong with these activities if they reflect reality: more experiments were really done; the variances decreased with repetition; a senior scientist really did take part in planning the experiments, analyzing the results, and working on the manuscript; and the reported methods were applied as widely and uniformly as stated. But perhaps some of these other experiments or tests were imaginary, or the senior scientist did not really participate or even know his name would be used. It's not the desire to strengthen a paper that's at fault—it's how it was done that counts.

Other manipulations are also unworthy. For example, leaving out crucial steps in the methods section to slow down competitors trying to use those techniques is engaging in misrepresentation (Jones 1980), although editors' urging to keep manuscripts short provides good camouflage. Relevant references may also be omitted, not just to save space, but also to suggest that the methods or results are more original than they are. Similarly, in reviewing manuscripts, it is unethical to hold a paper for a few months to allow one's own laboratory enough time to finish a competing project. So is raising extraneous objections to a research grant application in order to delay or sabotage its funding. Granting undeserved co-authorship may be merely a favor for a friend, colleague, or senior faculty member; putting a well-known name on the paper may be a trick to enhance editorial interest; or gift authorship may be used to disguise the fact that a convincing but fabricated experiment did not require anyone other than the first author to make it up.

Other manipulations are more complex. Data selection, like awarding authorship, has earned a bad reputation through its alleged role in cases of falsification. The range of motivations for it is similar to that for any other unethical research practice, from making a paper look better to proving a result that is not true. However, honest selection of data is an indispensable part of research in an effort to control quality, to reflect details of individual experiments, or to find a subset of all the results that can fit in restricted publication space and still demonstrate the validity of the conclusions.

Some researchers concerned about dishonest data selection have proposed publication of all the data, an idea guaranteed to make honest scientists and editors shudder. (Even with electronic data archives that allow publication of far more than the printed data, few scientists would find it useful to display their many unsuccessful results for public dissemination.) Legitimate data selection must be practiced with discretion, honesty, and rigor.

Unfortunately, there are common selection practices that are less serious than research misconduct but do involve deception of the editor and reader. No one who chooses a picture of a gel or a radiograph or a graph of experimental data to use in a publication does so randomly. One selects a "representative" image, but more likely representative of the best-looking results than of all the repetitions. Is this an ethically problematic practice? Or only when the result presented is actually not representative of the rest of the data?

The other side of this practice is suppression of results. Leaving out the results of one or two specific experiments or clinical observations, deleting a statistical outlier, presenting a structured subset of all the results, omitting data to help the statistical analysis achieve significance—these various levels of suppression range from appropriate to improper to fraudulent (but not in the order listed). Preparing for publication clearly stimulates data selection, good or bad.

These and other petty deceptions do not constitute federally condemned falsification, fabrication, and plagiarism, but they should be described as unethical research and publication practices. On the other hand, the reporting of steps that were not actually taken, numbers of replications that were not done, controls that were not performed, data that differ from those in the notebooks, or data from wholly imaginary experiments constitutes fabrication or falsification, is clearly over the line, and warrants a proper inquiry and investigation followed by censure.

Preventive Measures: The Role of Educational Institutions, Professional Societies, and Journal Editors

Do minor or common transgressions lead to serious violations of the norms of science? The histories of those who have committed research fraud show earlier but less serious unethical or deceitful practices. These people have "drifted" down the slippery slope of misbehavior (Douglas 1993, S81) and have been caught. But most individuals who violate some norm, whether through ignorance, willfulness, or impatience, do not go on to serious misconduct. Is the difference in the individuals or their environment? Is the best way to improve the outcome to educate individual scientists, modify their environment, or impose more oversight of their research and sanctions for the violations? Perhaps the best approach is multifaceted, involving all of the parties invested in the processes of research and publication—educational institutions, professional societies, and editors.

Two influences have determined the responses of educational institutions. While successfully resisting pressures to reduce the freedom and independence of researchers, grantee institutions have been required by U.S. federal regulations to develop mechanisms to investigate suspected wrongdoing and to impose appropriate sanctions (see chaps. 8 and 9). A more positive approach, education, has also been stimulated by federal regulation, based on the hope that greater awareness of ethical issues will improve behavior (see chap. 10). Purposeful modification of the environment is harder to achieve, but the increased emphasis on mentoring and the very existence of new courses on research ethics are changing the environment favorably, even as fiscal restraints, increasing competition for the federal dollar, and rampant entrepreneurial activity are having an admittedly negative effect on research ethics.

Unfortunately, the norms of publication practice and record keeping in the laboratory to support research claims are unlikely to be articulated in a faculty code of conduct; senior scientists and other institutional leaders seem to believe that these are basics that their colleagues are sure to know. Only a handful of institutions spell out details of good practice, including publication practices (Eastwood et al. 1989; Committee on Academic Responsibility 1992; Faculty of Medicine, Harvard University 1988, 1991; Stanford University 1999; University of Michigan Medical School 1989).

Likewise, although professional societies may have codes of ethics that describe the aspirations of their members to the responsible conduct of research (and practice), few have spelled out details concerning a wide range of publication practices. My own society, the Association of University Radiologists (Friedman 1993b), like a few others (Huth 1997), has a published policy on authorship, even though it does not have the intention or the mechanism to settle disputes. The term *research misconduct* does not appear in this document, since it describes good practices rather than bad practices, but other professional groups have been explicit in describing undesirable practices, notably repetitive publication and negligent statistical analysis (Australian Vice-Chancellors' Committee 1997). One of the most detailed statements I have seen was published as an editorial by the *American Journal of Obstetrics and Gynecology* (Specific inappropriate acts 1996). This statement surpasses most statements concerning misconduct, in that it specifies the range of sanctions that would be imposed for violations of the code.

Editors wield a great deal of influence on ethical practices in publication. Their power, however, is balanced by reciprocal obligations. Editors can find themselves with as many entanglements as authors, if not more. Since I have never been an editor (except of a supplement [Friedman 1993a]), I can distance myself from the ethical and legal dilemmas that confront editors regularly (see case histories in Council of Biology Editors [CBE] 1990). Editors are not usually required to disclose their conflicts of interest, but they are easy to imagine. They must balance allegiance to institutions, supporters, powerful colleagues, and advertisers with a fiduciary responsibility to the journal, the sponsoring society or publisher, the scientific reader, the public, and the authors (see chap. 11). Incidentally, this illustrates a phenomenon known also in the law: there may be conflicts *between* an individual's fiduciary interests.

The rules of objectivity in selecting manuscripts for publication are unwritten but widely understood. But it is tempting to choose "easy" or "tough" referees to influence whether a paper is accepted because of other interests. The competitiveness that is characteristic of leading scientists is also found in the leading journals. Rapid review and acceptance of "hot" papers is well recognized (Roberts 1991) but becomes ethically dubious when the object is to beat out the competition's publication. How scrupulous must the editor be in checking the statistics (a notorious weak spot) of a submission? In contrast to the low probability of recognizing that an investigator is dishonest, it *is* possible to tell whether the author is computationally correct, placing an onus on the editor to do so (Fienberg 1990; Stoto 1990). Are negative results less likely to be published than positive ones (biasing the literature)? Current research shows that authors *anticipate* that editors will find negative results less worthwhile and thus fail to submit such papers (Dickersin, Min, and Meinert 1992; Rennie and Flanagin 1992).

Editors have ethical responsibilities beyond supervising a critical selection system for papers in an ethical manner. Questions of research misconduct will arise in the work of reviewers, either through detection or commission, and editors must be prepared to deal with these cautiously but effectively. The editorial blacklist, mentioned in confidential tones when editors get together, is not sufficient to protect the scientific literature, nor is it compiled with much due process. Thus, journals are in a position similar to that of research institutions more than a decade ago, before federal agencies forced them to develop policies and procedures for responding to charges of research misconduct. Skillful improvisation when faced with a case is not as good as following guidelines or policies that are in writing, not only for efficacy, but also to minimize legal liability. Because institutions have been given by federal agencies the job of enforcing the good behavior of their employees, it is important that the institution be notified if questions of integrity arise during peer review of or by one of their faculty members. It is helpful if written rules direct the editor to do this (Specific inappropriate acts 1996). The journal staff is rarely able to mount a formal inquiry and investigation, and since the journal is not the employer, it lacks standing to compel cooperation by the individual. It is far better for the institution to exercise its rights and responsibilities in conducting a review of the charges, with the due process that is incorporated into its policies.

Editors are quite convinced of the central role of publication in the documentation of scientific progress; they do not need any persuasion. Regard for the validity of the written record motivates a great deal of effort in editing and peer reviewing and is the antepenultimate concern in the federal attack on misconduct (the ultimate concern is that the public will suffer from misapplication of false research findings; the penultimate concern is the waste of taxpayer dollars on invalid results). At least one editor has suggested that only *published* falsification, fabrication, and plagiarism should be counted as research misconduct, considerably reducing the range of activities that need be challenged and investigated.

There seems to be much greater indignation among misconduct investigation committee members in response to published lies, in contrast to false statements in grant applications or progress reports, meeting abstracts, or even in submitted manuscripts. A logical inconsistency arises, however: if fabricated research is detected as such before publication, blocking its acceptance, then it would fail to meet this narrow criterion of misconduct. To stave off publication fraud, however, one must be equally concerned about these prepublication transgressions, such as those I have briefly enumerated here; we cannot ignore deviations from good practice. Concern for the written record, therefore, must be acted on by setting and monitoring standards for the many complex and challenging aspects of doing and presenting research.

References

Australian Vice-Chancellors' Committee. 1997. Joint NHMRC/AVCC statement and guidelines on research practice. http://www.cs.rmit.edu.au/~jz/write/glrespra.htm. Site accessed 17 March 1999.

Committee on Academic Responsibility, Massachusetts Institute of Technology. 1992. *Fostering academic integrity.* Cambridge: Massachusetts Institute of Technology.

Council of Biology Editors (CBE), Editorial Policy Committee. 1990. *Ethics and policy in scientific publication.* Bethesda, Md.: Council of Biology Editors.

Dickersin, K., Y.-I. Min, and C. L. Meinert. 1992. Factors influencing publication of research results: Follow-up of applications submitted to two institutional review boards. *JAMA* 267:374–78.

Douglas, J. D. 1993. Deviance in the practice of science. *Academic Medicine* 68 (suppl to issue 9): S77–83.

Eastwood, S., P. H. Cogen, J. R. Fike, H. Rosegay, and M. Berens. 1989. BTRC guidelines on research data and manuscripts. San Francisco: Brain Tumor Research Center, University of California, San Francisco. Reprinted in *Responsible science: Ensuring the integrity of the research process,* Panel on Scientific Responsibility and the Conduct of Research, Committee on Science, Engineering, and Public Policy, National Academy of Sciences, National Academy of Engineering, Institute of Medicine, 2:206–22. Washington, D.C.: National Academy Press, 1993.

Engler, R. L., J. W. Covell, P. J. Friedman, P. S. Kitcher, and R. M. Peters. 1987. Misrepresentation and responsibility in medical research. *New England Journal of Medicine* 317:1383–89.

Faculty of Medicine, Harvard University. 1988. Guidelines for investigators in scientific research. In *Faculty policies on integrity in science,* 4–5. Boston: Harvard Medical School, 1996. See also http://www.hms.harvard.edu/integrity/scientif.html. Site accessed 17 March 1999.

———. 1991. Guidelines for investigators in clinical research. In *Faculty policies on integrity in science,* 6–7. Boston: Harvard Medical School, 1996. See also http://www.hms.harvard.edu/integrity/clinical.html. Site accessed 17 March 1999.

Fienberg, S. E. 1990. Statistical reporting in scientific journals. In Council of Biology Editors, Editorial Policy Committee, *Ethics and policy in scientific publication,* 202–6. Bethesda, Md.: Council of Biology Editors.

Friedman, P. J. 1990. Correcting the literature following fraudulent publication. *JAMA* 263:1416–19.

———, ed. 1993a. Integrity in biomedical research. *Academic Medicine* 68 (suppl to issue 9): S1–102.

———. 1993b. Standards for authorship and publication in academic radiology. Association of University Radiologists' Ad Hoc Committee on Standards for the Responsible Conduct of Research. *Radiology* 189:33–34; *Investigative Radiology* 28:879–81; *AJR American Journal of Roentgenology* 161:899–900.

Huth, E. J. 1997. Authorship standards: Progress in slow motion. *CBE Views* 20:127–32.

Jones, A. H. 1980. A question of ethics: Materials and methods. In *Proceedings of the 27th International Technical Communication Conference,* 2:W85–87. Washington, D.C.: Society for Technical Communication. Reprinted in *Technical communication and ethics,* ed. R. J. Brockmann and F. Rook, 45–47. Washington, D.C.: Society for Technical Communication, 1989.

Rennie, D., and A. Flanagin. 1992. Publication bias: The triumph of hope over experience. *JAMA* 267:411–12.

Roberts, L. 1991. The rush to publish. *Science* 251:260–63.

Specific inappropriate acts in the publication process. 1996. *American Journal of Obstetrics and Gynecology* 174:1–9.

Stanford University. 1999. Research policy handbook. http://www.stanford.edu/dept/DoR/RPH.html. Site accessed 17 March 1999.

Stoto, M. A. 1990. From data to analysis to conclusions: A statistician's view. In Council of Biology Editors, Editorial Policy Committee, *Ethics and policy in scientific publication,* 207–13. Bethesda, Md.: Council of Biology Editors.

University of Michigan Medical School. 1989. *Guidelines for the responsible conduct of research.* Ann Arbor: University of Michigan.

Douglas S. DeWitt

Until recently in my career as a professional scientist, I had not given much thought to scientific misconduct, publication ethics, or the peer-review process. And the idea that a group of prominent editors who met in Vancouver would tell me whether to put my department chair's name fourth, last, or not at all on my manuscripts would have struck me as funny. When I was asked to participate in the workshop that resulted in this text, I assumed it was because the organizers wanted a "real" scientist to offer a dose of reality to an otherwise theoretical and largely impractical discussion. But after I attended the workshop and then read the other chapters in this book, I was amazed at how practical and important the information is for real scientists.

A significant portion of a scientist's professional life is spent dealing with regulations, guidelines, and forms. We deal with regulations from our biohazard safety office (and, indirectly, from the federal Nuclear Regulatory Commission or state Bureaus of Radiation Control, the Occupational Safety and Health Administration, etc.) about how to safely handle and track radioactive and other hazardous materials. We have to cope with animal welfare requirements from the Department of Agriculture, the National Institutes of Health (NIH), and our own universities' animal care and use committees. We have to assure and document that our laboratory staff is trained to meet stringent regulations concerning general laboratory safety practices. Every funding agency from the NIH and the National Science Foundation to the Department of Defense to pharmaceutical companies has its own set of guidelines that must be met if we want to obtain and retain extramural funding. All of us recognize the importance of humane treatment of laboratory animals and of safe laboratory practices, so none of us seriously objects to animal welfare or biohazard safety regulations. But do we really need another complicated set of rules and guidelines, this time dealing with publication ethics? The answer is that we do.

Scientists are, overall, an honest bunch who can be trusted to make the right choice in an ethical conundrum. Unfortunately, we are influenced by forces that act in such a way as sometimes to obscure the right choice. For example, early in my career I was asked to review a manuscript for a senior faculty member, Dr. X, who did not want a formal review, just "some ideas to include with [his] own review." I provided a couple of pages of comments and didn't think anything of it until, several months later, I was given a revised version of the same manuscript (with the reviewers' comments) to review again. I was surprised to see that Dr. X had simply submitted my comments verbatim as his review. At the time I was flattered that he had liked my review enough to submit it as his own, but I realize now that what Dr. X had done was unethical. The reasons that Dr. X's behavior was unethical in this situation—as well as ethical considerations in many other situations—are clearly described and analyzed in the chapters in this book, which also offer guidance to help those of us faced with similar choices. Fortunately for those of us of a more practical than theoretical nature, most of the guidance and examples are based on actual rather than hypothetical situations.

An important reason for scientists to pay close attention to the ethics of scientific publication is that, as other industries have discovered, reaction and overreaction to well-publicized examples of occasional misconduct will add to the regulatory burden already borne by the scientific community. There seems to be a mild antiscience bias in the media and the entertainment industry, which often portray scientists unfavorably in films and on television. Cases of misrepresentation, plagiarism, and fraud will occur as long as human beings are involved in science, but it is our responsibility to demonstrate that the scientific community has done everything reasonable to minimize the opportunities for scientific misconduct and that we, as a community, react vigorously to incidents of unethical behavior once they are discovered. Conversely, no one wants a witch hunt, and alleged misconduct should be investigated fairly but expeditiously. Debra M. Parrish and C. K. Gunsalus provide very thorough descriptions of some of the mechanisms currently in place to deal with scientific and intellectual dishonesty (chaps. 8 and 9). Ideally, the scientific community will continue to monitor and regulate itself through our universities, journals, and professional societies.

In chapter 1, Anne Hudson Jones discusses the cases of Darsee (Culliton 1983) and Slutsky (Engler et al. 1987). These incidents disturb scientists who are involved in collaborative research, which now includes virtually all active investigators. Most of us are working on projects in which data are collected by several investigators, and most of us do not have the expertise to recognize falsified results from sophisticated techniques and analytical methods outside our own fields. Even projects being conducted by fellows in our own laboratories are difficult to monitor without our being present for each experiment.

A recent episode of plagiarism illustrates a kind of scientific misconduct to which most of us are vulnerable (Todd 1998). An invited editorial by Bhardwaj and Kirsch (1998) appeared in the August 1998 issue of *Anesthesiology*. Soon after it was published, the editor of *Anesthesiology* received a letter from James Cottrell saying that he believed that the editorial had been, in part, copied from a refresher course that Cottrell had presented at a large professional meeting the previous year. Cottrell wrote to the senior author of the editorial (Kirsch) as well as to the editor of *Anesthesiology* (Michael Todd). Kirsch gave the letter to the administration of the Johns Hopkins Medical Institutions, which ruled that much of the editorial had been plagiarized and that the authors should write letters of apology to the journal. The letters were published in *Anesthesiology* (Bhardwaj 1998; Kirsch 1998), along with an editorial by Todd (1998) explaining the situation and apologizing for the incident. The original editorial was withdrawn.

This example is interesting, not only because it could happen to nearly any busy investigator, but also because of the forthright way in which the incident was handled. On being made aware of the misconduct, Kirsch quickly notified the Johns Hopkins's Standing Committee on Discipline, which immediately investigated the incident. There was little that Kirsch, an extremely capable, conscientious physician-scientist, could have done to recognize the plagiarized sections of the editorial, which Bhardwaj had drafted. Kirsch had neither attended Cottrell's refresher-course lecture nor read Cottrell's text, and he trusted Bhardwaj, with whom he had worked for years. When he found out about the misconduct, he made no attempt to diminish or explain away the incident but turned the affair over to his university's research integrity committee. The letters of apology written by the authors were published in the next available issue of *Anesthesiology* (December 1998). Since the normal time lag for publication of a journal article is seven to 12 months after acceptance, the publication of Todd's editorial about the situation and the letters from Kirsch and Bhardwaj only a few months after their original editorial appearance shows a commendable commitment to academic honesty on the part of Todd and *Anesthesiology*. Despite the appropriate way in which this situation was handled, however, prevention is better than the best cure. Our best defense against being involved in such inadvertent plagiarism is to educate our trainees and colleagues, as discussed by Susan Eastwood and Addeane S. Caelleigh (chaps. 10 and 11).

Most, if not all, scientists would agree that falsifying data, stealing ideas, and plagiarism are unethical practices. One would find much less agreement, however, about authorship and publication policies. One observation from recent surveys of publication ethics, summarized by Richard Horton in chapter 2, is that there does not seem to be any consensus among scientists about who should or should not be an author—which is hardly surprising, since there does not seem to be a strong consensus about authorship policies among scientific journals. The guidelines offered by the International Committee of Medical Journal Editors (ICMJE) are an attempt to provide some consistency among biomedical journals but, as Horton notes, these guidelines are still evolving and are not universally accepted among medical and biological journals. More important, perhaps, is that most scientists have probably never heard of the "Uniform Requirements for Manuscripts Submitted to Biomedical Journals," the ICMJE, the Vancouver Group, or their authorship policies. This is an untested hypothesis, but Eastwood's survey suggests that it is correct, at least among trainees (Eastwood et al. 1996) (see chap. 10).

The same could be said about repetitive publications (chap. 5). Edward J. Huth describes ways in which a study can be sliced and diced into multiple publications, and he accurately describes the reasons this might be done, either appropriately or inappropriately. Publishing the same paper in two or more different places seems unethical, but splitting a large study with multiple end points into two smaller, more easily discussed papers seems less egregious. For example, we reported (DeWitt et al. 1997) the results of a screening study of three agents that, based on previous studies in other models of injury, might be expected to improve cerebral blood flow after head trauma and hemorrhage. The study was designed to compare different treatments to the same control groups, thereby minimizing animal use. The experimental design involved measuring the primary end points of cerebral blood flow, oxygen delivery to the brain, and electroencephalographic activity, as well as more than a dozen other variables such as blood pressure, blood oxygen and carbon dioxide levels, pH, and so forth in five groups of animals. When we were writing the manuscript, we considered splitting the data into two more manageable studies to allow for a more complete discussion of the implications of our data and the mechanisms involved in the effects, or lack of effects, that we observed. Ultimately, we decided that, since it had been designed and executed as one study, it should be published as one study, even if it resulted in a long manuscript.

These and other kinds of gray areas can best be addressed by developing a consistent policy toward authorship and publication issues. I am probably typical of most human beings and perhaps most scientists, in that I like tradition and am suspicious of change, but I am willing to conform to a consistent and reasonable new policy. The more important solution, however, is education (see below).

All scientists are involved in the peer-review process in scientific publishing as either producers or consumers or both. There are obvious areas of potential misconduct in the peer-review process (e.g., the Soman-Felig case [Broad 1980]), which are thoroughly discussed by Fiona Godlee and Craig Bingham in chapters 3 and 4. The less obvious areas, also discussed in chapters 3 and 4, are more difficult to address. It used to be a common practice for senior scientists, such as Dr. X, to give their junior associates grants and manuscripts to review and then to submit the reviews under the senior scientists' names. This practice is less common now, probably because many journals now include instructions to reviewers explicitly discouraging or forbidding such behavior. Similarly, blinded reviews help reduce bias, and signed reviews seem nicer and perhaps even a little more fair, although it is naïve to assume that the reviewer who will delay publication and steal ideas from competitors will not retaliate against colleagues who submit unfavorable, signed reviews.

These and other methods to improve the quality of the peer-review process may be unpopular at first but will probably ultimately be welcomed because all scientists have an interest in making the peer-review process for grant applications, as well as for manuscripts, as fair as possible. Unfortunately, the peer-review process for grant applications may not lend itself as well to some of the changes that work well for manuscript reviews. For example, blinded reviews are not practical for grant applications because the reviewer is charged with evaluating the quality of the applicants, in addition to the proposed research. Another change in the manuscript review policy that would meet some resistance among grant reviewers is the signed review. A negative grant review can have a profound effect on a scientist's career and, unlike a rejected manuscript, a grant application cannot routinely be buffed up and submitted elsewhere. It would be a brave reviewer who would submit a signed review that was very critical of a senior scientist who might sit on the very study section at which the re-viewer's grant might be judged. On the other hand, certain ethical guide-lines are the same for reviewing both manuscripts and grant applications. The confidentiality of the content of a grant application is extremely im-portant because the ideas in an application are often preliminary and, as such, are more vulnerable to theft than are ideas in a manuscript describing a completed study, which has probably been presented at a meeting in preliminary form.

Widespread acceptance of the use of the Internet to disseminate infor-mation by the scientific community may occur differently from accep-tance of changes in authorship or peer-review practices. Increasing aware-ness of the issues of publication ethics described in this book will probably proceed from journals, funding agencies, and senior scientists to midlevel and junior associates and then to trainees and students. In contrast, stu-dents and trainees are currently the people most comfortable with the world of virtual knowledge. I am more than passingly familiar with infor-mation retrieval from the Internet and the World Wide Web, but my 25-year-old secretary and my students are much better than I am. The medical students of the University of Texas Medical Branch's problem-based curric-ulum regularly use the Web to get patient case material, subject material from anatomy to biochemistry and pharmacology, as well as pathology slides and X-rays and other radiologic studies. Whether or not they are aware of it, these students are dealing with the "virtual" ethical issues described by Faith McLellan (chap. 7). The *Medical Journal of Australia* has demonstrated with its *eMJA* model that some scientists are willing to try a new format, while the failure of the World Journal Association (Bingham et al. 1998) (see chap. 4) suggests that acceptance of electronic journals, espe-cially those using unconventional review methods (i.e., postpublication, online peer review) lies in the future. It remains to be seen whether young physicians and scientists will be as receptive to contributing information to the Internet and the Web as they are to using them as sources.

To understand how scientists view other aspects of publication ethics, it is important to understand why one would become a professional re-searcher in the first place. Although I cannot speak for all scientists, my rea-sons include, not necessarily in any order, curiosity (i.e., the satisfaction of solving problems), money (i.e., a job, livelihood, food and shelter, etc.), a desire to help (we'd all like to think that our research helped make some-one's life better), and fame. I like to think that, in pursuit of these interests, I behave ethically, but I certainly cannot state, beyond a reasonable doubt, that I never violate someone's standards or guidelines. Even though governments, universities, professional societies, and journals have all defined research ethics, scientific misconduct, and publication standards, I wonder whether the average scientist could provide even the briefest summary of the ethical policies of his professional society or her university. Parrish discusses several definitions of misconduct (chap. 8), Annette Flanagin describes scientific conflicts of interest in general (chap. 6), and Godlee discusses potential conflict of interest in peer review (chap. 3), but, in fact, most of the topics in this book deal with conflicts of interest, and the complex issues and solutions are capably described elsewhere in this book. Perhaps the best approach is that of the *Lancet,* described in chapter 6, which states that authors should disclose information if "a non-disclosed commercial interest, should it be revealed later, would prove embarrassing to an author" (Politics of disclosure 1996, 627). Such a "sunshine rule"—broadened to include undisclosed information about experimental procedures, data-manipulation practices, personal and professional relationships, authorship assignment, and whatever might later prove embarrassing if generally known—would be a simple and useful guideline for most situations.

It is tempting to argue that it might be premature to launch a major educational campaign on publication ethics, since there does not seem to be a consensus on ethical issues in authorship, peer review, and the other areas discussed elsewhere in this text. Such an argument misses the point that the general concepts of publication ethics are well established, and these concepts can and should be practiced and taught to our trainees. As Eastwood notes (chap. 10), the NIH has required that all pre- and postdoctoral fellows in NIH-funded training centers receive training in responsible research conduct. Eastwood goes on to provide a reasonable blueprint for a training program designed to teach both ethical and effective conduct and reporting.

An important message from both Eastwood and Caelleigh (chap. 11) is that our students, employees, and young colleagues are quick to grasp the inequitable nature of the "do as I say, not as I do" approach. Lecturing on ethical research practices in the morning while showing our students how to slice their data into the least publishable unit (see chap. 5) in the afternoon gives them the impression that windows are broken in our ethical structures (see chap. 11). Most scientists realize that progress in research depends on trust. We have to trust each other, and the public, which funds much of our research, directly or indirectly, has to trust that the answers we provide are as true and honest as possible. Anything that the scientific community—including editors and ethicists—can do to demonstrate that such trust is warranted will foster further trust, will help the public feel comfortable about spending their money on research, and will reduce the likelihood that the scientific community will fall under additional burdensome governmental regulations.

References

Bhardwaj, A. 1998. Letter to the editor. *Anesthesiology* 89:1307–8.

Bhardwaj, A., and J. R. Kirsch. 1998. Anesthetic agents and hypothermia in ischemic brain protection. *Anesthesiology* 89:289–91.

Bingham, C. M., G. Higgins, R. Coleman, and M. B. Van Der Weyden. 1998. The *Medical Journal of Australia* Internet peer-review study. *Lancet* 352:441–45.

Broad, W. 1980. Imbroglio at Yale (I): Emergence of a fraud. *Science* 210:38–41.

Culliton, B. J. 1983. Coping with fraud: The Darsee case. *Science* 220:31–35.

DeWitt, D. S., D. S. Prough, T. Uchida, D. D. Deal, and S. M. Vines. 1997. Effects of nalmefene, CG3703, tirilazad, or dopamine on cerebral blood flow, oxygen delivery, and electroencephalographic activity after traumatic brain injury and hemorrhage. *Journal of Neurotrauma* 14:931–41.

Eastwood, S., P. A. Derish, E. Leash, and S. B. Ordway. 1996. Ethical issues in biomedical research: Perceptions and practices of postdoctoral research fellows responding to a survey. *Science and Engineering Ethics* 2:89–114.

Engler, R. L., J. W. Covell, P. J. Friedman, P. S. Kitcher, and R. M. Peters. 1987. Misrepresentation and responsibility in medical research. *New England Journal of Medicine* 317:1383–89.

Kirsch, J. R. 1998. Letter to the editor. *Anesthesiology* 89:1308.

The politics of disclosure. 1996. *Lancet* 348:627.

Todd, M. M. 1998. Plagiarism. *Anesthesiology* 89:1307.

The Other Two Cultures
How Research and Publishing
Can Move Forward Together

Frank Davidoff

Many of the problems documented in this volume arise from the basic fact that scientific research and scientific publishing are worlds apart—two cultures every bit as disparate as the two cultures of science and the humanities described by C. P. Snow 40 years ago (Snow 1959). Yet, at the same time, these two worlds literally cannot exist without each other. As a thought experiment, try to imagine research without publishing; it cannot be done. Now try to imagine publishing without research—even more obviously an absurdity. As we reflect on what to make of the rich information in this book, it may help to explore what makes those two worlds so very different and how the two manage to stay connected. Understanding those worlds—how they fit together, the push and pull between them—also puts us in better position to improve the relationship between them.

The World of Scientific Research

Research is a messy business. As I have suggested elsewhere, "researchers function in an uncertain universe where they are required continually to break the mould, wallow in the data, [and] filter out tiny signals from the mass of information" (Davidoff 1998d, 895). When they practice their craft, scientists are working in the role that Anne Hudson Jones has identified as "author-as-creator" (see chap. 1). Edward O. Wilson (1998, 64) described the process this way: "Scientists . . . do not think in straight lines. . . . Perhaps only openly confessional memoirs, still rare to nonexistent, might disclose how scientists actually find their way to a publishable conclusion." And, in fact, the memoirs of the great German physicist Helmholtz actually capture the sense of living and working in that world. Oliver Sacks (1995, 167) summarized Helmholtz's account as follows:

Helmholtz . . . uses the image of a mountain climb (he himself was an ardent alpinist), but describes the climb as anything but linear. One cannot see in advance, he says, a way up the mountain; it can only be climbed by trial and error. The intellectual mountaineer makes false starts, gets stuck, gets into blind alleys and cul-de-sacs, finds himself in untenable positions, has to backtrack, has to descend and to start again. Thus, slowly and painfully, with innumerable errors and corrections, he makes his zigzag way up the mountain.

As they beaver away at this work, scientists continually share information with each other; critique each others' ideas, methods, and data; and test hypotheses. This process takes place on the phone, at the lunch table, in the corridors, at seminars, in meetings, and now, of course, on the Internet. This intense, fluid communication is as much a part of science as designing and running the experiments themselves or applying for grant support. Fragments of this reflection-in-action (Schon 1987) are captured from time to time in meeting abstracts and, now, electronic files, but it is important to recognize that, when researchers produce such documents (part of the so-called *gray literature*), they do so as authors-as-creators, not authors-as-writers; they are *doing* research, *not publishing* it. Although not everyone agrees with this view (Smith 1999b), I submit that this kind of ongoing electronic exchange of information (the e-prints now used widely by physicists and others, which are cited almost *ad nauseum* as an exciting new form of publication) is, in fact, an expanded and enhanced version of gray literature: prepublication sharing of work-in-progress, not publication in any meaningful sense. It is, for one thing, exclusively a researcher-to-researcher activity; it is not intended for practitioners and other consumers of research results, and those others are excluded from it.

The difference between prepublication sharing of information and publication itself is not simply semantics or academic hairsplitting, and a good deal of confusion arises from failure to distinguish between these two outwardly similar but fundamentally different intellectual tasks. Sacks (1995, 167) captured the difference very clearly in describing Helmholtz's comments on this issue: "It is only when he [the scientist] reaches the summit or the height he desires that he will see that there was, in fact, a direct route, a 'royal road,' to it. In his publications . . . he takes his readers along this royal road, but this bears no resemblance to the crooked and tortuous processes by which he constructed a path for himself."

Wilson (1998, 64) refined and extended the insight, thus: "In one sense scientific articles are deliberately misleading. Just as a novel is better than the novelist, a scientific report is better than the scientist, having been stripped of all the confusions and ignoble thought that led to its composition. Yet such voluminous and incomprehensible chaff, soon to be forgotten, contains most of the secrets of scientific success." Among the most difficult and most important tasks required of scientists, then, is, first, to learn how to recognize when they have reached "the summit" (or at least the desired height)—that is, the publishable moment—and, second, having arrived at that point, to strip their reports of all the confusions and ignoble thought that led to their composition, the better to take their readers along the "royal road" to their conclusions. These are the tasks that scientists take on in their role of "author-as-writer" (see chap. 1); it is the role of peer reviewers and editors to help them get this important intellectual work done.

A major problem in making the traverse from research to publishing is, of course, that scientists frequently think they have reached the summit when they have not and, understandably, often have difficulty seeing or accepting that reality. The first task of editors and peer reviewers is to help authors judge whether a scientific work is, in fact, "ready for prime time," a task of enormous complexity. And since opinions on this point often differ, it is no wonder that the judgments of editors and peer reviewers are not always welcome. Moreover, even when a scientific work is fully matured, the process of transforming it into a publication—stripping away the chaff and hammering the residue into its new and hardly recognizable shape—is painful and challenging. It is no wonder, then, that many scientists whose performance is dazzling at the bench have great difficulty sitting down to write up their results for publication. And in this light it is even more understandable that editing and peer review are seen as problematic, since the second task of editors and peer reviewers is guiding the hammering and shaping of the material. Those who argue that every scientist can be her (or his) own publisher seem not to have grasped the reality of the transition that must be accomplished between the creation of a scientific work and its publication; they are, therefore, apparently quite unaware of either the importance or the difficulty of that transition.

The World of Scientific Publication

The world of scientific publication, by way of contrast, is an orderly one. By the time a manuscript describing scientific or scholarly work reaches an editor's desk, the information it contains is already highly structured, a distillate refined from the crude raw material of research. And it is into the fussy paper world of editing and publishing that the work must come, for as Wilson (1998, 59) wrote, "One of the strictures of the scientific ethos is that a discovery does not exist until it is safely reviewed and in print." This is an extraordinary statement. What does it mean, this being in print, that determines the very existence of scientific work?

In the narrowest sense, of course, *being in print* simply means that a printing press has put little black marks on paper that capture and convey the contents of a scientific or scholarly study. But, although the physical fact of being printed is not trivial (more on this below), it is obviously not enough to bring a study into existence. Many printed documents (the majority, probably) are not held to be scholarly or scientific; for example, having your scholarly work described in the newspaper is clearly not the same as being "in print" in Wilson's sense. (Yesterday's newspaper is useful mostly for wrapping fish.) Rather, being in print in the scholarly sense requires, first, that a piece of scientific work have reached a state of orderliness, completeness, and coherence suitable for public release and, second, that the information be captured in a stable medium that can be efficiently distributed, safely archived, and easily retrieved.

Why are these two characteristics of publishing necessary for a scientific work to exist? The first characteristic reflects completion of a process that begins when the authors-as-writers prepare to move their work out into the world: the getting rid of "voluminous and incomprehensible chaff," the stripping away of "confusions and ignoble thought" that make up the "deliberately misleading" act of writing up a study (Wilson 1998, 64); completion of the process is the precondition for final acceptance for publication. The relevant concerns at the point of acceptance include such questions as, Does the work include all the information it should: enough detail, all important facts and data, appropriate emphasis? Have all of the extraneous and redundant information and unnecessary detail been cut out? Is it organized logically and understandably? Do the data support the conclusions? Does the work as a whole hang together? In comparing the initial versions of high-quality biomedical manuscripts submitted to *Annals of Internal Medicine* with the final, accepted papers, Purcell, Donovan, and Davidoff (1998) found that, on average, nearly 50 substantive changes were required per paper before they were judged ready for publication. Interestingly, lack of information accounted for well over 40% of the changes, even though most manuscripts were too long, while too much information accounted for an additional 20% of the problems that led to changes. (The remainder of the changes were attributable to information that was inaccurate or misplaced.)

Although some journals may see themselves in the role of stenographer (i.e., doing little more than reporting and archiving the news), most editors and peer reviewers see themselves as deeply involved in the process of shaping scientific knowledge (Vandenbroucke 1998). This final shaping of a study is more than just aesthetic: it is a crucial part of research, since it often reveals gaps, incompleteness, and inconsistencies in the work that were simply unappreciated before the stripping away and shaping were accomplished. Importantly, this final shaping is also largely responsible for transforming a scientific work from something that, in its prepublication form, is of use exclusively to other researchers (i.e., producers of research) into something accessible to consumers of research results (i.e., practitioners and the general public).

Some parallels with other creative work are apropos. For example, the notebooks of Beethoven or Aaron Copeland may be of intense interest to other composers, as well as scholars of music history, but the consumers (i.e., the general listening public) do not want to see (or hear) the nascent fragments and blind starts—the chaff—from those prepublication sources. They want the finished (finally accepted) product; anything less finished would be irrelevant, confusing, disappointing. The analogy is more than superficial; scientific publishing has a performance aspect that is not to be taken lightly: it is a public display, is expected to meet certain aesthetic as well as intellectual standards, and will be subjected to postperformance critical review (in correspondence to the authors and the journal).

As usual, however, there is a dark side, for as Godlee points out (see chap. 3), skeptics see the selection and final shaping of manuscripts, including peer review, as little more than censoring by opinionated editors who are responsible to no one. To many of those same skeptics, the Internet will be the liberator. Before everyone rushes out to abandon publishing as we know it, however, Vandenbroucke (1998, 2005–6) has suggested we consider the following scenario:

> Imagine that from this day, we abolish all edited journals by decree, and we invite anyone who thinks that he or she has a relevant fact or opinion to put it somewhere on the Internet. Tomorrow a mass outpouring of facts begins.
>
> The first consequence would be that this mass of facts . . . would be so overwhelming and at the same time so conflicting that the poor general practitioner would not know what to make of them, and cease to look at them.
>
> Within a few days after the abolishment of edited journals . . . we will be receiving commercial e-mail messages from some young unknowns who tell us that they have the time as well as the technical resources to retrieve the informa-

tion for us. They will add that, of course, since so much information on the Internet is nonsensical, they also will obligingly sieve out the nonsense. . . . Because they are not conversant with all aspects of medicine, they will invoke the help of some trusted friends to read the retrieved information and judge its quality. Within a week, my best guess, our edited journal system will be born again, inclusive of peer review.

Does this scenario convince us that the editing and peer review are more than just perverse historical accidents? Of course not. But Vandenbroucke does make a reasonable case that editing and peer review, in some form, are a necessary and natural consequence of the messiness, the fluidity, the fuzziness of research; that if the editorial shaping of research did not exist, we would have to invent it.

As to the second characteristic of publishing—the requirement for a stable medium, efficient distribution, safe archiving, and easy retrieval—it is also fair to ask how something so technical, so dry, so mundane can determine the very existence of something so intellectual, so serious, as science? The broadest possible answer (which is an essentially Bayesian view) is that, while scholarly scientific work is created by individual researchers, science is essentially a vast, collective, cumulative undertaking. The published body of all scientific work makes up a kind of collective mind; it is also immortal and continually (or at least intermittently) refines itself, but only on condition that the published record exists and is easily and fully accessible. Thus, to the extent the record is unstable, hidden, or not retrievable, science suffers from a kind of collective dementia.

From that point of view, the current enthusiasm for storing scientific information only in electronic formats is disturbing. Egyptian papyrus records are as clear now as they were when they were written five thousand years ago (Parkinson and Quirke 1995); computer programming done at the beginning of my six-month sabbatical at MIT had already become unusable by the end of that time because the programming language changed—"rotten code," in the local computer patois. At the rate the technology is evolving, how likely is it that all the information currently stored in computer files will be readable 100, 50, or even 20 years from now? For the integrity of science, it is a major mistake to take for granted the medium in which science is published and stored, to think of it as a trivial or peripheral issue. Marshall McLuhan (1964) said it well: "The medium *is* the message" (my italics); science *is* publication.

Printing signals the existence of science in another important way:

printed information exists in three dimensions. You can touch, and feel, and turn over the printed page; it has a sheen, a pattern, even a scent. Although the usual printed journal is far from Chinese calligraphy, printing, like calligraphy, "addresses the eye and is an art of space" (Wilson 1998, 118). In contrast, information published electronically (quite apart from the widely appreciated difficulty of using it in bed or in the bathroom) exists in two dimensions only, and even that existence is ephemeral, since the information vanishes if the power goes off or if lightning fries your modem.

But the medium is only the beginning. Even the information in printed documents in effect does not exist if users cannot locate the information they need within them or retrieve it when they have located it. Unfortunately, just as the importance of the medium in which science is published and stored is widely deprecated, systems for information search and retrieval are also not considered a matter of serious intellectual concern. It is time, then, for another thought experiment. Envision a world in which scholarly publications contain all the same scientific content they do now in the form of individual papers, but books and journals bear no titles, volume numbers, or years of publication; the articles and chapters are arranged in no particular order and have no page numbers; librarians shelve volumes at random; and indexes, electronic or otherwise, do not exist. In such a world, science as we know it would essentially not exist.

In addition to providing a stable storage medium, therefore, publication makes possible an ordered, integrated information meta-structure that allows the rapid, accurate, and efficient retrieval of scattered scientific content, a process that is as important, in its way, as any other single element of the scientific enterprise. It is probably not an overstatement to assert that document identifiers, those innocent-looking, rather boring elements of reference citations, are as essential to the existence and the evolution of science as DNA is to living organisms. A pithy phrase of the biologist S. J. Singer says it well: "I link, therefore I am" (quoted in Wilson 1998, 110).

In summing up the nature of scientific publication, it may help to borrow an epistemologic model of meta-diagnosis proposed by Diamond and Forrester (1983), which provides an important general framework for scientific meaning. In contrast to the usual simplistic judgment that a patient either does or does not have disease X, their model views diagnosis as a set of judgments at three separate but interrelated levels. The first characterizes the patient's biomedical state and is captured in an expression such as, "There's a 40% chance you have disease X." The second characterizes the mind of the clinician caring for the patient and is captured in an expression such as, "There's a 10% chance I know what I'm talking about." And the third characterizes the knowledge available to the larger system of all clinicians (the degree of orderliness in that system, sometimes defined by its converse, or entropy) and is captured in an expression such as, "With the information available from this patient, the confidence among all doctors that they know what they're talking about ranges from 2% to 35%, with most estimates at around 15%."

And so it is with science: the original investigation itself by the author-as-creator provides information directly about the phenomenon being studied, the published report expresses the author-as-writer's interpretation of and confidence in that information, and the aggregate of all published studies of the same subject makes it possible to estimate the amount of information available on that subject in the entire scientific corpus. The technique of the *systematic review* now used increasingly in biomedical research directly addresses the third concern (Cook and Mulrow 1998).

Scientific Publishing as an Intellectual Act

As a purely intellectual matter and quite apart from ethical considerations, any act that threatens scientific publishing (in the largest sense of the term) pragmatically threatens the very existence of science. The list of threats is not long, but each is potentially serious, and each can appear in many guises, which is not surprising given the sheer intellectual complexity of research and of publishing and the intricacies of the relationship between the two.

The chapters in this volume eloquently catalogue the most telling of those acts: research fraud, conflict of interest, misrepresentation of authorship, arbitrary and capricious editorship, misuse of peer review, repetitive publication. The analysis above suggests that, in figuring out how best to deal with those threats, it may help to separate them into those that belong on one side or the other of the line or, more properly, the gray zone that separates the world of research from that of publishing. Thus, research fraud involves authors-as-creators and hence belongs primarily on the research side; issues of authorship, editorship, peer review, and repetitive publication involve authors-as-writers, editors, and peer reviewers and hence rest primarily on the publishing side; while conflict-of-interest issues exist on both sides of the divide.

At the same time, it would be naïve to conclude that, simply because a damaging behavior occurs primarily in one of those worlds, the other is exonerated from doing something about it. Indeed, given the total interdependence of the two worlds, there is no escaping the need for both to be part of the solution. But sorting the problems into research-related and publishing-related misconduct helps to decide where authority and responsibility for handling misconduct now rest in the current system and where they belong in an ideal system. Although authority (the power to decide) and responsibility (being in a position to collect both blame and credit) are often thought of as inseparable attributes, they are actually quite independent. Effective systems assign them very carefully, since authority without responsibility promotes autocracy, while responsibility without authority produces frustration.

Take the problem of conflict of interest in research (I am talking here primarily about financial conflict, although in many instances other conflicts—e.g., personal loyalty, intellectual passion—may be at least as important, if not more so) (Spece, Shimm, and Buchanan 1996). Since in this case the actual site of the conflict is in the research world (the conflicts of interest for editors and peer reviewers obviously exist in the publishing world), the responsibility for dealing with it rests primarily with those directly involved with the research: researchers themselves, the researchers' institutions, and funding sources. For example, researchers have the responsibility for not being drawn into situations where their objectivity could be compromised by financial incentives, and they have the authority to do so: they can just say no. Researchers' institutions have both the responsibility and the authority to require that contracts between researchers and funding sources do not compromise academic freedom. Funding sources have the same authority, but sometimes have other responsibilities (e.g., industry sources have obligations to stockholders) that conflict with the responsibility to uphold academic freedom.

What sort of authority and responsibility lie with editors and peer reviewers in matters of research-related conflict of interest? Editors have virtually no direct authority to prevent financial conflicts of interest in research, but they do share some of the responsibility for dealing with them. Thus, at a minimum, journal editors have a responsibility to promote widespread understanding of important distinctions among the various types of conflict. For example, their editorial policies need to recognize that, while financial ties always create dual commitments, they do not necessarily or automatically create true conflict—that is, meaningful bias; likewise, their editorial policies need to be tuned to the reality that the financial ties between funding sources and individual researchers differ importantly from the ties between funding sources and research projects (International Committee of Medical Journal Editors [ICMJE] 1998; Davidoff 1997). Journal editors also have the authority to require disclosure of information that makes these potentially biasing relationships clear to everyone, and while such disclosure obviously carries no direct authority over what researchers and funders can and cannot do, it can reinforce the authority of researchers and their institutions in limiting the creation of incentives that bias.

In contrast, take misattribution of authorship. Here is a problem that clearly occurs in the publishing world, and journal editors consequently have the primary responsibility for minimizing it. Although in principle editors also have the authority to do so, they have thus far asserted that authority only to the extent of articulating a policy on authorship but have not yet found a way to enforce that policy (ICMJE 1998). Do academic institutions share at least some of the responsibility to protect the integrity of authorship? Most people would agree they do, since authorship carries considerable weight in the conduct of research. Do they have the authority to do so? Here people disagree: only a minority of medical schools in the United States have exercised this authority by creating and enforcing institutional authorship policies (see chap. 1), while faculty in other schools have resisted such policies as an intrusion on academic freedom, insisting that the criteria for authorship can be determined only on a disciplinary, or departmental, or individual research group basis.

But what of the responsibility of researchers themselves to "do right" by authorship? Richard Horton's analysis (see chap. 2) is telling in this regard, starting, as it does, with the characteristic of *attribution,* which he points out carries with it both credit and responsibility for the work; it requires participation in the doing, writing, and approving of the paper. The increasing number of different investigators and disciplines required by much current scientific research unfortunately carries with it pressure to *attribute* authorship to ever larger numbers of "contributors" (Rennie, Yank, and Emanuel 1997). At the same time, each participant is involved with an increasingly narrow slice of the project, which makes it increasingly hard to assign overall responsibility for the project to any one of them. It is precisely this increasing fragmentation of the roles of authors-as-creators and authors-as-writers that has motivated the recent proposal that every published study needs to designate one or more "guarantors" who would be responsible for the integrity of the whole (Rennie, Yank, and Emanuel 1997).

Horton argues that authorship is further characterized by *authority*. In most institutions, at least, the researchers themselves are the ones—and the only ones—who decide who will be an author, who will not, and in what order their names will appear on the byline. It is not difficult to conclude that the combination of decreasing responsibility (attribution) combined with rigidly defended autonomy (authority) among researchers has contributed importantly to abuses of authorship, a phenomenon that, as Horton points out, seems at present to be a concern for editors but not for the researchers themselves.

Horton also makes the case for two additional characteristics of authorship: *animus*, the combination of motivation with interpretive intent, and *agency*, the understanding of who creates the text. Animus, it seems, is an issue primarily when authors cannot agree among themselves, which may make "something of a nonsense of that part of the ICMJE definition [of authorship] calling for public responsibility to be accepted by all authors" (see chap. 2). Animus hardly seems to be a fundamental characteristic of authorship, but rather a dimension of human feeling, and all the more reason to require that one or more authors speak for the integrity of the entire work. Agency refers to the insight that the meaning of a text is created not by the authors who wrote the text, but by the reader from the text; that, in effect, science does not exist until it is read. Agency can therefore be looked at as simply a postmodern extension of our earlier assertion that science does not exist until it is published.

Agency is clearly a very real and important consideration, but as a characteristic of authorship it is problematic. First, readers are receivers, not producers, of information. As human beings rather than automatons, of course readers interpret, respond to, make meaning out of the information in published papers, but doing so hardly makes them authors, any more than hearing a Beethoven piano sonata makes listeners into composers because they have made meaning out of the performance. Agency is therefore a characteristic of *readership,* not *authorship*. Second, and more to the point, if it is really readers who create meaning, then authors, peer reviewers, and editors no longer need to feel much responsibility for the quality of the information contained in the text, hardly something we want to see happen.

Biomedical Publishing as a Social Act

The worlds of biomedical research and biomedical publishing circulate around each other in a kind of intellectual solar system, each in its own orbit but bound inseparably together by the gravitational pull of science. As Addeane S. Caelleigh makes very clear (see chap. 11), however, that self-contained intellectual system is firmly embedded in a larger social and moral universe. It is only by understanding the larger universe that many of the ethical problems facing biomedical publishing begin to make sense and meaningful approaches to managing those problems can be expected to emerge.

Thus, Caelleigh's community model, including the corrosive effects of certain kinds of publicly visible damage (broken windows and fare jumpers), the power of the hidden curriculum, and the like, provide important insights into both mechanisms and solutions. And both Caelleigh and Huth (see chap. 5) touch on a critical, but often neglected, aspect of social models—namely, the problem of scale. In brief, they argue that it is difficult to know how best to deal with a social problem, ethical or otherwise, unless you know how big it is. (In this connection, it is worth noting that, in the realm of law, the recent adoption of *screens,* or *Chinese walls,* as a mechanism for separating lawyers within the same firm with potential conflicts of interest was driven by the growth in size of law firms [Wolfram 1996].) Thus, in exploring the nature of repetitive publication, Huth estimates that repetitive papers appear at a rate of somewhere between 0.017 and 306 per 1,000 papers published. The rate makes a difference: a larger figure (over 30%) might very well call for more drastic measures than a figure five orders of magnitude smaller. Caelleigh, reflecting on how established editors might best meet their obligations to newly appointed colleagues, in like fashion calculates that the so-called MEDLINE community of editors might have as many as 360 neophyte editors per year, a nontrivial number that defines a nontrivial task.

It is hard to disagree with the conclusion that, all other things being equal, solutions work better when they are suited, in size as well as shape, to the problems they are designed to solve. True, even a rare sort of transgression can warrant drastic remedial and preventive measures if it is sufficiently egregious. (The major actions taken in response to the unethical behavior of Darsee and Slutsky are cases in point. The strength of the reaction seems to have been justified by a legitimate concern that these researchers had smashed a very obvious window in the edifice of science and that many more rock-throwers would materialize unless the window was fixed, immediately and publicly.) But Caelleigh is right on target in reminding us about "the usual small amount of deviancy that turns up in any human activity" and the consequent importance of keeping most ethical problems in proportion by viewing them as normal aberrations rather than ethical catastrophes.

Responses to the ethical problems associated with peer review are illustrative. As documented by Godlee (see chap. 3), peer reviewers do unethical things: they plagiarize the ideas from manuscripts sent to them for review, delay reviews of work by competitors, and give favorable reviews of papers by friends and colleagues. Authors are blinded to the identity of the peer reviewers for most scientific journals, which has led some people to the not unreasonable conclusion that the ability of peer reviewers to hide behind the mask of anonymity encourages corruption among them, an ethical concern compounded by asymmetry, since authors' identities are almost always revealed to peer reviewers. The response of some journals to these ethical concerns has been to abandon blinded peer review (Smith 1999a).

But consider the scope of the problem in quantitative terms: taking the four thousand MEDLINE biomedical journals commented on by Caelleigh and making conservative assumptions that the majority of these journals are published monthly, that each issue contains between ten and 20 peer-reviewed articles, and that each article is read by two peer reviewers, the total number of biomedical peer reviews is somewhere between one and two million annually. Yet the number of serious ethical breaches by peer reviewers is small; only a handful are well documented or frequently cited. Underreporting is likely, of course, but even assuming one or two serious breaches of peer-review ethics per journal per year, the rate would still be a fraction of 1%. Is this rate meaningfully above the "usual small amount of deviancy that turns up in any human activity"? And is it ethical, does it even make common sense, to sacrifice the potential advantages of blinded peer review as a response to a problem of this magnitude? Given the central importance of blinding as a method reducing bias in all scientific endeavor (Kaptchuk 1998; Davidoff 1998a); and given that at least one well-controlled study found that blinding improves the quality of peer review (McNutt et al. 1990), while other studies show no effect; and given that other approaches to the problem are available, including establishing standards for peer review and requiring training for peer reviewers, the unblinding of peer review is at best a highly debatable option.

Returning now to the general issue of the social universe, the complexities of social systems make it unlikely that any particular factor such as scale or any single model will be adequate to understand adequately how such systems really function. Thus, while the community model provides important insights into the ethical problems of scientific publishing, at least five other social models with known explanatory power are worth considering here.

The Moral Syndromes of Public Life

The work of the social geographer and critic Jane Jacobs (1992) provides two sets of moral precepts (syndromes)—about 15 in each set—that govern the two principal systems of survival in public life: taking (think conquest, taxes, and tithes) and trading (think contracts, investments, and capital). Governments, the military, churches, and to some degree the professions have been governed by the taking, or guardian, moral syndrome whose precepts include: shun trading, be obedient and disciplined, be exclusive, respect hierarchy, exert prowess, adhere to tradition, treasure honor, be fatalistic, and deceive for the sake of the task. Commerce, in contrast, is governed by the moral syndrome of trading, whose precepts include: come to voluntary agreements, dissent for the sake of the task, collaborate easily with strangers and aliens, compete, respect contracts, use initiative and enterprise, be open to inventiveness and novelty, be optimistic, and be efficient, among others.

Most scientific researchers are part of the academic community, which lives by several of the guardian precepts, particularly the admonition to shun trading. At the same time, rigorous scientific research requires intellectual honesty, inventiveness, optimism, and dissent—all precepts that are very much part of the commercial moral syndrome and a challenge to the guardian moral syndrome. Thus, right from the start, scientific researchers discover that they are required to function in two distinct and mutually incompatible moral worlds, a circumstance that violates "syndrome integrity" and that ordinarily produces serious tensions and ethical distortions (Davidoff 1998b). The introduction of financial incentives into the biomedical research community, apart from being a source of potential intellectual bias, forces researchers into a further and even more major violation of guardian-syndrome integrity, which probably accounts for much of the disruptiveness of such incentives.

Academic life is characterized by another important social and moral force, one that it shares with clinical medicine: gift relationships, based on gift exchange (Hyde 1983; Davidoff 1998c). The species of *gift exchange* referred to here is a ritualized social system in which gifts are given without expectation of immediate return in kind; they then circulate through a so-ciety, ultimately returning to the original giver, usually increased in value. Commercial exchange—the immediate, exact, and reckoned exchange of goods and cash—and gift exchange are mutually incompatible systems. It was gift exchange, rather than commercial exchange, that served as the principal form of social connection in many societies, particularly smaller ones, over the centuries.

Gift exchange has also long been an important part of the social system in which research is carried out (Biagioli 1998), and while commercial exchange has replaced gift exchange in most aspects of modern life, both clinical medicine and scientific research still contain many elements of gift relationships. For example, most scientific research is still supported by grants from private foundations or public agencies—the modern form of giving, which has largely replaced support from wealthy individual patrons—rather than contracts; researchers owe nothing material to the granting agencies in return. Researchers give, rather than sell, their re-search results to journals for publication, on the way to giving them to the general public; they do not expect to be paid for doing so, at least not directly; rewards, material or academic, eventually arrive, although they generally come later, indirectly, and in an amount that bears little relation to their initial contribution. In contrast, as Hyde pointed out (1983), al-though scientific research or writing done as "work for hire" returns imme-diate and well-defined financial rewards, it receives little or no academic credit. Finally, it is also true that most research training is given, not sold. Thus, while the giving of gifts in certain circumstances can and does create substantial ethical problems (Hyde 1983), we are not on firm or consistent moral ground in condemning gift authorship out of hand while at the same time living comfortably in a research system based largely on gifts and gift relationships.

Systems Thinking

A *system* is "a collection of interdependent elements that interact to achieve a common purpose" (Nolan 1998, 294). While that rather abstract definition smacks of managerial or engineering jargon, from it flows an integrating view of complex organizations known as *systems thinking,* a network of working principles that are as applicable to scientific publishing as they are to corporations, governments, or any other social system (Senge 1990). An overriding principle of systems thinking is that *every system is perfectly designed to achieve the results it actually gets;* an important corollary of this principle is that it is the structure of the system, more than the performance of individuals within it, that largely determines the performance of the system.

From the systems-thinking point of view, misattribution of authorship, repetitive publication, and salami science (least publishable units) all persist because they are elements in a reinforcing feedback loop, or circle of causality, analogous to the more familiar vicious circles (or virtuous circles), one that has evolved to produce exactly these practices. In this circle, promotions and tenure committees count the number of publications rather than their quality; faculty therefore make it their business to publish the largest possible number of papers; some of these same faculty with large bibliographies make up the promotions committees, which assures that the standard for promotion will continue to be the number of publications; and the cycle continues. Although journals might help break the circle by requiring authors to disclose their contributions to the work (Rennie, Yank, and Emanuel 1997), systems thinking suggests that these particular violations of publication ethics will diminish only when promotions committees explicitly discard the number of publications as a criterion for promotion (as a few have begun to do) and focus more seriously and intensively on the quality of their faculties' work.

Note in this (slightly oversimplified) example that persistence of these ethical problems is not ascribed to the actions of a few unethical people, nor is the solution more and better ethics education or more severe punishment of transgressors. Although nothing in systems thinking would exclude these latter activities as reinforcers, the primary intervention is a *change in the structure of the system.* Whether the goal is general, as in quality improvement (Berwick and Nolan 1998), or specific, as in error reduction (Leape 1994), the systems-thinking approach asserts that it is more productive in the long run to redesign the system itself, rather than chase after individual incompetent performers; or, in statistical terms, there is more to gain by shifting the entire performance curve upward rather than repeatedly lopping off the outliers.

Complex Adaptive Systems

A complex adaptive system is a collection of individual agents who have freedom to act in ways that are not always predictable and whose actions are interconnected such that one agent's actions change the context for the others (Kauffman 1995). The properties of such systems include

- adaptable elements: the elements of the system can change themselves.
- nonlinearity: small changes can have big effects.
- emergent behavior: continual creativity is a natural state of the system.
- not predictable in detail: forecasting is inherently an inexact, yet boundable, art.
- context and embeddedness: there are systems within systems, and that matters.
- co-evolution: the system proceeds forward through constant tension and balance. (Plsek 1998)

Scientific publication certainly qualifies as a complex adaptive system, and some of the more vexing aspects of ethical problems in scientific publication become more understandable when viewed through the lens of the complex adaptive-systems model. For example, it is likely that at least some authors will "game" a system in which editors require them to describe their contributions to research projects (adaptable elements), and academic departments often behave quite autonomously despite being units within medical centers and universities, which greatly complicates the development of authorship policies (context and embeddedness).

Students of the problem have suggested strategies that are more likely to be effective in changing complex adaptive systems than are traditional ones. These include techniques such as finding new metaphors for understanding the problem (Caelleigh's community model of scientific publishing is an excellent example) or using simple rules rather than always trying to plan out and guide things in great detail. For example, John C. Bailar (1997) suggested that the simple rule, "Disclosure is almost a panacea" would be more effective than many of the complex, almost Kafkaesque rules and regulations created in response to problems in publication ethics. Other techniques include using paradox and tension as excellent opportunities for real change, launching many diverse experiments in system change, and finding ways to work with naturally occurring networks and forces within systems, rather than trying to force changes.

The Diffusion of Innovations

The rate at which new and better ways of doing things are adopted is often exasperatingly slow. How and why innovations diffuse (or do not) has been the subject of serious inquiry for decades, and the diffusion process is understood in considerable depth, as described in Everett Rogers's (1995) now classic work. Diffusion happens in five stages: (1) *knowledge:* knowledge about the innovation spreads; (2) *persuasion:* people become persuaded as to its value; (3) *decision:* people decide to adopt the innovation; (4) *implementation:* the innovation is actually put into use; (5) *confirmation:* people look for reinforcement for continuing with the innovation. The cast of characters in this drama includes Innovators, Early Adopters, an Early Majority, a Late Majority, and, last but not least, the Laggards. The qualities of the innovation itself contribute to the outcome; thus, an innovation spreads in proportion to its *relative advantage* (how much better it is than what it is replacing), *compatibility* (consistency with existing values, experiences, needs), *complexity* (difficulty in being understood and used), *trialability* (degree to which it can be tried out in limited experiments), and *observability* (visibility of the results of using the innovation). The process is complex, involving channels of communication, networks, and change agents; it can be derailed by many things, including lack of access to communication channels, lack of leadership, disenchantment, and the like. And the outcomes of diffusion are complex, uncertain, sometimes even perverse (a characteristic, as we have seen, of complex adaptive systems).

Most important of all, diffusion of innovations is an intensely social process: the best ideas may go nowhere if the social process fails, and weak or even destructive ideas can spread rapidly if social conditions are favorable. The relevance of all this to the ethics of scientific publishing is clear. For example, the disclosure of authorship contributions is an innovation whose diffusion has followed the classic pattern: innovators put forth knowledge about the concept in print and at meetings, including those at Nottingham in 1996 (Horton and Smith 1996) and Berkeley in 1998; a few early adopters were persuaded as to its validity, decided to use it, and implemented it (Horton 1997; Smith 1997); an early majority of adopters (now including some five general medical journals) may be emerging; and analysis of the early data on contributorship may help to confirm its value (Yank and Rennie 1999).

But disclosure of contributorship is an innovation that is far from fully established; it could easily fail to spread further, lose momentum, be extinguished, or be dropped. Those interested in making sure disclosure becomes a universal standard would do well, therefore, to study Rogers carefully, learn in depth and detail what encourages the spread of good ideas and what damps them out, and take the actions that will confirm and extend the diffusion process.

Murder

On the face of it, murder seems an unlikely social model for understanding and managing the ethical breaches in scientific publication. But murder is, after all, the ultimate in antisocial behavior, and those who are not held to account when they violate ethical codes—whether the violation is research fraud, misattribution of authorship, or repetitive publication—are said to be "getting away with murder." A deep understanding of the essential nature of murder may therefore have useful things to teach about the nature of all breaches of the social contract.

Language, appropriately enough, provides the principal clue, for the word *murder* originally "denoted *secret* murder, which in Germanic antiquity was alone regarded as (in the modern sense) a crime, open homicide being considered a private wrong calling for blood-revenge or compensation" (*OED* 1989). It is secrecy, then, rather than violence per se that makes the act of murder so heinous; secret acts are cowardly, guilty acts; a murderer, being anonymous, is not an individual and is therefore less than human; and the devil you don't know is always more threatening than the devil you know. By the same token, detection—finding out "whodunit"—is ultimately a moral act, since it converts the unknown, a faceless creature who cannot be called to account, into the known: a flesh-and-blood killer now answerable for his or her crime (Davidoff 1996). The power of disclosure—transparency, clarity, exposure—as a mechanism, perhaps as a panacea, for preventing and setting right breaches of publication ethics is thus revealed. We would do well to take the lesson seriously.

Conclusions

Science does not exist until it is published. It is the symbiotic relationship of two separate and distinct worlds—research and publishing—that makes scientific publishing possible. Authors-as-creators work in the messy world of research, relying heavily as they do so on prepublication networks of information exchange. The difference, both quantitative and qualitative, between that prepublication, e-print communication, on the one hand, and scientific publication, on the other, is vast. Prepublication gray literature consists largely of work in progress: nascent, partly formed fragments. A publishable work is one that has reached a high state of orderliness, completeness, and coherence; it is *not* simply an extension of a scientific work-in-progress along an unbroken information continuum.

When a study reaches the state of development that makes it ready for publication, researchers shift to the role of authors-as-writers and begin the benign yet "deliberately misleading" process of converting the tortuous and erratic course of research into a meaningful, publishable article; stripping away the "voluminous and incomprehensible chaff," the "confusions and ignoble thought" that constitute research (Wilson 1998, 64). That material is then sent across the divide that separates the messy world of research from the orderly world of publishing. Editors and peer reviewers continue the process of moving a paper into final publishable form, one that will become part of a stable, tangible, cumulative scientific record, a highly structured network of information that is accessible not only to other researchers but also to the practitioners and other consumers of scientific results.

Understanding the distinctions between research and publishing as intellectual tasks is helpful in understanding where and how ethical distortions in scientific publishing occur. It is even more helpful in seeing where authority and responsibility now reside, and where they should reside, for both prevention and remediation of ethical breaches. But scientific publishing is also a social act; that is, the intellectual worlds of research and publishing are contained within a larger social and moral universe. In this universe, the scale of an ethical problem matters. Moreover, several social models—including community dynamics, the moral syndromes of public life, the reframing of issues through systems thinking, the subtleties of complex adaptive systems, the mechanisms for diffusion of innovations, and even the deeper meaning of murder as a violation of the social contract—all provide important insights into how ethical problems in scientific publishing come to be and how we might manage them better. Unless we draw on these insights, unless we achieve a *consilience*—that is, "a 'jumping together' of knowledge by the linking of facts and fact-based theory across disciplines to create a common groundwork of explanation" (Wilson 1998, 8)—I suspect we will still be wrestling 50 years from now with the same patchwork, after-the-fact, fundamentally unsatisfactory solutions to the same vexing ethical problems we are struggling with today.

References

Bailar, J. C. 1997. Peer review, misconduct, and progress in science. Paper presented at the 3d International Congress on Biomedical Peer Review and Global Communications, 19 September, Prague.

Berwick, D. M., and T. W. Nolan. 1998. Physicians as leaders in improving health care: A new series in *Annals of Internal Medicine*. *Annals of Internal Medicine* 128:289–92.

Biagioli, M. 1998. The instability of authorship: Credit and responsibility in contemporary biomedicine. *FASEB Journal* 12:3–16.

Cook, D., and C. Mulrow, eds. 1998. *Systematic reviews: Synthesis of best evidence for health care decisions*. Philadelphia: American College of Physicians.

Davidoff, F. 1996. Mystery, murder, and medicine: Reading the clues. In *Who has seen a blood sugar? Reflections on medical education*, 91–95. Philadelphia: American College of Physicians.

———. 1997. Where's the bias? *Annals of Internal Medicine* 126:986–88.

———. 1998a. Masking, blinding, and peer review: The blind leading the blinded. *Annals of Internal Medicine* 128:66–68.

———. 1998b. Medicine and commerce. 1: Is managed care a "monstrous hybrid"? *Annals of Internal Medicine* 128:496–99.

———. 1998c. Medicine and commerce. 2: The gift. *Annals of Internal Medicine* 128:572–75.

———. 1998d. Publication and promotion: Intelligence work. *Lancet* 352:895–96.

Diamond, G. A., and J. S. Forrester. 1983. Metadiagnosis: An epistemologic model of clinical judgment. *American Journal of Medicine* 75:129–37.

Horton, R. 1997. The signature of responsibility. *Lancet* 350:5–6.

Horton, R., and R. Smith. 1996. Time to redefine authorship. *BMJ* 312:723.

Hyde, L. 1983. *The gift: Imagination and the erotic life of property*. New York: Random House.

International Committee of Medical Journal Editors (ICMJE). 1998. Statement on project-specific industry support for research. *Canadian Medical Association Journal* 158:615–16.

Jacobs, J. 1992. *Systems of survival: A dialogue on the moral foundations of commerce and politics*. New York: Random House.

Kaptchuk, T. J. 1998. Intentional ignorance: A history of blind assessment and placebo controls in medicine. *Bulletin of the History of Medicine* 72:389–433.

Kauffman, S. A. 1995. *At home in the universe: The search for laws of self-organization and complexity*. New York: Oxford University Press.

Leape, L. L. 1994. Error in medicine. *JAMA* 272:1851–57.

McLuhan, M. 1964. *Understanding media: The extensions of man*. New York: McGraw-Hill.

McNutt, R. A., A. T. Evans, R. H. Fletcher, and S. W. Fletcher. 1990. The effects of blinding on the quality of peer review: A randomized trial. *JAMA* 263:1371–76.

Nolan, T. W. 1998. Understanding medical systems. *Annals of Internal Medicine* 128:293–98.

Oxford English Dictionary (OED). 2d ed. 1989. s.v. "murder."

Parkinson, R. B., and S. Quirke. 1995. *Papyrus*. London: British Museum Press.

Plsek, P. 1998. An organization is not a machine! Principles for managing complex adaptive systems. IHI Forum Mini-Plenary Presentation, Orlando, Fla., December.

Purcell, G. P., S. L. Donovan, and F. Davidoff. 1998. Changes to manuscripts during the editorial process: Characterizing the evolution of a clinical paper. *JAMA* 280:227–28.

Rennie, D., V. Yank, and L. Emanuel. 1997. When authorship fails: A proposal to make contributors accountable. *JAMA* 278:579–85.

Rogers, E. M. 1995. *Diffusion of innovations.* 4th ed. New York: Free Press.

Sacks, O. 1995. Scotoma: Forgetting and neglect in science. In *Hidden histories of science,* ed. R. B. Silvers, 141–87. London: Granta Books.

Schon, D. A. 1987. *Educating the reflective practitioner: Toward a new design for teaching and learning in the professions.* San Francisco: Jossey-Bass.

Senge, P. 1990. *The fifth discipline: The art and practice of the learning organization.* New York: Doubleday.

Smith, R. 1997. Authorship: Time for a paradigm shift? *BMJ* 314:992.

———. 1999a. Opening up *BMJ* peer review: A beginning that should lead to complete transparency. *BMJ* 318:4–5.

———. 1999b. What is publication? A continuum. *BMJ* 318:142.

Snow, C. P. 1959. *The two cultures.* New York: Cambridge University Press.

Spece, R. G., Jr., D. S. Shimm, and A. E. Buchanan, eds. 1996. *Conflicts of interest in clinical practice and research.* New York: Oxford University Press.

Vandenbroucke, J. P. 1998. Medical journals and the shaping of medical knowledge. *Lancet* 352:2001–6.

Wilson, E. O. 1998. *Consilience: The unity of knowledge.* New York: Knopf.

Wolfram, C. E. 1996. Screening. In *Conflicts of interest in clinical practice and research,* ed. R. G. Spece Jr., D. S. Shimm, and A. E. Buchanan, 137–57. New York: Oxford University Press.

Yank, V., and D. Rennie. 1999. Disclosure of researcher contributions: A study of original research articles in *The Lancet. Annals of Internal Medicine* 130:661–70.

Selected Key Resources

Research Integrity and Scientific Misconduct

Bailar, J. C. 1986. Science, statistics, and deception. *Annals of Internal Medicine* 104:259–60.

Broad, W., and N. Wade. 1982. *Betrayers of the truth: Fraud and deceit in the halls of science.* New York: Simon & Schuster.

Commission on Research Integrity (CRI), Ryan Commission. 1995. *Integrity and misconduct in research: Report of the Commission on Research Integrity to the Secretary of Health and Human Services, the House Committee on Commerce, and the Senate Committee on Labor and Human Resources.* Washington, D.C.: Department of Health and Human Services, Public Health Service. See also http://www.faseb. org/opar/cri.html. Site accessed 8 April 1999.

Committee on Publication Ethics (COPE). 1998. The COPE report, 1998. London: BMJ Books.

DeBakey, L., and S. DeBakey. 1975. Ethics and etiquette in biomedical communication. *Perspectives in Biology and Medicine* 18:522–40.

de Solla Price, D. J. 1963. *Little science, big science.* New York: Columbia University Press.

———. 1964. Ethics of scientific publication. *Science* 144:655–57.

Douglas, J. D. 1993. Deviance in the practice of science. *Academic Medicine* 68 (suppl to issue 9):S77–83.

Engler, R. L., J. W. Covell, P. J. Friedman, P. S. Kitcher, and R. M. Peters. 1987. Misrepresentation and responsibility in medical research. *New England Journal of Medicine* 317:1383–89.

The ethics of scholarly publishing: A special issue. 1993. *Scholarly Publishing* 24:193–280.

Fienberg, S. E. 1990. Statistical reporting in scientific journals. In Council of Biology Editors, Editorial Policy Committee, *Ethics and policy in scientific publication,* 202–6. Bethesda, Md.: Council of Biology Editors.

Friedman, P. J. 1990. Correcting the literature following fraudulent publication. *JAMA* 263:1416–19.

——, ed. 1993. Integrity in biomedical research. *Academic Medicine* 68 (suppl to issue 9):S1–102.

Hackett, E. J. 1993. A new perspective on scientific misconduct. *Academic Medicine* 68 (suppl to issue 9):S72–76.

Kevles, D. J. 1998. *The Baltimore case.* New York: Norton.

LaFollette, M. C. 1992. *Stealing into print: Fraud, plagiarism, and misconduct in scientific publishing.* Berkeley and Los Angeles: University of California Press.

Lee, Y. T., R. Yalow, and S. Weinberg. 1993. Ethical research: Principles and practices. In *Ethics, values, and the promise of science: Forum proceedings,* 21–24. Research Triangle Park, N.C.: Sigma Xi.

Lock, S. 1995. Lessons from the Pearce affair: Handling scientific fraud. *BMJ* 310:1547–48.

Lock, S., and F. Wells, eds. 1996. *Fraud and misconduct in medical research.* 2d ed. London: BMJ Publishing Group.

Macrina, F. L. 1995. *Scientific integrity: An introductory text with cases.* Washington, D.C.: American Society for Microbiology.

Medawar, P. B. 1996. *The strange case of the spotted mice, and other classic essays on science.* Oxford: Oxford University Press.

Parrish, D. 1999. Scientific misconduct and correcting the scientific literature. *Academic Medicine* 74:221–30.

Petersdorf, R. G. 1986. The pathogenesis of fraud in medical science. *Annals of Internal Medicine* 104:252–54.

Pritchard, I. A. 1993. Integrity versus misconduct: Learning the difference between right and wrong. *Academic Medicine* 68 (suppl to issue 9):S67–71.

Reiser, S. J. 1993. Overlooking ethics in the search for objectivity and misconduct in science. *Academic Medicine* 68 (suppl to issue 9):S84–87.

Relman, A. S. 1983. Lessons from the Darsee affair. *New England Journal of Medicine* 308:1415–17.

——. 1990. Publishing biomedical research: Role and responsibilities. *Hastings Center Report,* May/June, 23–27.

Sigma Xi. 1986. *Honor in science.* Research Triangle Park, N.C.: Sigma Xi.

Stewart, W. W., and N. Feder. 1987. The integrity of the scientific literature. *Nature* 325:207–14.

Wenger, N. S., S. G. Korenman, R. Berk, and H. Liu. 1998. Punishment for unethical behavior in the conduct of research. *Academic Medicine* 73:1187–94.

Statements and Policies of Disciplinary Organizations and Journals

American Chemical Society (ACS), Publications Division. 1996. Ethical guidelines. http://pubs.acs.org/instruct/ethic.html. Site accessed 6 November 1998.

American Diabetes Association (ADA), Publications Policy Committee. 1992. Duplicate publication in American Diabetes Association journals: Challenges and recommendations. *Diabetes Care* 15:1059–61.

American Federation for Clinical Research (AFCR). 1990. Guidelines for avoiding conflict of interest. *Clinical Research* 38:239–40.

American Psychological Association (APA). 1992. Ethical principles of psychologists and code of conduct. *American Psychologist* 47:1597–1628. See also http://www.apa.org/ethics/code.html. Site accessed 4 January 1999.

Association of American Medical Colleges (AAMC). 1990. Guidelines for dealing with faculty conflicts of commitment and conflicts of interest in research. *Academic Medicine* 65:488–96. See also http://www.aamc.org/research/dbr/coi.htm. Site accessed 8 November 1998.

——, Ad Hoc Committee on Misconduct and Conflict of Interest in Research. 1992. *Beyond the "framework": Institutional considerations in managing allegations of misconduct in research*. Washington, D.C.: Association of American Medical Colleges.

Association of American Universities (AAU). 1988. *Framework for institutional policies and procedures to deal with fraud in research*. No. 4. Washington, D.C.: Association of American Universities, National Association of State University and Land-Grant Colleges, Council of Graduate Schools. Reissued 10 November 1989.

Friedman, P. J. 1993. Standards for authorship and publication in academic radiology. Association of University Radiologists' Ad Hoc Committee on Standards for the Responsible Conduct of Research. *Radiology* 189:33–34; *Investigative Radiology* 28:879–81; *AJR American Journal of Roentgenology* 161:899–900.

Institute of Medicine (IOM), Committee on the Responsible Conduct of Research. 1989. *The responsible conduct of research in the health sciences*. Washington, D.C.: National Academy Press. See also IOM report of a study on the responsible conduct of research in the health sciences. 1989. *Clinical Research* 37:179–91.

Jorgensen, A. 1995. *Society policies on ethics issues*. Washington, D.C.: Council of Scientific Society Presidents.

National Academy of Sciences (NAS), Committee on the Conduct of Science. 1989. *On being a scientist*. Washington, D.C.: National Academy Press.

——, Institute of Medicine. 1989. *Responsible conduct of research in the health sciences: Report of a study*. Washington, D.C.: National Academy of Sciences.

——, Panel on Scientific Responsibility and the Conduct of Research. 1992. *Responsible science: Ensuring the integrity of the research process*. Vol. 1. Washington, D.C.: National Academy Press.

——. 1993. *Responsible science: Ensuring the integrity of the research process*. Vol. 2. Washington, D.C.: National Academy Press.

Policy on scientific misconduct. 1996. *International Journal of Radiation Oncology, Biology, and Physics* 35:4.

Royal College of Physicians (RCP). 1991. *Fraud and misconduct in medical research: Causes, investigation, and prevention*. London: Royal College of Physicians.

Society for Neuroscience. 1998. Responsible conduct regarding scientific communication ("guidelines"). http://www.sfn.org/guidelines/guidelines-Final.doc. Site accessed 23 May 1999.

Specific inappropriate acts in the publication process. 1996. *American Journal of Obstetrics and Gynecology* 174:1–9.

Statements and Policies of Universities and Medical Schools

Committee on Academic Responsibility, Massachusetts Institute of Technology. 1992. *Fostering academic integrity*. Cambridge: Massachusetts Institute of Technology.

Faculty of Medicine, Harvard University. 1988. Guidelines for investigators in scientific research. In *Faculty policies on integrity in science,* 4–5. Boston: Harvard Medical School, 1996. See also http://www.hms.harvard.edu/integrity/scientif.html. Site accessed 17 March 1999.

——. 1991. Guidelines for investigators in clinical research. In *Faculty policies on integrity in science,* 6–7. Boston: Harvard Medical School, 1996. See also http://www.hms.harvard.edu/integrity/clinical.html. Site accessed 8 April 1999.

——. 1996. *Faculty policies on integrity in science*. Boston: Harvard Medical School. See also http://www.hms.harvard.edu/integrity/index/html. Site accessed 8 April 1999.

——. 1996. Policy on conflicts of interest and commitment. In *Faculty policies on integrity in science,* 12–19. Boston: Harvard Medical School. See also http://www.hms.harvard.edu/integrity. Site accessed 8 April 1999.

Guidelines and resource material for the ethical conduct and reporting of research and procedures for handling allegations of unethical research activities at the University of Louisville School of Medicine. 1988. Louisville: University of Louisville School of Medicine. See also http://www.louisville.edu/research/ethics.htm. Site accessed 8 April 1999.

Guidelines for the responsible conduct of research at Yale University School of Medicine. 1991. New Haven: Yale University School of Medicine. See also http://info.med.yale.edu/sciaffr/grants/guidelin.htm. Site accessed 8 April 1999.

Investigator/authorship guidelines of Rush Medical College. 1996. Chicago: Rush Medical College.

Stanford University. 1999. Research policy handbook. http://www.stanford.edu/dept/DoR/RPH.html. Site accessed 17 March 1999.

University of Illinois at Urbana-Champaign. 1998. Code of policies and regulations applying to all students. http://www.uiuc.edu/admin_manual/code/. Site accessed 17 February 1999.

University of Michigan Medical School. 1989. *Guidelines for the responsible conduct of research*. Ann Arbor: University of Michigan.

Government Reports and Policies

Australian Vice-Chancellors' Committee. 1997. Joint NHMRC/AVCC statement and guidelines on research practice. http://www.cs.rmit.edu.au/~jz/write/glrespra.htm. Site accessed 17 March 1999.

Commission on Research Integrity (CRI), Ryan Commission. 1995. *Integrity and misconduct in research: Report of the Commission on Research Integrity to the Secretary of Health and Human Services, the House Committee on Commerce, and the Senate Committee on Labor and Human Resources.* Washington, D.C.: Department of Health and Human Services, Public Health Service. See also http://www.faseb.org/opar/cri.html. Site accessed 17 February 1999.

Danish Committee on Scientific Dishonesty (DCSD). 1996. *The Danish Committee on Scientific Dishonesty: Annual report 1995.* Copenhagen: Danish Research Councils. See also http://www.forskraad.dk/publ/rap-uk/index.html. Site accessed 31 March 1999.

———. 1998. *The Danish Committee on Scientific Dishonesty: Annual report 1997.* Copenhagen: Danish Research Councils. See also http://www.forskraad.dk/spec-udv/uvvu/ann-report97/index.htm. Site accessed 31 March 1999.

———. 1999. *The Danish Committee on Scientific Dishonesty: Guidelines for good scientific practice.* Copenhagen: Danish Research Agency. See also http://www.forskraad.dk/spec-udv/uvvu/guidelines/index.htm. Site accessed 12 July 1999.

Food and Drug Administration (FDA), Department of Health and Human Services. 1998. Financial disclosure by clinical investigators [Docket No. 93N-0445] 21 CFR part 54. See also http://www.fda.gov. Site accessed 5 March 1999.

National Academy of Sciences (NAS), Panel on Scientific Responsibility and the Conduct of Research. 1992. *Responsible science: Ensuring the integrity of the research process.* Vol. 1. Washington, D.C.: National Academy Press.

———. 1993. *Responsible science: Ensuring the integrity of the research process.* Vol. 2. Washington, D.C.: National Academy Press.

National Health and Medical Research Council (NHMRC). 1997. Joint NHMRC/AVCC statement and guidelines on research practice. http://www.health.gov.au/nhmrc/research/nhmrcavc.htm. Site accessed 31 March 1999.

National Institutes of Health (NIH). 1992. Reminder and update: Requirement for instruction in the responsible conduct of research in National Research Service Award institutional training grants. *NIH Guide for Grants and Contracts* 21:2–3.

———. 1997. Guidelines for the conduct of research in the intramural research programs of NIH. 3d ed. http://www.nih.gov/news/irnews/guidelines.htm. Site accessed 12 January 1999.

National Science Foundation (NSF). 1991. Misconduct in science and engineering: Final rule. *Federal Register* 56:22286–90.

———. 1995. Investigator financial disclosure policy. *Federal Register* 60:35820–23. See also http://frwebgate1.access.gpo.gov/cgi-bin/waisgate.cgi?WAISdocID=7165820026+0+0+0&WAISaction=retrieve. Site accessed 26 March 1999.

Office of Research Integrity (ORI), Public Health Service. 1993. NIH strengthens responsible conduct of research requirement in training grant applications. *ORI Newsletter* 1:1, 8. See also http://ori.dhhs.gov/newsltrs.htm. Site accessed 13 July 1999.

——. 1995. ORI model policy and procedures for responding to allegations of scientific misconduct. http://ori.dhhs.gov/models.htm. Site accessed 24 May 1999.

——. 1999. ORI guidelines for editors: Managing research misconduct allegations. http://ori.dhhs.gov/ori_guidelines_for_editors.htm. Site accessed 14 July 1999.

Public Health Service (PHS), Department of Health and Human Services. 1995. Objectivity in research. *Federal Register* 60:35810–19. (42 CFR part 50 and 45 CFR part 94.) See also http://frwebgate3.access.gpo.gov/cgi-bin/waisgate. cgi?WAISdocID=694491288+0+0+0WAISaction=retrieve. Site accessed 26 March 1999.

U.S. Department of Health and Human Services. 1989. Responsibility of PHS awardee and applicant institutions for dealing with and reporting possible misconduct in science. 42 CFR part 50: subpart A. http://ori.dhhs.gov/89rule.htm. Site accessed 5 March 1999.

U.S. House. 1990. Subcommittee on Human Resources and Intergovernmental Relations of the Committee on Government Operations. *Are scientific misconduct and conflicts of interest hazardous to our health?* 101st Cong., 2d sess., H.R. 101–688. Washington, D.C.: Government Printing Office.

Authorship

Australian Vice-Chancellors' Committee. 1997. Authorship. Chap. 3 in Joint NHMRC/AVCC statement and guidelines on research practice. http://goanna. cs.rmit.edu.au/~jz/write/glrespra.htm#g3 . Site accessed 14 July 1999.

Biagioli, M. 1998. The instability of authorship: Credit and responsibility in contemporary biomedicine. *FASEB Journal* 12:3–16.

Bhopal, R. J., J. M. Rankin, E. McColl, L. H. Thomas, E. F. Kaner, R. Stacy, P. H. Pearson, B. G. Vernon, and H. Rodgers. 1997. The vexed question of authorship: Views of researchers in a British medical faculty. *BMJ* 314:1009–12.

Burman, K. D. 1982. "Hanging from the masthead": Reflections on authorship. *Annals of Internal Medicine* 97:602–5.

Caelleigh, A. S. 1991. Credit and responsibility in authorship. *Academic Medicine* 66:676–77.

Danish Committee on Scientific Dishonesty (DCSD). 1999. Guidelines concerning authorship. Chap. 6 in *The Danish Committee on Scientific Dishonesty: Guidelines for good scientific practice.* Copenhagen: Danish Research Agency. See also http:// www.forskraad.dk/spec-udv/uvvu/guidelines/author.htm. Site accessed 12 July 1999.

DeBakey, L., and S. DeBakey. 1975. Ethics and etiquette in biomedical communication. *Perspectives in Biology and Medicine* 18:522–40.

de Solla Price, D. J. 1981. Multiple authorship. *Science* 212:986.

Fine, M. A., and L. A. Kurdek. 1993. Reflections on determining authorship credit and authorship order on faculty-student collaborations. *American Psychologist* 48:1141–47.

Flanagin, A., and D. Rennie. 1995. Acknowledging ghosts. *JAMA* 273:73.

Fotion, N., and C. C. Conrad. 1984. Authorship and other credits. *Annals of Internal Medicine* 100:592–94.

Friedman, P. J. 1993. Standards for authorship and publication in academic radiology. Association of University Radiologists' Ad Hoc Committee on Standards for the Responsible Conduct of Research. *Radiology* 189:33–34; *Investigative Radiology* 28:879–81; *AJR American Journal of Roentgenology* 161:899–900.

Fye, W. B. 1990. Medical authorship: Traditions, trends, and tribulations. *Annals of Internal Medicine* 113:317–25.

Goodman, N. W. 1994. Survey of fulfillment of criteria for authorship in published medical research. *BMJ* 309:1482.

Horton, R. 1997. The signature of responsibility. *Lancet* 350:5–6.

[Huth, E. J.] 1983. Responsibilities of coauthorship. *Annals of Internal Medicine* 99:266–67.

Huth, E. J. 1986. Abuses and uses of authorship. *Annals of Internal Medicine* 104:266–67.

———. 1986. Guidelines on authorship of medical papers. *Annals of Internal Medicine* 104:269–74.

International Committee of Medical Journal Editors (ICMJE). 1997. Uniform requirements for manuscripts submitted to biomedical journals. *Annals of Internal Medicine* 126:36–47. See also http://www.acponline.org/journals/resource/unifreqr.htm. Site accessed 18 April 1999.

Kennedy, D. 1985. *On academic authorship*. Washington, D.C.: American Council of Learned Societies.

Relman, A. S. 1990. Responsible science—responsible authorship: Discussion. In Council of Biology Editors, Editorial Policy Committee, *Ethics and policy in scientific publication*, 199. Bethesda, Md.: Council of Biology Editors.

Rennie, D., and A. Flanagin. 1994. Authorship! Authorship! Guests, ghosts, grafters, and the two-sided coin. *JAMA* 271:469–71.

Rennie, D., V. Yank, and L. Emanuel. 1997. When authorship fails: A proposal to make contributors accountable. *JAMA* 278:579–85.

Riesenberg, D., and G. D. Lundberg. 1990. The order of authorship: Who's on first? *JAMA* 264:1857.

Riis, P., and D. Andersen. 1996. Authorship and co-authorship. Chap. 2 in *The Danish Committee on Scientific Dishonesty: Annual report 1995*. Copenhagen: Danish Research Councils. See also http://www.forskraad.dk:80/publ/rap-uk/kap05.html. Site accessed 17 February 1999.

Schiedermayer, D. L., and M. Siegler. 1986. Believing what you read: Responsibilities of medical authors and editors. *Archives of Internal Medicine* 146:2043–44.

Shapiro, D. W., N. S. Wenger, and M. F. Shapiro. 1994. The contributions of authors to multiauthored biomedical research papers. *JAMA* 271:438–42.

Smith, R. 1997. Authorship is dying: Long live contributorship. *BMJ* 315:744–48.

Wilcox, L. J. 1998. Authorship: The coin of the realm, the source of complaints. *JAMA* 280:216–17.

Yank, V., and D. Rennie. 1999. Disclosure of researcher contributions: A study of original research articles in *The Lancet*. *Annals of Internal Medicine* 130: 661–70.

Zuckerman, H. A. 1968. Patterns of name ordering among authors of scientific papers: A study of social symbolism and its ambiguity. *American Journal of Sociology* 74:276–91.

Peer Review

Adams, M. D., and J. C. Venter. 1996. Should non-peer-reviewed raw DNA sequence data release be forced on the scientific community? *Science* 274:534–36.

Bingham, C. M., G. Higgins, R. Coleman, and M. B. Van Der Weyden. 1998. The *Medical Journal of Australia* Internet peer-review study. *Lancet* 352:441–45.

Black, N., S. van Rooyen, F. Godlee, R. Smith, and S. Evans. 1998. What makes a good reviewer and a good review for a general medical journal? *JAMA* 280:231–33.

Dickersin, K., Y-I. Min, and C. L. Meinert. 1992. Factors influencing publication of research results: Follow-up of applications submitted to two institutional review boards. *JAMA* 267:374–78.

Evans, A. T., R. A. McNutt, S. W. Fletcher, and R. H. Fletcher. 1993. The characteristics of peer reviewers who produce good-quality reviews. *Journal of General Internal Medicine* 8:422–28.

Godlee, F., and T. Jefferson. 1999. *Peer review*. London: BMJ Books.

Goodman, S. N., J. Berlin, S. W. Fletcher, and R. H. Fletcher. 1994. Manuscript quality before and after peer review and editing at *Annals of Internal Medicine*. *Annals of Internal Medicine* 121:11–21.

Guarding the guardians: Research on editorial peer review. Selected proceedings from the First International Congress on Peer Review in Biomedical Publication. 1990. *JAMA* 263 (theme issue):1317–1441.

Harnad, S. 1995. Re: Peer commentary vs. peer review. http://cogsci.ecs.soton.ac .uk/~harnad/Hypermail/Theschat/0007.html. Site accessed 19 March 1999.

Horrobin, D. F. 1990. The philosophical basis of peer review and the suppression of innovation. *JAMA* 263:1438–41.

Judson, H. F. 1994. Structural transformations of the sciences and the end of peer review. *JAMA* 272:92–94.

Kassirer, J. P., and E. W. Campion. 1994. Peer review: Crude and understudied, but indispensible. *JAMA* 272:96–97.

Lock, S. 1986. *A difficult balance: Editorial peer review in medicine*. Philadelphia: ISI Press.

McNutt, R. A., A. T. Evans, R. H. Fletcher, and S. W. Fletcher. 1990. The effects of blinding on the quality of peer review: A randomized trial. *JAMA* 263:1371–76.

Peer Review Congress III. 1998. *JAMA* 280 (theme issue):213–302.

Peer review in scientific publishing: Papers from the First International Congress on Peer Review in Biomedical Publication (sponsored by the American Medical Association). 1991. Chicago: Council of Biology Editors.

Protocol for Internet peer review study II. 1998. *Medical Journal of Australia.* http://www.mja.com.au/public/information/iprs2doc.html#rules. Site accessed 19 March 1999.

The Second International Congress on Peer Review in Biomedical Publication. 1994. *JAMA* 272 (theme issue):91–173.

Smith, R. 1999. Opening up *BMJ* peer review: A beginning that should lead to complete transparency. *BMJ* 318:4–5.

Repetitive Publication

American Diabetes Association (ADA), Publications Policy Committee. 1992. Duplicate publication in American Diabetes Association journals: Challenges and recommendations. *Diabetes Care* 15:1059–61.

Council of Biology Editors (CBE), Editorial Policy Committee. 1996. Redundant publication. *CBE Views* 19:76–77.

Flanagin, A., R. M. Glass, and G. D. Lundberg. 1992. Electronic journals and duplicate publication: Is a byte a word? *JAMA* 267:2374.

Huston, P., and D. Moher. 1996. Redundancy, disaggregation, and the integrity of medical research. *Lancet* 347:1024–26.

Huth, E. J. 1986. Irresponsible authorship and wasteful publication. *Annals of Internal Medicine* 104:257–59.

National Library of Medicine (NLM). 1998. Fact sheet: Errata, retraction, duplicate publication, and comment policy. http://www.nlm.nih.gov/pubs/factsheets/errata.html. Site accessed 12 January 1999.

Relman, A. S. 1981. The Ingelfinger rule. *New England Journal of Medicine* 305:824–26.

Susser, M., and A. Yankauer. 1993. Prior, duplicate, repetitive, fragmented, and redundant publication and editorial decisions. *American Journal of Public Health* 83:792–93.

Conflict of Interest

American Federation for Clinical Research (AFCR). 1990. Guidelines for avoiding conflict of interest. *Clinical Research* 38:239–40.

Angell, M., and J. P. Kassirer. 1996. Editorials and conflicts of interest. *New England Journal of Medicine* 335:1055–56.

Anything to declare? 1993. *Lancet* 341:728.

Association of American Medical Colleges (AAMC). 1990. Guidelines for dealing with faculty conflicts of commitment and conflicts of interest in research. *Academic Medicine* 65:488–96. See also http://www.aamc.org/research/dbr/coi.htm. Site accessed 8 November 1998.

Bero, L. 1998. Disclosure policies for gifts from industry to academic faculty. *JAMA* 279:1031–32.

Blumenthal, D., E. G. Campbell, M. S. Anderson, N. Causino, and K. S. Louis. 1997. Withholding research results in academic life science: Evidence from a national survey of faculty. *JAMA* 277:1224–28.

Food and Drug Administration (FDA), Department of Health and Human Services. 1998. Financial disclosure by clinical investigators [Docket No. 93N-0445] 21 CFR part 54. See also http://www.fda.gov. Site accessed 5 March 1999.

Frankel, M. S. 1996. Perception, reality, and the political context of conflict of interest in university-industry relationships. *Academic Medicine* 71:1297–1304.

Friedman, P. J. 1992. The troublesome semantics of conflict of interest. *Ethics & Behavior* 2:245–51.

Glass, R. M., and M. Schneiderman. 1997. A survey of journal conflict of interest policies. Paper presented at the 3d International Congress on Biomedical Peer Review and Global Communications, 18 September, Prague. http://www.ama-assn.org/public/peer/apo.htm. Site accessed 8 November 1998.

Huth, E. J. 1996. Conflicts of interest in industry-funded clinical research. In *Conflict of interest in clinical practice and research,* ed. R. G. Spece Jr., D. S. Shimm, and A. E. Buchanan, 389–406. New York: Oxford University Press.

International Committee of Medical Journal Editors (ICMJE). 1998. Statement on project-specific industry support for research. *Canadian Medical Association Journal* 158:615–16.

Koshland, D. E., Jr. 1992. Conflict of interest policy. *Science* 257:595.

National Science Foundation (NSF). 1995. Investigator financial disclosure policy. *Federal Register* 60:35820–23. See also http:// frwebgate1.access.gpo.gov/cgi-bin/waisgate.cgi?WAISdocID=7165820026+0+0+0&WAISaction=retrieve. Site accessed 26 March 1999.

The politics of disclosure. 1996. *Lancet* 348:627.

Rennie, D. 1997. Thyroid storm. *JAMA* 277:1238–43.

Rothman, K. J. 1991. The ethics of research sponsorship. *Journal of Clinical Epidemiology* 44 (suppl 1):25S–28S.

———. 1993. Conflict of interest: The new McCarthyism in science. *JAMA* 269:2782–84.

Spece, R. G., Jr., D. S. Shimm, and A. E. Buchanan, eds. 1996. *Conflicts of interest in clinical practice and research.* New York: Oxford University Press.

Electronic Publication

Alexander, J. E., and M. A. Tate. 1999. Evaluating web resources. http://www.science.widener.edu/~withers/inform.htm. Site accessed 23 March 1999.

———. 1999. *Web wisdom: How to evaluate and create information quality on the Web.* Mahwah, N.J.: Lawrence Erlbaum Associates.

Boyer, C., M. Selby, J.-R. Scherrer, and R. D. Appel. 1998. The Health on the Net

Code of Conduct for medical and health Websites. *Computers in Biology and Medicine* 28:603–10.

Ginsparg, P. 1996. Winners and losers in the global research village. http://xxx.lanl.gov/blurb/pg96unesco.html. Site accessed 19 March 1999.

Harnad, S. 1991. Post-Gutenberg galaxy: The fourth revolution in the means of production of knowledge. *Public-Access Computer Systems Review* 2:39–53. See also ftp://cogsci.ecs.soton.ac.uk/pub/harnad/harnad91.postgutenberg. Site accessed 19 March 1999.

——. 1995. Implementing peer review on the Net: Scientific quality control in scholarly electronic journals. In *Electronic publishing confronts academia: The agenda for the year 2000*, ed. R. Peek and G. Newby, 103–18. Cambridge: MIT Press. See also ftp://cogsci.ecs.soton.ac.uk/pub/harnad/harnad95.peer.review. Site accessed 19 March 1999.

Health on the Net Foundation. 1997. Health on the Net (HON) code of conduct (HONcode) for medical and health Web sites. Version 1.6. http://www.hon.ch/HONcode/Conduct.html. Site accessed 23 March 1999.

International Committee of Medical Journal Editors (ICMJE). 1992. Statements on electronic publication and on peer-reviewed journals. *Annals of Internal Medicine* 116:1030.

Jadad, A. R., and A. Gagliardi. 1998. Rating health information on the Internet: Navigating to knowledge or to Babel? *JAMA* 279:611–14.

Kassirer, J. P. 1992. Journals in bits and bytes: Electronic medical journals. *New England Journal of Medicine* 326:195–97.

——. 1995. The next transformation in the delivery of health care. *New England Journal of Medicine* 332:52–54.

Kassirer, J. P., and M. Angell. 1995. The Internet and the *Journal*. *New England Journal of Medicine* 332:1709–10.

LaPorte, R. E., E. Marler, S. Akazawa, F. Sauer, C. Gamboa, C. Shenton, C. Glosser, A. Villasenor, and M. Maclure. 1995. The death of biomedical journals. *BMJ* 310:1387–90.

Odlyzko, A. M. 1994. Tragic loss or good riddance? The impending demise of traditional scholarly journals. http://www.-mathdoc.ujf-renoble.fr/textes/Odlyzko/amo94/amo94.html. Site accessed 25 March 1999.

Richardson, M. L., M. S. Frank, and E. J. Stern. 1995. Digital image manipulation: What constitutes acceptable alteration of a radiologic image? *AJR American Journal of Roentgenology* 164:228–29.

Silberg, W. M., G. D. Lundberg, and R. A. Musacchio. 1997. Assessing, controlling, and assuring the quality of medical information on the Internet: *Caveant lector et viewor:* Let the reader and viewer beware. *JAMA* 277:1244–45.

Varmus, H. 1999. E-BIOMED: A proposal for electronic publications in the biomedical sciences. http://www.nih.gov/welcome/director/ebiomed/ebi.htm. Site accessed 8 July 1999.

Winograd, S., and R. N. Zare. 1995. "Wired" science or whither the printed page? *Science* 269:615.

Copyright and Other Legal Matters

Alford, W. P. 1995. *To steal a book is an elegant offense: Intellectual property law in Chinese civilization.* Stanford: Stanford University Press.

Godwin, M. 1987. Copyright crisis: Copyright holders, with some reason, fear the Net's threat to intellectual property, but the laws being proposed go too far in restricting rights. *Internet World,* March, 100–102.

Li, X., and L. Xiong. 1996. Chinese researchers debate rash of plagiarism cases. *Science* 274:337–38.

Mallon, T. 1989. *Stolen words: Forays into the origins and ravages of plagiarism.* New York: Ticknor & Fields.

Nimmer, M. B. 1963. *Nimmer on copyright.* New York: Matthew Bender.

Parrish, D. 1994. Scientific misconduct and the plagiarism cases. *Journal of College and University Law* 21:517–54.

U.S. Code. http://www4.law.cornell.edu/uscode. Site accessed 31 March 1999.

World Intellectual Property Organization (WIPO). 1996. Diplomatic conference on certain copyright and neighboring rights questions: WIPO copyright treaty. http://www.wipo.org/eng/diplconf/index.htm. Site accessed 23 March 1999.

Clinical Trials

Begg, C., M. Cho, S. Eastwood, R. Horton, D. Moher, I. Olkin, R. Pitkin, D. Rennie, K. F. Schulz, D. Simel, and D. F. Stroup. 1996. Improving the quality of reporting of randomized controlled trials: The CONSORT statement. *JAMA* 276:637–39.

Dickersin, K., S. Chan, T. C. Chalmers, H. S. Sacks, and J. Smith Jr. 1987. Publication bias and clinical trials. *Controlled Clinical Trials* 8:343–53.

Horton, R. 1997. Medical editors trial amnesty. *Lancet* 350:756.

Making clinical trialists register. 1991. *Lancet* 338:244–45.

Institutional Processes and Policies

Angell, M. 1986. Publish or perish: A proposal. *Annals of Internal Medicine* 104:261–62.

Association of American Medical Colleges (AAMC), Ad Hoc Committee on Misconduct and Conflict of Interest in Research. 1992. *Beyond the "framework": Institutional considerations in managing allegations of misconduct in research.* Washington, D.C.: Association of American Medical Colleges.

Gunsalus, C. K. 1993. Institutional structure to ensure research integrity. *Academic Medicine* 68 (suppl to issue 9):S33–38.

——. 1998. How to blow the whistle and still have a career afterwards. *Science and Engineering Ethics* 4:51–64.

——. 1998. Preventing the need for whistleblowing: Practical advice for university administrators. *Science and Engineering Ethics* 4:75–94.

Korenman, S. G., R. Berk, N. S. Wenger, and V. Lew. 1998. Evaluation of the research norms of scientists and administrators responsible for academic research integrity. *JAMA* 279:41–47.

Olswang, S. G., and B. A. Lee. 1984. Scientific misconduct: Institutional procedures and due process considerations. *Journal of College and University Law* 11:51–63.

Parrish, D. 1997. Improving the scientific misconduct hearing process. *JAMA* 277:1315–19.

Education

Bird, S. J. 1993. Teaching ethics in the sciences: Why, how and what. In *Ethics, values, and the promise of science*, 228–32. Research Triangle Park, N.C.: Sigma Xi.

Booth, V. 1993. *Communicating in science*. 2d ed. New York: Cambridge University Press.

Committee on Science, Engineering, and Public Policy. 1995. *Reshaping the graduate education of scientists and engineers*. Washington, D.C.: National Academy Press.

Council of Biology Editors (CBE), Editorial Policy Committee. 1990. *Ethics and policy in scientific publication*. Bethesda, Md.: Council of Biology Editors.

Day, R. A. 1998. *How to write and publish a scientific paper*. 3d ed. Phoenix: Oryx Press.

Eastwood, S., P. A. Derish, E. Leash, and S. B. Ordway. 1996. Ethical issues in biomedical research: Perceptions and practices of postdoctoral research fellows responding to a survey. *Science and Engineering Ethics* 2:89–114.

Fischbach, R., ed. 1994. *Educating for the responsible conduct of research: NIH policy and other mandates*. Boston: PRIM&R.

Friedman, P. J. 1990. Research ethics: A teaching agenda for academic medicine. *Academic Medicine* 65:32–33.

Glantz, S. A. 1992. *Primer of biostatistics*. 3d ed. New York: McGraw-Hill.

Greenhalgh, T. 1997. *How to read a paper: The basics of evidence based medicine*. London: BMJ Publishing Group.

Hafferty, F. W., and R. Franks. 1994. The hidden curriculum, ethics teaching, and the structure of medical education. *Academic Medicine* 69:861–71.

Hoshiko, T. 1993. Responsible conduct of scientific research: A one-semester course for graduate students. *American Journal of Physiology* 264:S8–10.

Hundert, E. M., F. Hafferty, and D. Christakis. 1996. Characteristics of the informal curriculum and trainees' ethical choices. *Academic Medicine* 71:624–33.

Huth, E. J. 1999. *Writing and publishing in medicine*. 3d ed. Baltimore: Williams & Wilkins.

Iverson, C., A. Flanagin, and P. Fontanarosa. 1998. *American Medical Association*

Manual of Style: A Guide for Authors and Editors. 9th ed. Baltimore: Williams & Wilkins.

Kalichman, M. W., and P. J. Friedman. 1992. A pilot study of biomedical trainees' perceptions concerning research ethics. *Academic Medicine* 67:769–75.

Korenman, S. G., and A. C. Shipp. 1994. *Teaching the responsible conduct of research through a case study approach: A handbook for instructors.* Washington, D.C.: Association of American Medical Colleges.

Krulwich, T. A., and P. J. Friedman. 1993. Integrity in the education of researchers. *Academic Medicine* 68 (suppl to issue 9):S14–18.

Lo, B. 1993. Skepticism about teaching ethics. In *Ethics, values, and the promise of science: Forum proceedings,* 151–56. Research Triangle Park, N.C.: Sigma Xi.

Medawar, P. B. 1981. *Advice to a young scientist.* New York: Harper & Row.

National Institutes of Health (NIH). 1992. Reminder and update: Requirement for instruction in the responsible conduct of research in National Research Service Award institutional training grants. *NIH Guide for Grants and Contracts* 21:2–3.

Ordway, S., S. Eastwood, and P. Derish. 1994. *A guide to publishing biomedical research.* San Francisco: Department of Neurological Surgery, University of California, San Francisco.

Swazey, J. P. 1993. Teaching ethics: Needs, opportunities, and obstacles. In *Ethics, values, and the promise of science: Forum proceedings,* 233–42. Research Triangle Park, N.C.: Sigma Xi.

Woodford, F. P., ed. 1986. *Scientific writing for graduate students.* Bethesda, Md.: Council of Biology Editors.

———. 1999. *How to Teach Scientific Communication.* Reston, Va.: Council of Biology Editors.

Zeiger, M. 1991. *Essentials of writing biomedical research papers.* New York: McGraw-Hill.

Statements and Policies of Editors' Organizations

Council of Biology Editors (CBE), Editorial Policy Committee. 1996. Redundant publication. *CBE Views* 19:76–77.

———. 1999. Policy of journal referral of possible misconduct. Revised draft. http://www.cbe.org/cbe/DraftPolicies.html. Site accessed 8 July 1999.

———. 1999. Policy on journal access to data. Revised draft. http://www.cbe.org/cbe/DraftPolicies.html. Site accessed 8 July 1999.

———. 1999. Policy on responsibilities and rights of editors of peer-reviewed journal. Revised draft. http://www.cbe.org/cbe/DraftPolicies.html. Site accessed 8 July 1999.

International Committee of Medical Journal Editors (ICMJE). 1988. Retraction of research findings. *Annals of Internal Medicine* 108:304.

———. 1992. Statements on electronic publication and on peer-reviewed journals. *Annals of Internal Medicine* 116:1030.

——. 1997. Uniform requirements for manuscripts submitted to biomedical journals. *Annals of Internal Medicine* 126:36–47. See also http://www.acponline.org/
journals/resource/unifreqr.htm. Site accessed 18 March 1999.

——. 1998. Statement on project-specific industry support for research. *Canadian
Medical Association Journal* 158:615–16. See also http://www.cma.ca/cmaj/
vol-158/issue-5/0615e.htm. Site accessed 25 September 1999.

Index

Library of Congress Cataloging-in-Publication Data

Ethical issues in biomedical publication / edited by Anne Hudson Jones and
Faith McLellan.

    p. cm.

  Includes bibliographical references and index.

  ISBN 0-8018-6314-7 (hb : acid-free paper) — ISBN 0-8018-6315-5 (pbk. :
acid-free paper)

    1. Medical publishing—Moral and ethical aspects.   I. Jones, Anne
Hudson.   II. McLellan, Faith.

R118.E889   2000

174'.2—dc21   99-044900